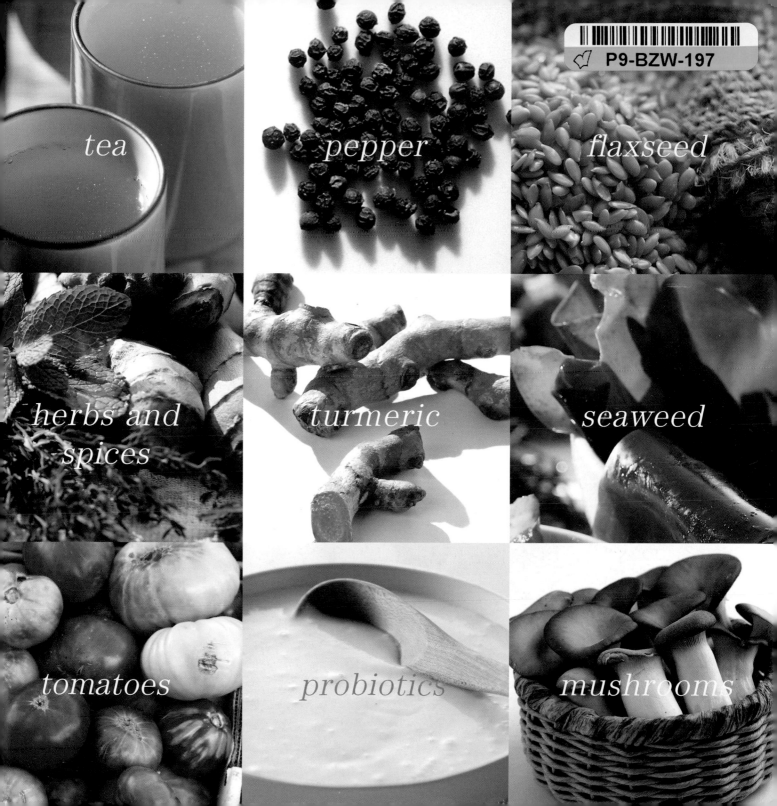

tea

pepper

flaxseed

herbs and spices

turmeric

seaweed

tomatoes

probiotics

mushrooms

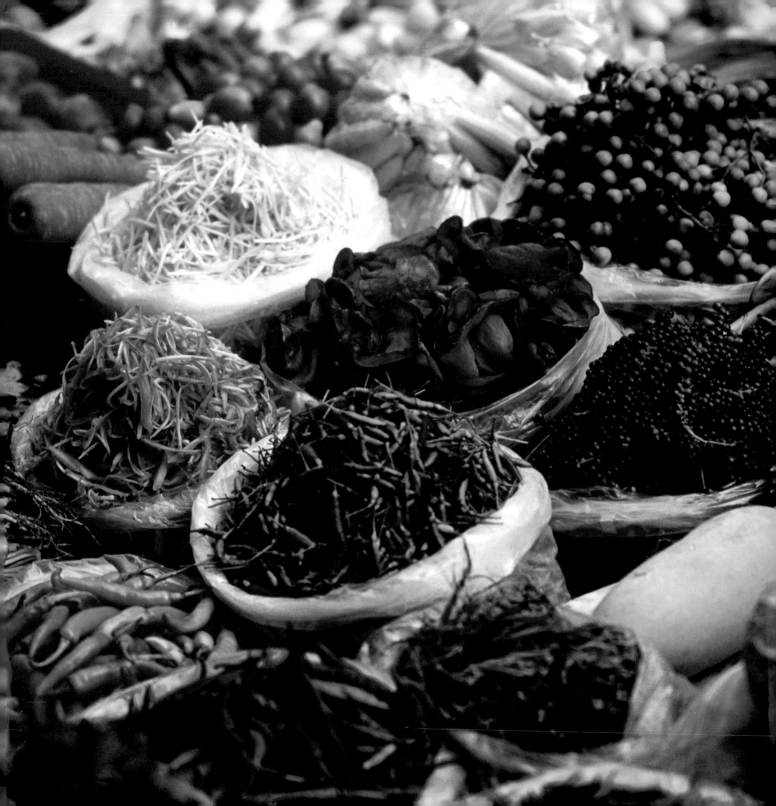

COOKING WITH FOODS THAT FIGHT CANCER

RICHARD BÉLIVEAU, PH.D.

DENIS GINGRAS, PH.D.

TRANSLATED BY MILÉNA STOJANAC AND GORDON McBRIDE

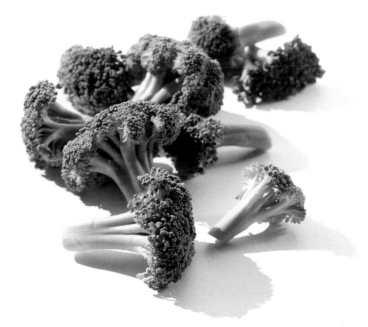

MOLECULAR MEDICINE LABORATORY

HÔPITAL SAINTE-JUSTINE ET UNIVERSITÉ DU QUÉBEC À MONTRÉAL

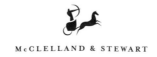

McCLELLAND & STEWART

Original title: Cuisiner avec les aliments contre le cancer
Copyright © 2006 Éditions du Trécarré
Published under arrangement with Éditions du Trécarré, une division de Quebecor Média inc., Outremont, Quebec, Canada

English-language edition copyright © 2007 McClelland & Stewart Ltd.
English-language translation copyright © 2007 Éditions du Trécarré
Translation by Miléna Stojanac and Gordon McBride

Library and Archives Canada Cataloguing in Publication

Béliveau, Richard, 1953–
      Cooking with foods that fight cancer / Richard Béliveau and Denis Gingras.

Originally published in French under title: Cuisiner avec les aliments contre le cancer.
Includes bibliographical references and index.

ISBN 978-0-7710-1136-8

      1. Cancer – Diet therapy – Recipes. 2. Cancer – Prevention.
3. Cancer – Nutritional aspects.   I. Gingras, Denis   I. Title.

RC271.D52B4413 2007   641.5'631   C2007-901812-2

We acknowledge the financial support of the Government of Canada through the Book Publishing Industry Development Program (BPIDP) and that of the Government of Ontario through the Ontario Media Development Corporation's Ontario Book Initiative. We further acknowledge the support of the Canada Council for the Arts and the Ontario Arts Council for our publishing program.

Original French-language edition
Design: Cyclone design communications, Caroline Desrosiers
Editorial: Nathalie Guillet
Copyediting: Dominique Issenhuth, Linda Nantel
Proofreading: Anik Charbonneau, Dominique Issenhuth, Carole Mills
Index: Diane Baril
Author photo on page 5 : Robert Etcheverry
Recipe photos: Tango
Food stylist: Jacques Faucher
Accessories stylist: Luce Meunier
Accessories: Stokes, Anglo Canada
Nutritionist: Frances Boyte

Additional photos
Photos on pages 1, 3, 47, 48, 59, 60, 62, 63, 67, 68, 70, 71, 77, 78, 81, 83, 88, 91, 98, 101, 104, 106, 107, 108, 110, 113, 114, 117, 118 and 119 : Tango
Photos on pages 114 (tea fields) and 119 (cacao tree) : Getty Images
Photo on page 117 (vineyards) : Bureau interprofessionnel des vins de Bourgogne/N. Eschmann

Printed and bound in Canada

McClelland & Stewart Ltd.
75 Sherbourne Street
Toronto, Ontario
M5A 2P9
www.mcclelland.com

3 4 5 6 7   12 11 10 09 08

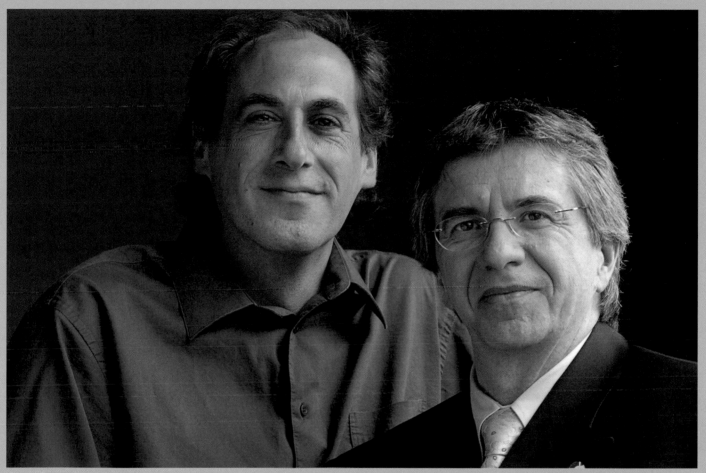

Denis Gingras (left) and Richard Béliveau.

This book is dedicated to all persons suffering from cancer.

TABLE OF *contents*

Recipes

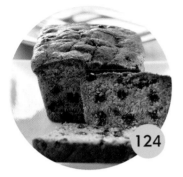

124

BREAKFASTS AND BRUNCHES

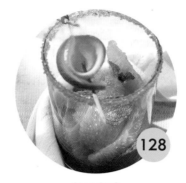

128

SNACKS

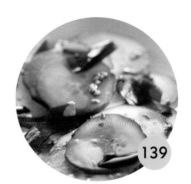

139

APPETIZERS

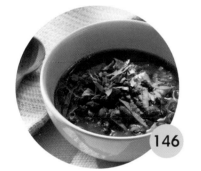

146

SOUPS AND BROTHS

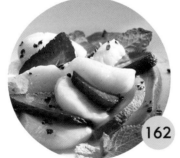

162

FIRST COURSES

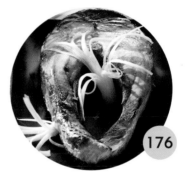

176

MAIN DISHES

SAUCES AND SEASONINGS

212

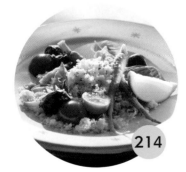

214

SIDE DISHES

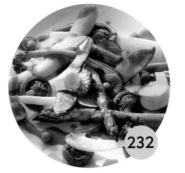

232

SALADS

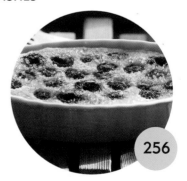

256

DESSERTS

FORE*words*

THE FONDATION SERGE-BRUYÈRE was founded in 2004, in memory of a great chef who left his mark on Quebec gastronomy. Its goal is twofold: first, to recognize the culinary *savoir-faire* of the talented professionals now working in this field, and second, in particular, to provide support to a younger generation by awarding scholarships, offering encouragement, and promoting the culinary philosophy and ideals of Serge Bruyère.

Many of the foundation's chefs donate their time to our fundraising activities, and I would like to acknowledge them here. They have all devoted time and energy to create the recipes in this book while respecting the principles and values outlined by the authors. A heartfelt thank-you to all of these colleagues!

Our chefs make no pretension of teaching cooking skills or revolutionizing dietary customs; instead, they endeavour to respond to the growing preoccupation of all those who wish to learn more about diet and nutrition without giving up the pleasures of fine cooking.

Serge Bruyère once said: "In cooking, as in the arts, simplicity is the sign of perfection." In other words, it's best to cook simply, with fresh, high-quality ingredients! In the countryside where I grew up, plentiful nature surrounded us. Farmers passed on their land and their passion for that land and for what it gave them from one generation to the next. Respect for local products was absolute and non-negotiable. Today, we feel the need to return to this bounty, all too often poorly treated, in order to relearn the authentic flavours of childhood, to rediscover the soul of farm-fresh products with emotion, by trial and error, during a private moment at home or in the noisy solitude of the professional kitchen.

To all of you in your kitchens, I wish happiness and long life.

JEAN SOULARD
President, Fondation Serge-Bruyère
Executive Chef at the Fairmont Le Château Frontenac

Fondation
SERGE - BRUYÈRE

I WOULD LIKE TO CONGRATULATE Drs. Richard Béliveau and Denis Gingras as well as Éditions du Trécarré for the tremendous success of their first book, *Foods That Fight Cancer* (originally *Les aliments contre le cancer*). Along with tens of thousands of other readers, I heard this book's message as an earth-shaking revelation: here was well-documented, irrefutable scientific proof, clearly explained by renowned cancer researchers to a lay audience, that the right foods properly used really had the power to help prevent this terrible disease. *Foods That Fight Cancer* is an invaluable tool box, a treasure chest of ideas and tips, for better taking charge of one's health. Now, with *Cooking With Foods That Fight Cancer*, the pleasure principle takes its place in the tool chest . . .

The book you are reading is what results when people set out to create a network of cancer prevention knowledge. This is the first time so many different and complementary areas of expertise have been put together to better inform the reading public. In joining their expertise to that of cancer researchers and nutritionists, the chefs became more aware of the importance of fruits, vegetables, whole grains, and "good" fats, and came up with ideas to better integrate these products and principles into their art and work. Similarly, the presence of top chefs with unique expertise in the art of preparing food with an eye to bringing out all of its subtleties allows the scientists to establish a collection of delicious, original, and healthful recipes while reaching out to a vast public of amateurs who are nonetheless fond of fine dining.

Cooking With Foods That Fight Cancer also represents a coalition of the generous, since the medical researchers, nutritionists, and chefs involved all share the desire to help their neighbour. The Fondation Serge-Bruyère is exemplary in this regard; its educational mission stresses the importance of a cuisine built around local products of quality, a value dear to the late Serge Bruyère. This cookbook, to which I had the honour of contributing several recipes, is proof that one can protect one's health while eating meals fit for royalty!

ANNE L. DESJARDINS
Author; health and lifestyle journalist specializing in fine dining and gastronomy; cancer survivor

FORE*word*

THE CANCER RESEARCH SOCIETY has funded the innovative and promising research done by Dr. Béliveau and his team for a number of years now because we believe it represents an important path for the future in our fight against cancer. Cancer is in constant progression in our society. Since 1987, the number of yearly cancer cases has jumped by 54.4 per cent, with a 58.5 per cent hike in breast cancer incidence and a devastating 121.5 per cent increase in the number of prostate cancer cases. Although these statistics can be partly explained by the greying of the population, we must be conscious that environment and lifestyle choices are inextricably linked to such tragic numbers. The lesson here is that we *can* change the situation. Over one third of cancers may be prevented. It's up to us to act! The Cancer Research Society is on the front lines, investing in this research avenue through the Environment-Cancer Fund (ECF), which will finance other projects focusing on the link between the way we live and the development of cancer . . . Because an ounce of prevention is worth a pound of cure!

Cancer prevention can be accomplished by making simple changes, modifying lifestyle habits that have an impact on health. Blueberries, cranberries, flaxseed, cabbage, and green tea are back, to better enrich our meals. To these we now add mushrooms, herbs and spices, and many other foods with heretofore unsuspected virtues.

Although the basic research described here may seem sealed-off and abstract, it performs a vital function: it inevitably gives rise to knowledge that allows us to better comprehend the phenomena around us. The key to taking effective action against a foe as pernicious as cancer, research also lets us better understand the causes and mechanisms of this disease.

Using simple language, this book offers us access to precious concepts that would normally circulate among a small circle of research and health professionals. And yet the public has an unmistakable thirst for this kind of information, which allows it to reclaim power over individual lives. A treat for the eye, soon to be a treat for the tastebuds, this book is sure to find its place in our homes and kitchens, nourishing conversations and conversions to tasty, healthy meals.

Enjoy!

GILLES LÉVEILLÉ
Executive Director
The Cancer Research Society

IF YOU WANT TO LIVE LONG, LIVE BETTER.

INTRO*duction*

The human being is the only animal that sees the act of feeding itself as both a necessary condition for survival and an essential dimension of well-being. The importance we give to food and diet is beautifully illustrated in Chinese script, one of the most ancient known to humanity; the character that designates the word "food," 食, is a combination of 良, meaning "to improve," and 人, or "human." "Improving the human" with the help of food also seems to have been on the minds of early Greek philosophers: *diata*, the root of the word "diet," means "*art de vivre.*" According to Epicurus, this art of living implied a constant search for balance, a balance that optimized both pleasure and health. The incredible number of foods identified in nature over the course of history, especially foods of plant origin, testify to this search for balance. The fruits, vegetables, roots, shoots, cereals, and nuts that we still eat today have played an essential role in the evolution of culinary traditions associated with the rise of different civilizations as well as in the prevention of disease.

Human preoccupation with food and nourishment probably arose from an acute awareness of the precarious character of existence and our vulnerability as living, mortal beings. All throughout human evolution, this consciousness has motivated people to provide for their descendants, of course, but it has also spurred them to create ever greater works of art, or indulge in reckless conquests and rash political alliances that would guarantee them widespread fame; in other words, live on after their death. Human life is not just survival, the simple propagation of genes. Life means building, acting, creating, sculpting our environment so that a brief existence is justified by the memory that future generations will have of what their ancestors accomplished.

Concretely, this quest for success has always been directly dependent on health; guaranteeing a human being the longest life possible allows him or her to use to greatest advantage the time needed to accomplish his or her objectives. We should not be too surprised that enjoying good health has always preoccupied and often obsessed us. We often forget that today's high-tech medicine, such an important part of modern life, is a relatively recent phenomenon in the history of humanity; its remarkable progress goes back barely half a century. In practice, humans have always had to compensate for the lack of medical resources by avoiding getting sick! This prevention-based attitude grew out of a profound understanding of the impact of diet on well-being.

We believe there are important lessons to be learned from the relationship between food and the preventive effect it has on disease. Many of the principal diseases afflicting society today — the large numbers of cancers, diabetes, or cardiovascular disease cases — are often directly linked to lifestyle, and may thus in many instances be avoided. Prevention is extremely important; every year, 36 million individuals the world over lose their lives to these diseases. If we do nothing, it is estimated that the next generation will have a lower life expectancy than that of the previous one for the first time in history. This drop is directly attributable to the steep increase in diseases linked to lifestyle habits, such as diet. Even if we assume that progress in medical science will eventually succeed in relieving many of the negative aspects associated with these chronic illnesses, it remains that life expectancy, probably the most important measuring stick for an individual in good health, will be adversely affected.

We also believe, however, that the current situation is far from irreversible; on the contrary, there is great reason for hope. Over the past few years, we have witnessed growing interest in the relationship between diet and the development of certain cancers. More and more people are becoming concerned by the nature and quality of the food on their plate and the ways this food may be used on a daily basis to improve quality of life and reduce the risk of being affected by serious diseases such as cancer. These concerns prove that the special relationship between human beings and the food they eat is not some vague concept or a holdover from the past; quite the opposite. The nature of food is an important issue for many people.

It is in this spirit that we have created this new book. We wish to review the ways in which a healthful diet may actively participate in human well-being and the prevention of disease, but we would also like to offer the reader some concrete ways of putting these principles into practice on a daily basis, using quick, easy, inexpensive, and delicious recipes. As you will see, preventing cancer by paying special attention to the nature of what we eat opens the door to a new world of flavours and textures, where the pleasures of eating well go hand in hand with health.

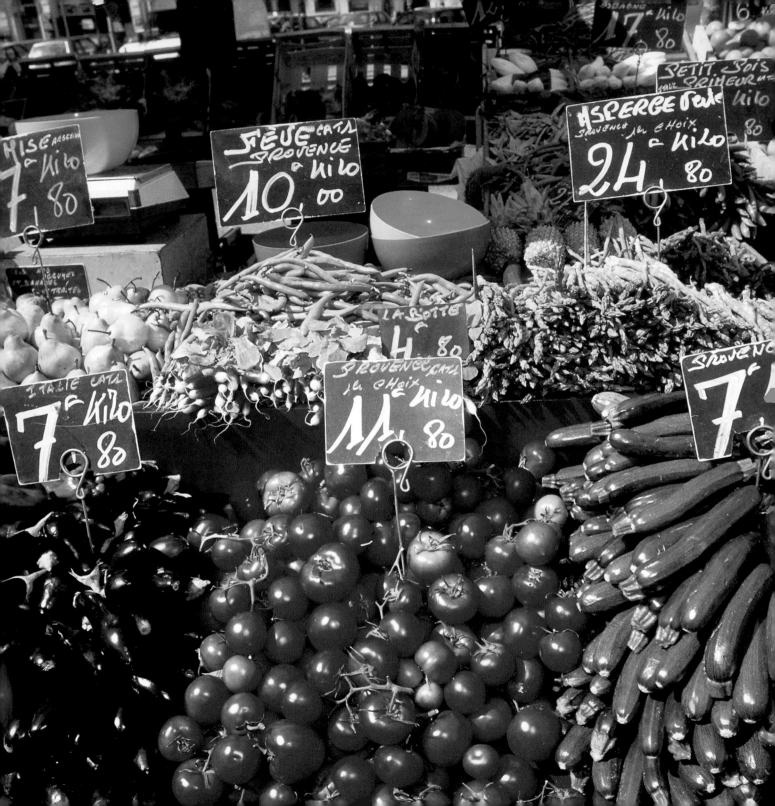

PART *one*

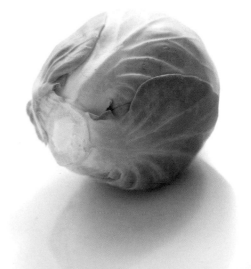

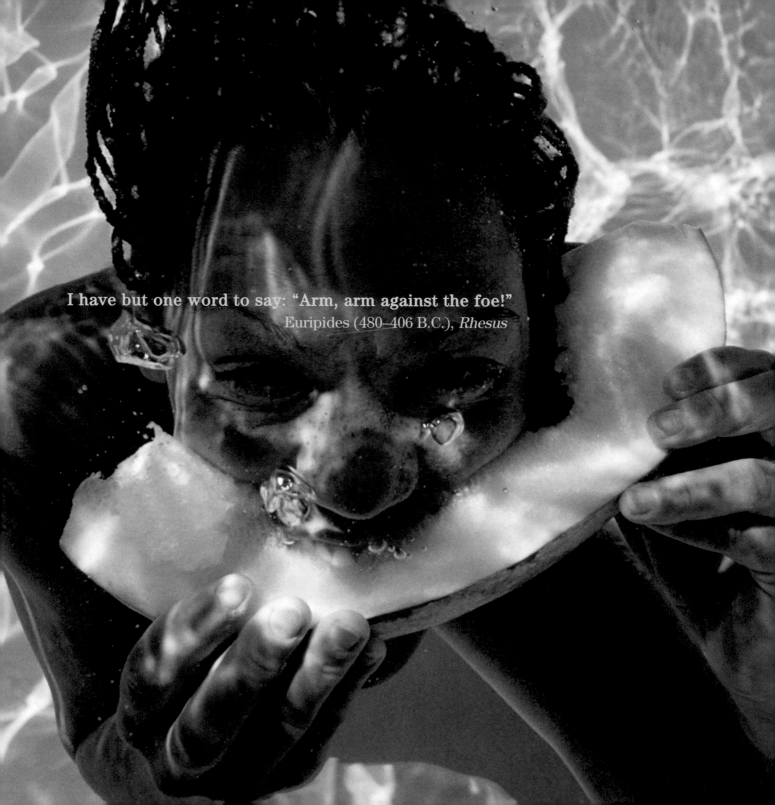

I have but one word to say: "Arm, arm against the foe!"
Euripides (480–406 B.C.), *Rhesus*

CHAPTER 1

The Fight Against Cancer :
A Daily Struggle

In Canada, as in many other regions of the globe, cancer has become the major public health problem, overtaking for the first time cardiovascular disease as the chief cause of mortality. The

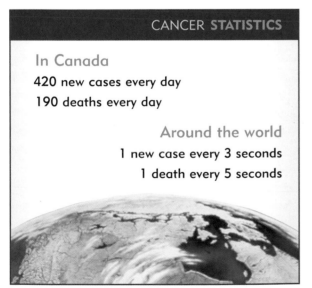

CANCER STATISTICS

In Canada

420 new cases every day
190 deaths every day

Around the world

1 new case every **3** seconds
1 death every **5** seconds

Table 1

statistics associated with cancer are of a dizzying magnitude (Table 1) : around the world, a new case of cancer is diagnosed every three seconds and every five seconds a person dies from the disease. Nothing lets us foresee that this trend will reverse itself over the next few years; it is now estimated that two people in five will see their life disrupted by cancer, and in spite of all the strength, the willpower, and the hope they devote to this struggle, barely half of them will survive five years into their diagnosis. Cancer is a complex disease that remains very difficult to treat effectively, even today, especially when it is diagnosed at an advanced stage, as is sadly all too often the case. Even though progress in surgery, radiotherapy, and chemotherapy now allows us to successfully treat certain cancers, others, very common ones, have survival rates not exceeding 25 per cent and are responsible for the deaths of thousands of people every year.

CANCER: ALL TOO OFTEN A QUESTION OF LIFESTYLE

We generally have a fatalistic approach to cancer, as if these terrible statistics described an immutable situation that we have to submit to without any possibility of intervention. Yet fighting cancer cannot be reduced to waiting until the disease has reached a clinically advanced stage requiring surgery, radiotherapy, and chemotherapy: it's possible to take a active stand against the disease by adopting certain behaviours that allow us to fight cancer at its source and thus prevent its appearance (Figure 1). In fact, a detailed analysis of the principal causes of cancer reveals that close to two-thirds are directly linked to specific lifestyle choices and may therefore be avoided. Giving up smoking, which is alone responsible for a third of all cancers, is the best example of the positive impact that certain lifestyle modifications may have. But beyond tobacco use, other lifestyle aspects, particularly with respect to the composition of diet, also have important repercussions on the risk of being affected by multiple cancers. The potential of cancer prevention is enormous; prevention is a weapon whose importance in the fight against this disease must be understood.

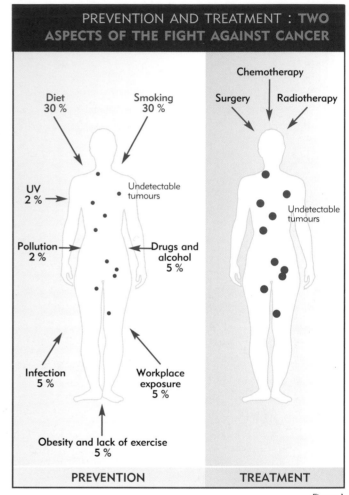

Figure 1

THE IMPACT OF DIET ON CANCER

There is now no doubt that the nature of diet plays a determining role in the risk of developing cancer. All of the estimates prepared by different international organizations of experts in the field, especially those of the World Cancer Research Fund, corroborate the fact that about a third of cancers are directly linked to poor diet, generally characterized by a lack of foods of plant origin, such as fruits and vegetables. The principal cancers that now affect Western societies all contain a component of nutritional origin, in a proportion that is especially

			Capable of being prevented through diet	
Rank (Incidence)	Type of tumour	Global incidence (per million)	Conservative (pessimistic) estimate (%)	Liberal (optimistic) estimate (%)
1	Lung	1,320	20	33
2	Stomach	1,015	66	75
3	Breast	910	33	50
4	Colorectal	875	66	75
5	Mouth and pharyngeal	575	33	50
6	Liver	540	33	66
7	Cervical	525	10	20
8	Esophageal	480	50	75
9	Prostate	400	10	20

THE IMPACT OF DIET ON **CANCER INCIDENCE**

Source: *Food, Nutrition and the Prevention of Cancer : A Global Perspective.* World Cancer Research Fund, American Institute for Cancer Research.

Table 2

high for cancers of the digestive system: three-fourths of these cancers are directly attributable to diet (Table 2). These statistics are particularly striking for colon cancer, the second cause of mortality after lung cancer. In much the same way as lung cancer is associated with smoking (85 per cent of lung cancers are caused by tobacco use), the incidence of colon cancer is linked to the food we eat: about 75 per cent of cases are intimately linked to nutrition and diet. Moreover, several studies conducted on migrant populations have shown that a high proportion of other widespread cancers, such as breast cancer and prostate cancer, also contain an important component of nutritional origin; this characteristic would seem to contribute significantly to the elevated incidence of these cancers in the West (see inset, page 18).

The high incidence of colon, breast, and prostate cancers typical of industrialized societies is an example that is as tragic as it is eloquent; it speaks to the major part played by diet in the development of cancer, and underscores the extent to which the modification of diet, through the addition of foods capable of protecting us against cancer, represents an incontrovertible objective of any strategy in the fight against this disease.

WHEN DR. JEKYLL BECOMES MR. HYDE . . .

A clinically detectable cancer is not an instantaneous phenomenon, one that appears overnight, or from one day to the next; it is the end result of a long process, during which normal cells undergo a series of transformations. Little by little, they become capable of sidestepping our defence

DIET AND THE PREVENTION OF BREAST CANCER

Twelve per cent of North American women, or one woman in nine, will one day be affected by breast cancer. Even though much attention has been accorded over the last few years to the presence of mutations in the genes that cause this type of cancer (the BRCA1 and BRCA2 genes), we must keep in mind that these mutations are present in only one woman in 300 (0.3 per cent), although they are present in a much higher proportion in Ashkenazi Jewish women: one woman in 40 (3 per cent) is a carrier of the defective gene. On the other hand, research indicates that other lifestyle aspects, especially the nature of diet, play a predominant role in the development of this disease. For example, numerous studies have shown that Asian women, who have one of the lowest incidences of breast cancer in the world, experience a quadrupling in breast cancer rates upon emigrating to the West; this increase is directly linked to changes made in diet.

Western and Asian diets differ in several aspects; it has often been speculated that these differences are responsible for the increase in breast cancer risk once an Asian woman adopts a Western lifestyle and diet. For example, it has become more and more established that the regular consumption of soy-based foods by Asian women significantly lowers the risk of breast cancer, especially if it begins at an early age, before or during puberty. In the same manner, the ubiquity of marine algae (see chapter 5) and cruciferous vegetables on Asian menus contributes to the discrepancies observed in the incidence of different cancers between East and West.

The nature of fats in diet seems to be another factor that renders Western women more vulnerable to developing breast cancer. A surplus of saturated fats, coupled with the lack of polyunsaturated omega-3 fatty acids (see chapter 7) and monounsaturated fatty acids that are typical of Western diet, strongly increases this risk. Among other outcomes, the excessive consumption of saturated fats often leads to obesity, a state that, according to recent studies, doubles the risk of this deadly disease. These observations illustrate the importance of diet in the prevention of breast cancer, and suggest that changes in Western diet, such as eating more soy-based foods during childhood and adolescence, and more cruciferous vegetables and omega-3 fatty acids as an adult, may have a concrete impact on prevention.

systems and invading their host tissues. We can compare the transformation of a normal cell into a cancer cell with that of a child who becomes a criminal as an adult. No one is born with a criminal temperament. It is the accumulation of bad influences and physical and/or psychic traumas that change an individual's social behaviour and nudge

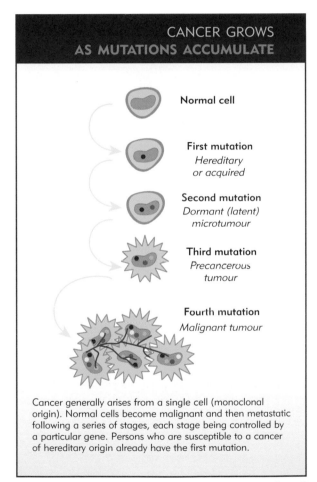

CANCER GROWS AS MUTATIONS ACCUMULATE

Normal cell

First mutation
Hereditary or acquired

Second mutation
Dormant (latent) microtumour

Third mutation
Precancerous tumour

Fourth mutation
Malignant tumour

Cancer generally arises from a single cell (monoclonal origin). Normal cells become malignant and then metastatic following a series of stages, each stage being controlled by a particular gene. Persons who are susceptible to a cancer of hereditary origin already have the first mutation.

Figure 2

him or her toward criminality. The same is true of cancer: most cancers originate in very "normal" cells that have been subjected to "trauma," a triggering event that "transforms" their personality by modifying their genetic material (DNA). These traumas are called **mutations**. Mutations are relatively frequent phenomena: the arrival in the body of various carcinogenic substances, viruses, radiation, or free radicals represents different events that damage DNA, possibly leading to delinquent behaviour by an affected cell. In certain cases, these delinquent cells are transmitted by heredity: persons who inherit delinquent cells possess from birth cells that have already been modified.

One fact must be understood: whether hereditary or acquired, delinquent cells are not yet cancerous; they only have the potential to become cancerous. They still must benefit from an environment that encourages and supports the transformation toward a cancerous state. In practice, as we shall see in greater detail in the following chapter, the cellular environment in which precancerous cells are found is generally unfavourable to their growth, and the cell that seeks to become a cancer cell must overcome numerous obstacles to succeed in its mission. It must learn to reproduce itself without external help, hide itself from the watchful surveillance of the immune system, and, very importantly, acquire a blood vessel network that will supply it with the nutrients and oxygen it needs. Each of these steps represents a gruelling task; each step requires a new mutation destined to provide the cell with a new growth advantage that, if successful, makes the cell even more dangerous. In other words, it is only after a series of mutations that the transformed cell acquires sufficient strength to grow and invade the tissue in which it finds itself, and eventually spread throughout the body as metastases (Figure 2).

Attaining the full-blown cancer stage, we see, is a difficult process for a normal cell. It is possible for us to take advantage of this arduous journey to prevent the development of cancer. With the

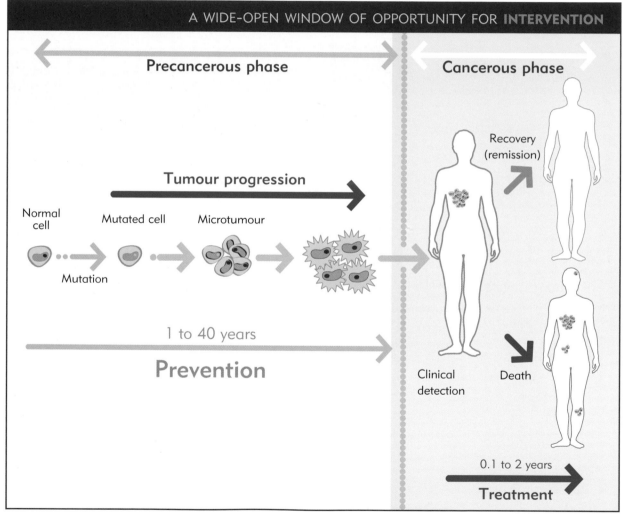

A WIDE-OPEN WINDOW OF OPPORTUNITY FOR **INTERVENTION**

Precancerous phase

Cancerous phase

Tumour progression

Normal cell   Mutated cell   Microtumour

Mutation

Recovery (remission)

1 to 40 years

Prevention

Clinical detection

Death

0.1 to 2 years

Treatment

Figure 3

exception of some particularly harmful mutations (those often responsible for cancers in young children), the majority of persons who are exposed to mutations or who have a hereditary predisposition to cancer may avoid developing the disease by adopting a lifestyle destined to block delinquent cells from acquiring new mutations, these new personality traits that make them so dangerous. This is precisely where diet comes in. The foods we eat every day may significantly stimulate the creation of an environment that is supremely hostile to the growth of cells seeking to become cancerous, thwarting them in their quest for the necessary characteristics that will let them attain a mature state.

CANCER, A DISEASE THAT MUST BE FOUGHT WHEN VULNERABLE

The difficulties encountered by precancerous cells make the appearance of a clinically detectable cancer a slow process, one stretching out over many years or even decades, during which the precancerous cells are extremely fragile (Figure 3). Six years, on average, are needed for a mutation-transformed cell to reproduce itself sufficiently to cause the formation of a precancerous tumour with a volume of 1 cubic millimetre, a microtumour containing several hundreds of thousands of cells that are still harmless and undetectable. In practice, many precancerous cells succeed in reaching the microtumour stage during the course of our lives; the truth is that we are not affected by them.

For example, one-third of women in their forties live with breast microtumours, and more than 40 per cent of men of the same age have microscopic prostate tumours. These innocuous tumours may remain dormant for long periods, as long as the precancerous cells they contain do not succeed in acquiring the other mutations that will cause them to progress to a mature stage. However, once this stage is reached, tumour growth accelerates and, in several months or several years, the tumour will reach a clinically detectable stage that will necessitate rapid medical intervention to prevent its spreading throughout the body as metastases (Figure 3).

We can compare cancer to a complicated puzzle whose every piece comes from a mutation necessary for the progression of the disease (Figure 4). Acquiring all the pieces of the puzzle is a long and difficult test for precancerous cells; once all the pieces have been assembled, however, they are rapidly fitted together, and the disease progresses at an accelerated rate, finally attaining an extremely dangerous stage that leads all too often to the death of the afflicted person.

We must therefore take advantage of the window of opportunity during which we can intervene; a window created by the long period necessary for the development of the tumour. We intervene by continuously attacking the precancerous cells in order to prevent them from assembling the pieces needed to complete this fatal puzzle. This prevention is all the more feasible since we have at our disposal certain lifestyle factors that actively contribute to restricting the development of these tumours by creating a set of hostile conditions that stop them cold and condemn them to remain in a latent and benign state. Of all these factors, not one plays as important a role as diet.

REFUSING TO GREET CANCER AT THE DOOR
Plants are without a doubt the foods with the greatest potential of lowering the risk of developing a whole slew of cancers. More than two hundred epidemiological studies have shown that persons who consume abundant quantities of foods of plant origin (fruits, vegetables, cereals, spices, and green tea) are about two times less at risk of developing cancer than people who only occasionally eat such foods. This preventive effect is linked in large part to the exceptional phytochemical compound content of these foods. Phytochemicals are anti-cancer molecules that are able to block many of the processes used by precancerous cells to grow.

Cruciferous vegetables (the cabbage family), for example, and the Alliaceae (the garlic family) contain phytochemical compounds that accelerate the elimination of carcinogenic substances from the body, and that also have the potential to inhibit the development of cancer cells by forcing them to self-destruct by apoptosis. Other foods, such as berries or green tea, contain molecules that are capable of preventing microtumours from forming the blood vessel network they need to continue growth (the process by which the blood vessel network is created is known as angiogenesis). These are only a few examples among many others; many, many foods of plant origin – oranges, or soy, for example, and even chocolate, which is plant-derived – contain phytochemical compounds capable of hindering the progression of cancer by disrupting the activity of key enzymes involved in the growth of precancerous cells. The identification and characterization of the anti-cancer molecules present in food is today a field of intense research activity, as seen by the tens of thousands of scientific publications published in the last few years on the role of these molecules in cancer prevention.

A diet containing large amounts of foods rich in anti-cancer molecules allows us to take full

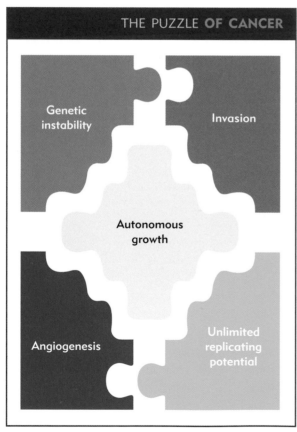

THE PUZZLE **OF CANCER**

Genetic instability

Invasion

Autonomous growth

Angiogenesis

Unlimited replicating potential

Figure 4

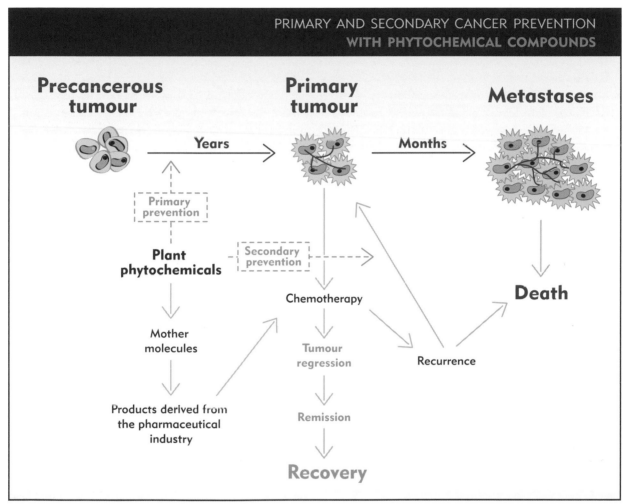

PRIMARY AND SECONDARY CANCER PREVENTION
WITH PHYTOCHEMICAL COMPOUNDS

Precancerous tumour

Primary tumour

Metastases

Years

Months

Primary prevention

Plant phytochemicals

Secondary prevention

Chemotherapy

Death

Mother molecules

Tumour regression

Recurrence

Products derived from the pharmaceutical industry

Remission

Recovery

Figure 5

advantage of the long latency period that is necessary for precancerous cells to attain a mature stage (to become cancerous); we must attack relentlessly, thus preventing these cells from completing the series of mutations that are essential for them to grow and progressively invade their host tissue (Figure 5). This preventive role of diet is not limited to blocking the appearance of a tumour (primary prevention); it also allows us to counteract the growth of residual cancer cells that may have survived a chemotherapy session and that may yet develop into tumours (recurrence), threatening

NATURE, A SOURCE OF ANTI-CANCER COMPOUNDS

Plants cannot run away from their aggressors and have thus had to evolve in such a way as to develop a considerable chemical arsenal to survive under hostile conditions. This "chemical war" is made possible by the high content in plants of molecules with powerful antibacterial, insecticidal, or fungicidal activity that allow them to successfully fight off their aggressors. These molecules are often present in exceptional quantities in the skin (or peel) of plants, where, in the case of fruits in particular, they serve to safeguard the integrity of the genetic material present in the fruit pit, thus ensuring the propagation of the species. The best example of this mechanism is that of the resveratrol contained in the skin of grapes. Resveratrol is a molecule that acts as a powerful fungicide to control the colonization of grapes by microscopic fungi. As a complement to their crucial role in plant survival, many of these compounds also have significant anti-cancer effects that we can exploit daily to preventive ends.

In addition to these food-based molecules, many studies in ethnopharmacology (a science that seeks to identify naturally occurring active molecules by seeking inspiration from the traditional use of plants as medicine) have shown that the plant world is an incredible vault of compounds with beneficial properties, several of them showing particularly strong activity against cancer cells. Certain complex anti-cancer molecules derived from plants are very effective and may be used as is (taxol, vincristine, and vinblastine) to treat advanced-stage cancer or to serve as a jumping-off point for the synthesis of even more powerful derivatives (etoposide, irinotecan, docetaxel). This therapeutic use of plant-derived anti-cancer molecules is neither rare nor marginal: more than 60 per cent of the drugs now used in clinical chemotherapy to save numerous lives are derived in one way or another from plant sources!

once again the life of the affected person. In other words, falling back on a diet rich in foods of plant origin is the equivalent of subjecting precancerous cells to a kind of daily, non-toxic chemotherapy, during which the constant presence of anti-cancer molecules confounds the attempts of precancerous cells to grow to an advanced stage.

The anti-cancer properties associated with compounds present in foods of plant origin are in no way abstract or theoretical; on the contrary, the presence of molecules capable of interfering with the development of cancer is a widespread phenomenon among plants, the majority of drugs used today in chemotherapy deriving from plant sources (see inset, page 24). In the same vein, many compounds of nutritional origin that show inhibitory activity on certain phenomena associated with the development of cancer currently serve as models for the pharmaceutical industry, which hopes to create comparable cancer-fighting molecules (Figure 5).

This approach becomes even more intriguing when we realize that, in certain cases, the plant-derived molecules already show similar activity to that of the synthetic molecules created in pharmaceutical labs! For instance, we have recently observed that luteolin and apigenin, two molecules that are particularly abundant in herbs such as mint, thyme, and parsley, powerfully inhibit the activity of a key enzyme activated by the growth factor PDGF and involved in the establishment of new blood vessels in tumours. Luteolin and apigenin possess an activity comparable to that of Gleevec®, a new, extremely effective chemotherapy drug that over the past few years has become the gold standard in the treatment of certain types of leukemia (Figure 6). These observations illustrate the extent to which the food we eat every day contains a complete array of anti-cancer molecules capable of blocking the development of cancer and thus becoming an effective rampart against this disease.

THE ADVANTAGES OF A SUSTAINED LIGHTNING ATTACK

There are many advantages to be had in exploiting a nascent cancer's long latency period by treating it with plant-derived anti-cancer phytochemicals and thus effectively preventing its development (Figure 7). From a strictly quantitative point of view,

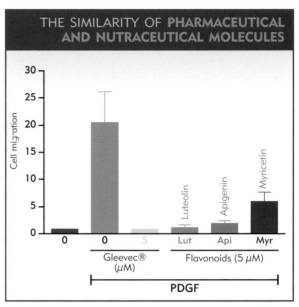

Figure 6

it is much easier to eliminate a few thousand cells present in a benign microtumour than it is to eradicate the *billions* of cancer cells that make up the mature tumour. For example, a very effective anti-cancer molecule, one that would be capable of destroying 99.9 per cent of cancer cells present, will be able to kill a microtumour, but a greater number of cancer cells will inevitably survive when a more advanced-stage tumour is treated. The treatment is more effective when the precancerous cells are in a vulnerable state; they are then much less apt to modify their genes (mutate) in order to form the blood vessel network capable of supplying their energy needs and synthesize the proteins that enable them to resist the attack of anti-cancer molecules. In other words, the smaller and more immature the tumour, the better our chances of destroying it.

We may conclude this first chapter by stressing that the multiple phytochemical compounds contained in foods of plant origin are real treasures ; the anti-cancer molecules they contain are chemotherapy agents capable of preventing the development of cancer directly at its source by blocking precancerous cells from procuring the elements necessary to their maturation. This preventive effect will be amplified if we undertake profound changes in lifestyle so that precancerous tumours do not benefit from conditions that might support their development. Cancer is a wily, obstinate, and resourceful enemy, constantly on the lookout for the smallest breach or weakness that will help it obtain what it needs to grow ; and it is determined to grow. This Machiavellian enemy must be deprived of the environment that allows it to express its immense destructive potential.

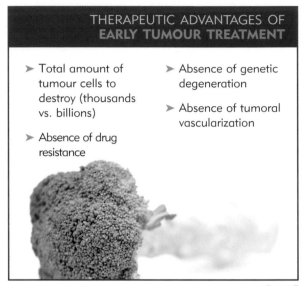

THERAPEUTIC ADVANTAGES OF
EARLY TUMOUR TREATMENT

➤ Total amount of tumour cells to destroy (thousands vs. billions)

➤ Absence of drug resistance

➤ Absence of genetic degeneration

➤ Absence of tumoral vascularization

Figure 7

In summary...

- Making lifestyle changes designed to prevent cancer constitutes an effective weapon in reducing the incidence of cancer.

- Foods of plant origin play a key role in cancer prevention by way of their exceptional content in various anti-cancer molecules that block the development of cancer at the source.

- This prevention may be compared to a preventive kind of non-toxic chemotherapy, in which the anti-cancer molecules present in certain foods prevent precancerous cells from acquiring the strength necessary to reach an advanced stage.

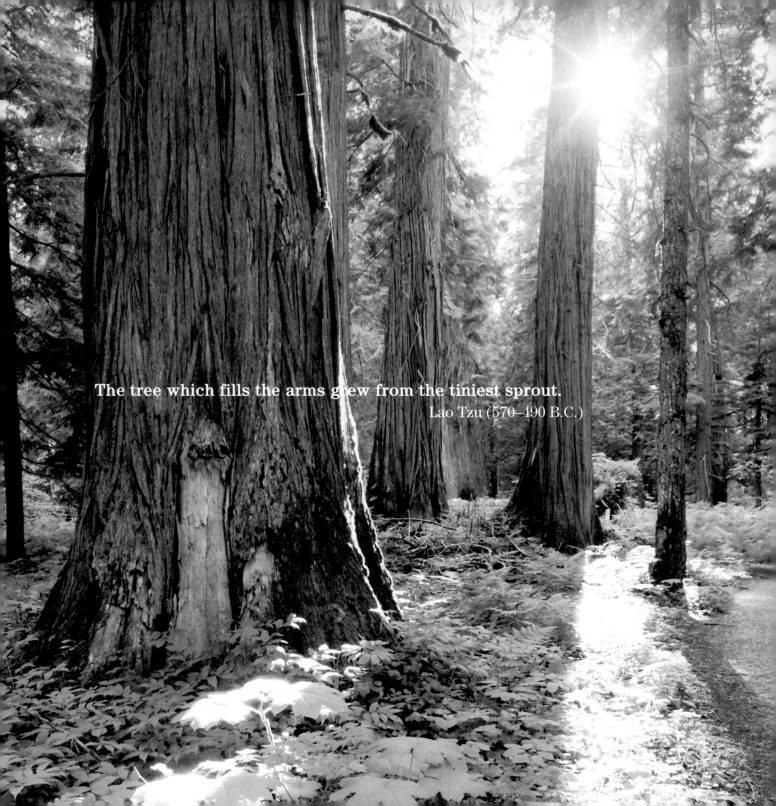

The tree which fills the arms grew from the tiniest sprout.
Lao Tzu (570–490 B.C.)

CHAPTER 2

Cancer, a Question of Context

Cancer prevention is not only a matter of firing wildly on immature cancer cells using the anti-cancer compounds present in certain foods for ammunition. In spite of their genetic instability, meaning their predisposition to cause gene mutations more quickly than their normal counterparts, cancer cells cannot succeed alone in invading their host tissue. They must count on an environment favourable to this growth, a receptive context that will supply them with the nutrients essential to their progression and encourage the constant quest for mutations that are necessary to the successful outcome of their mission. It is up to us to thwart the creation of such a pro-cancer environment in order to effectively prevent the development of cancer.

A SEED DEEP IN THE SOIL

In a way, the development of cancer may be compared to that of a seed in the soil, a seed that seems vulnerable on first glance, but that under favourable conditions gains the ability to take advantage of all the nutrients in its environment to grow to frightening maturity (Figure 8). In the case of a plant, we know that the seed must be able to count on an adequate supply of sunlight and water, two factors that are indispensable to the assimilation of the nutrients present in soil. It's the same with cancer: nascent microtumours, whether of hereditary origin or acquired over the course of life, are incapable by themselves of benefiting from the nutritious elements in their host environment. In fact, the environment in which precancerous cells develop, known as the stroma, is composed of a very large number of non-cancerous cells, particularly conjunctive tissue cells, making for a milieu that is hostile to the presence of microtumours: it carries a kind of anti-cancer character stamp that blocks their development. Microtumours are thus completely dependent on other factors that can "activate" the stroma, forcing it to modify its status quo so they

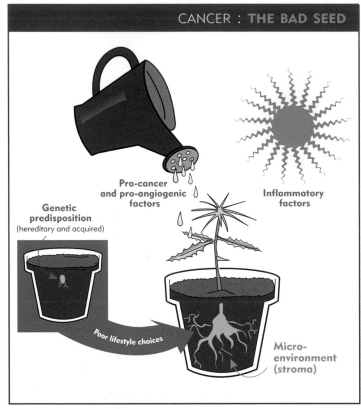

CANCER : THE BAD SEED

Pro-cancer and pro-angiogenic factors

Inflammatory factors

Genetic predisposition (hereditary and acquired)

Poor lifestyle choices

Micro-environment (stroma)

Figure 8

function of stromal cells, forcing them to secrete different substances which, on the one hand, allow the microtumour to clear a path to the tissue interior and, on the other hand, contribute to its progression by supplying it with a new blood vessel network to satisfy its energy needs.

However, growth stimulated by pro-cancer and pro-angiogenic factors would be a lot slower if the microtumour were not able to count on a second type of pro-cancer factor. Carrying the plant analogy further, this factor may be compared to sunlight; it accelerates the process by providing an important source of powerful stimulants: the inflammatory cells of our own immune system. In other words, like water and sunlight in the case of a plant, pro-cancer and inflammatory factors act in concert to permit precancerous cells to take the nutrients necessary to their growth from their immediate environment.

Preventing cancer implies attacking the seeds, the nascent tumours, to prevent them from multiplying uncontrollably and invading the whole environment. It also implies modifying this environment in order to purge it of elements able to create a climate favourable to tumour growth. This two-pronged preventive approach is essential, as many aspects of our lifestyle, and especially diet, may actively contribute to accelerating the development of cancer by supporting the creation of that "favourable milieu." Nothing better illustrates the influence of this environment than the crucial role played by inflammation in the progression of cancer.

can absorb from it the nutrients they need for growth.

Two types of pro-cancer factors present in the immediate environment of precancerous cells are especially important in the development of cancer. The first, which may be compared to watering a seed, seeks to embed the seed in the surrounding soil, so that the seed establishes its presence there where it is able to count on a constant supply of nutrients. These pro-cancer factors modify the

INFLAMMATION, THE ALLY THAT CAN BECOME AN ENEMY

The immune system comprises all the phenomena that allow us to defend ourselves against aggressors, whether they are of pathogenic origin (bacteria and viruses), chemical in nature, or traumatic. It may be compared to an army, with its own elite squadrons of crack troops specializing in taking out the enemy with precise surgical strikes. The "inflammation" squadron, a division charged with the rapid neutralization of intruders, is a front-line actor. The cells in this squadron, particularly special white blood cells known as macrophages, are labelled "inflammatory" because they release very reactive molecules designed to eliminate potential pathogens trying to invade the body; the reactive molecules in turn cause irritation that is easily noticed, in the form of redness, swelling, or itching. The inflammatory reaction also triggers the repair of damaged tissues, thanks to the numerous growth factors secreted by inflammatory cells which accelerate the arrival of healthy cells and favour the formation of new blood vessels. Normally, this reaction is of short duration, since the continued presence of inflammatory cells becomes extremely irritating for the affected tissues. When the reaction persists, however, a state of chronic inflammation sets in, which can cause intense pain at the inflammation site. As we shall see, chronic inflammation may also be promoted by certain lifestyle factors (smoking, obesity, caloric surplus, lack of sufficient omega-3 fatty acids). Even though this type of chronic inflammation does not necessarily cause apparent symptoms, it does create a context favourable to the growth of cells present in the inflamed environment; a particularly dangerous situation if the tissue contains microtumours composed of precancerous cells. True opportunists, precancerous cells will use the growth factors secreted by inflammatory cells and the new blood vessel network created near the inflammation site to grow into a mature tumour.

CANCER, AN INFLAMMATORY DISEASE

The inflammation caused by the immune system is a phenomenon essential to the body's integrity; without it, we would be completely at the mercy of the numerous pathogens present in our external environment (see inset, page 31). When the inflammation becomes too intense, however, or when it occurs over too long a period of time, it can cause the development of different pathologies and even encourage the progression of diseases such as cancer. The close association between inflammation and cancer was already known to the pathologists who first became interested in cancer. In fact, the abundant presence of macrophages and other immune cells in tumours is a fundamental characteristic of a large number of

THE LINKS BETWEEN CANCER AND INFLAMMATION

➤ Many types of tumours prefer to appear in inflamed tissues.

➤ The immune cells that cause chronic inflammation are found in abundance in tumours.

➤ The chemical mediators that control inflammation are produced by tumours.

➤ The inhibition of inflammatory mediators prevents the development of cancer.

➤ Genetic variants of inflammatory genes change the probability of developing cancer as well as the seriousness of the developing tumour.

➤ The long-term use of anti-inflammatory agents reduces the risk of certain cancers.

Table 3

cancers; generally speaking, the more important this presence, the more dangerous a stage the tumour has reached.

The importance of inflammation in the cancer story is also well illustrated by the close relationship between various pathologies caused by chronic inflammation and the devastating increase in the risk of cancer associated with these inflammatory conditions (Table 3). We have known for quite a while that chronic inflammation, whether caused by repeated exposure to toxic substances (cigarette smoke, asbestos fibres), certain bacteria or viruses (*Helicobacter pylori*, the hepatitis virus), or the presence of a longstanding metabolic imbalance, considerably increases the risks of developing a cancer of the organs affected by inflammation (Table 4). For example, the inflammation caused by the continuous presence of *H. pylori* in the stomach increases by a factor of three to six the risk of stomach cancer, while ulcerative colitis, an inflammatory disease of the large intestine, increases by a factor of ten the risk of developing

colon cancer. These relationships are far from isolated cases: researchers estimate that *one cancer in six* on the planet is directly linked to the

INFLAMMATORY DISEASES THAT MAY PREDISPOSE US TO CANCER

Intestinal inflammation ➤	Colorectal cancer
Gastritis caused by ➤ *H. pylori*	Gastric cancer
Salpingitis ➤	Ovarian cancer
Schistosomiasis ➤	Bladder cancer
H. pybri ➤	MALT lymphoma
Hepatitis B and C ➤ viruses	Liver cancer
HHV-8 ➤	Kaposi's sarcoma
Silica ➤	Bronchial carcinoma
Asbestos ➤	Mesothelioma
Barrett's metaplasia ➤	Esophageal cancer
Thyroiditis ➤	Thyroidal papillary carcinoma
Prostatis ➤	Prostate cancer

Table 4

presence of a chronic inflammatory condition.

INFLAMMATION: SITUATION ESCALATION!

The mechanisms by which pre-cancerous cells use inflammation to grow to maturity are complex. They testify to the extraordinary ability of cancer to use all the elements present in its immediate environment to achieve its goals.

Cancer cells secrete messages destined for the inflammatory cells in their vicinity, provoking these cells into releasing a large number of growth factors and enzymes that allow the cancer to clear a pathway through tissue, as well as molecules essential to the formation of a blood vessel network, and therefore indispensable to the progression of cancer (Figure 9). All of these growth factors and enzymes normally accelerate healing and re-establish balance in damaged tissues, but for a precancerous tumour looking to improve its chances of growth, they are gifts from heaven!

These factors also promote the survival of cancer cells by activating a key protein, nuclear factor κB (NFκB). NFκB plays a crucial role in the growth of these cells by considerably increasing the production of cyclooxygenase-2 (COX-2), a very important enzyme involved in the production of inflammatory molecules; an excess of COX-2 increases the number of macrophages and immune cells at the inflammation site. We are witnessing the establishment of a vicious circle in which the growth factors produced by macrophages are used by the cancer cells to survive and grow; the growing cancer cells provoke the further production of large numbers of inflammatory molecules, leading to the recruitment of even more macrophages. This explains why inflammation is such an important aspect of the progression of cancer: by creating an environment rich in growth factors and by the fact of their continued presence, inflammatory cells provide the conditions that allow precancerous cells to accelerate their attempts at mutation and acquire the new properties essential for them to continue growing.

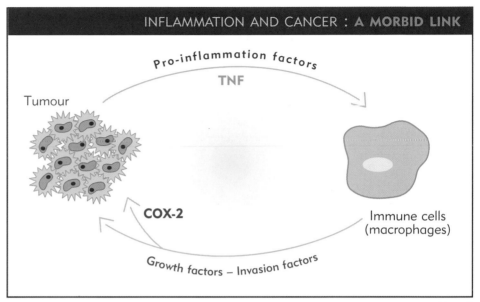

INFLAMMATION AND CANCER : A MORBID LINK

Pro-inflammation factors

TNF

Tumour

COX-2

Immune cells (macrophages)

Growth factors – Invasion factors

Figure 9

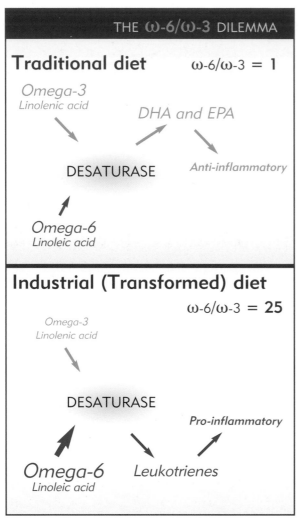

THE ω-6/ω-3 DILEMMA

Traditional diet   ω-6/ω-3 = 1

Omega-3
Linolenic acid

DHA and EPA

DESATURASE

Anti-inflammatory

Omega-6
Linoleic acid

Industrial (Transformed) diet

ω-6/ω-3 = 25

Omega-3
Linolenic acid

DESATURASE

Pro-inflammatory

Omega-6
Linoleic acid   *Leukotrienes*

Figure 10

a much lower risk of developing certain types of cancers, especially colon cancer. However, these drugs have serious side effects on the cardio-vascular system (effects that led to the removal of Vioxx® from the market) which limit their use as preventive agents. Nevertheless, the protective effect exhibited by these anti-inflammatory molecules indicates that reducing inflammation represents a very promising avenue in cancer prevention.

The chronic inflammation so essential to the development of cancer is not always caused by external aggressions; it may also be brought on by diet. The excessive consumption of transformed foods loaded with sugars and harmful fats, asso-ciated with a lack of foods of plant origin, especially fruits and vegetables, is a highly efficient way of creating pro-inflammatory conditions, a chronic state that promotes the development of cancer.

THE OMEGA-3 FATTY ACID DEFICIT

Polyunsaturated fats may be divided into two large classes: omega-3s and omega-6s. These two types of fats are called "essential" because they are indispensable to proper body function; our bodies, however, are incapable of manufacturing them, and they must be obtained from food. Omega-3 and omega-6 fatty acids participate in the formation of cellular membranes, the development of brain activity, and the manufacture of substances necessary to blood pressure regulation, blood vessel elasticity, and the inflammatory and immune responses.

In the body, omega-6s are transformed into leukotrienes, pro-inflammatory molecules that

REDUCING INFLAMMATION THROUGH DIET

Over the last few years, studies have shown that regular users of anti-inflammatory drugs that inhibit COX-2 activity (such as Vioxx® and Celebrex®) have

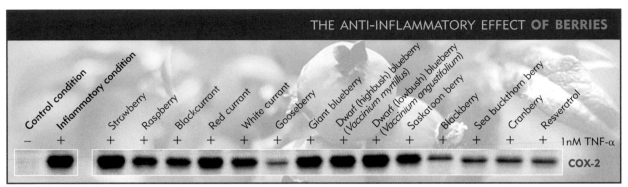

THE ANTI-INFLAMMATORY EFFECT **OF BERRIES**

Control condition · Inflammatory condition · Strawberry · Raspberry · Blackcurrant · Red currant · White currant · Gooseberry · Giant blueberry · Dwarf (highbush) blueberry (*Vaccinium myrtillus*) · Dwarf (lowbush) blueberry (*Vaccinium angustifolium*) · Saskatoon berry · Blackberry · Sea buckthorn berry · Cranberry · Resveratrol

1nM TNF-α

COX-2

Figure 11

promote coagulation and cell growth, two phenomena linked to defence against pathogens and the repair of lesions caused by cell tearing (wounds). Omega-3s are transformed into docosahexaenoic acid (DHA) and eicosapentaenoic acid (EPA), two types of polyunsaturated fats that prevent these phenomena from getting out of hand and causing damage to surrounding affected tissue, thanks to their anti-inflammatory, anti-coagulant, and anti-proliferative activity (Figure 10). The proper omega-3/omega-6 balance in a diet is therefore essential to ensuring adequate control of inflammatory processes.

Omega-6s and omega-3s are transformed into active molecules with the help of the same enzymatic system (desaturase). The human body has adapted itself over the course of evolution to function with a diet balanced in polyunsaturated fatty acids; the balance leans toward the production of EPA and DHA, creating an anti-inflammatory environment. However, as a result of the important changes introduced by the industrialization of food, especially the heavy use of vegetable oils rich in omega-6s, this

balance has been disturbed and no longer exists: most of us consume about twenty-five times more omega-6s than omega-3s. This imbalance carries important consequences in terms of cancer prevention, since an excess of omega-6s tends to tip the balance toward inflammation. As we shall see in the chapter on flaxseed, it now seems certain that increasing intake of omega-3 fatty acids while lowering that of omega-6s, in order to re-establish the proper balance and prevent the creation of a chronically inflamed environment, is an important prerequisite for interfering with the development of cancer. In the same line of thought, certain fatty fish, such as salmon, mackerel, herring, and sardines, contain significant quantities of EPA and DHA; eating them regularly is another effective way of lessening inflammation.

THE PLANT DEFICIT

Certain foods of plant origin possess powerful anti-inflammatory properties, and their absence or inadequate presence in Western diet contributes to the creation of an inflammatory climate that

Cancer, a Question of Context | **Chapter 2**

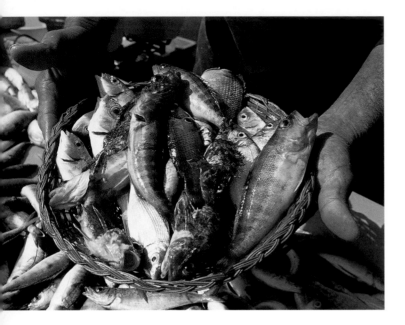

favours the onset of cancer. For example, the resveratrol present in red wine and the curcumin in turmeric (see chapter 8) are molecules capable of blocking a crucial step in the synthesis of COX-2 by cancer cells; this property plays an important part in their ability to interfere with the growth of certain types of cancer cells. Many plants seem to share this anti-inflammatory property. Recent research carried out in our laboratory suggests that adding gooseberry, blackberry, or cranberry extracts to prostate cancer cells inhibits the sharp rise in COX-2 induced by TNF, a powerful molecule involved in the appearance of inflammation (Figure 11). Knowing the important role played by inflammation in the development of cancer, we must stress that the anti-inflammatory properties shown by many foods can only have a very positive impact on the prevention of cancer.

We should try to see the growth of cancer not as an isolated phenomenon, but as a process whose success depends directly on a set of favourable conditions supplied by the host. This strong dependence of cancer on environment is in fact a weakness, a chink in its armour, that we can exploit to our advantage. Cancer creates nothing; it is an outright parasite that remains in a vulnerable state as long as it finds itself in inhospitable territory. When conditions become favourable, as we have seen, cancer deploys ingenious methods to better exploit its immediate environment, and is constantly on the lookout for new mutations that allow it to grow. In the absence of such conditions, however, cancer has no resources to fall back on and does not succeed in achieving its full potential. Anonymous and impotent, it is condemned to a life in hiding.

It is therefore vital to not only keep chronic inflammation to a minimum by adopting a diet richer in plants, but also to avoid at all costs the factors that favour chronic inflammation. In this context, the excessive consumption of transformed foods that are loaded with harmful fats and sugars, and the obesity which may be its outcome, are the principal lifestyle factors that promote inflammation and the progression of microscopic tumours toward an advanced stage.

In summary...

- Cellular environment is very important to the progression of cancer. This environment supplies precancerous cells with many elements that allow these cells to better implant themselves in their host tissue.

- Among these environmental factors, the immune system cells responsible for chronic inflammation participate actively in the growth of cancer by supporting the survival and growth of precancerous cells, as well as allowing them to acquire a blood vessel network that provides for their energy needs.

- The presence in diet of an abundance of foods of plant origin as well as significant amounts of omega-3 fatty acids plays a crucial part in reducing inflammation, an indispensable feature of cancer prevention.

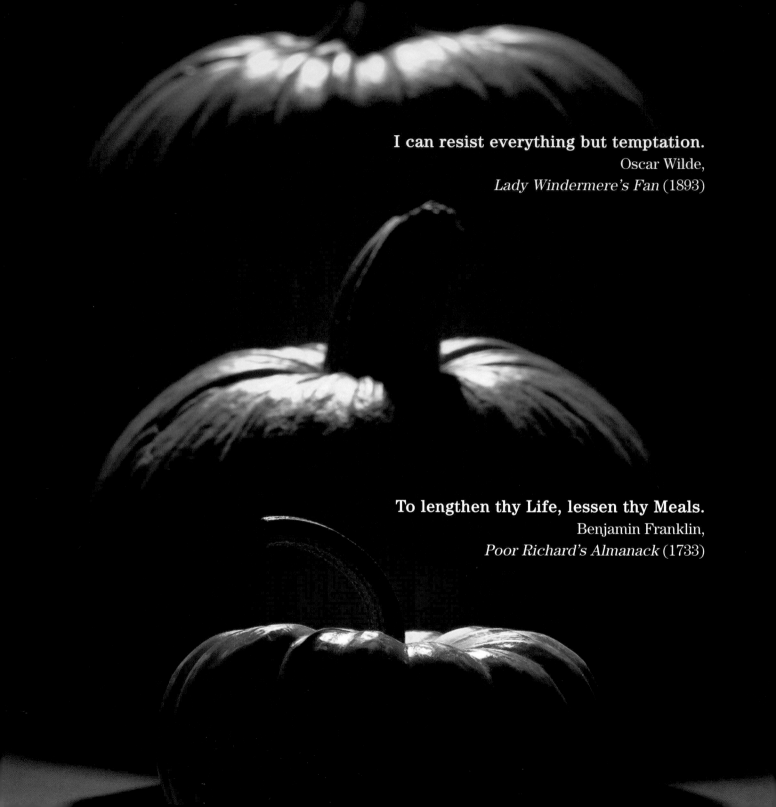

I can resist everything but temptation.
Oscar Wilde,
Lady Windermere's Fan (1893)

To lengthen thy Life, lessen thy Meals.
Benjamin Franklin,
Poor Richard's Almanack (1733)

CHAPTER 3

Obesity, a Sizable Problem

Scarcely a century ago, the principal diet-related problem threatening our society was malnutrition. The inevitable deficiencies in nutrients and the vitamins associated with them were directly responsible for the premature death of thousands of people. A century later, diet still provokes disquiet and fears, albeit completely different ones this time around, at least in wealthier nations. Today, over-eating and generally poor food quality constitute a major public health problem because they are responsible for chronic diseases that reduce the quality of life and life expectancy of an ever-growing number of individuals. This incredible reversal illustrates not only the crucial role of food in maintaining good health, but also the fragility and the complexity of their relationship. Paying attention to the specifics of diet in order to re-establish a balance compatible with sustained good health is guaranteed to have a positive impact on the prevention of diseases such as cancer.

THE BAD SIDE OF THE HORN OF PLENTY

According to Greek legend, a special horn grew from the forehead of Amalthea, the goat nurse of Zeus. Blessed with magical powers, the horn was capable of producing meals and beverages at will; the modern word "cornucopia," or horn of plenty, refers to this myth. Today, we dine on feasts worthy of the gods of Olympus: never, since the appearance of the human species on Earth, have we enjoyed such easy access to such a wealth and variety of food. There has been extraordinary progress; in 2 million years of human history, obtaining the necessary foods for survival has represented an immense challenge which has called for many adaptations. This progress is directly related to the Industrial Revolution, marked by the development of new manufacturing and refining processes, as well as by intensive agri-cultural production, all of which facilitate access to considerable quantities of food at reasonable cost for the great majority of the world's people today.

The abundance and the diversity of fresh fruits and vegetables available year-round and the sheer number of foods arriving from the four corners of the globe have widened our cultural horizons and allowed us to indulge in a quantity and variety of food that would have been the envy of our ancestors.

Unfortunately, this abundance is not always synonymous with quality. The past few decades have witnessed the birth of a new industrial sector, centred on the large-scale production of energy-rich foods designed for quick consumption. The arrival of "junk" food has had enormous consequences not only on eating patterns, but also on the relationship of individuals to the food they eat. These days, there is no real need to cook or to take the trouble of sitting down to dinner: it is possible to feed oneself quickly and efficiently in any location, in one's car or in front of the television set. Food has become a consumer good like any other, a widely available product that has been standardized within an inch of its life to appeal to the largest possible cross-section of the population. The pleasure associated with discovering new flavours and textures has

THEN AND NOW: A SIZABLE PROBLEM

	1960	2000
Average women's clothing size sold	8	14
Muffin	75 g	170 g
Bottle of cola	200 ml	500 ml
Bag of potato chips	30 g	85 g
Hamburger	40 g	40 to 225 g

Table 6

become secondary, replaced by the base feeling of satisfying one's hunger . . . until the next mealtime (see inset, page 42).

And there is a whole lot available to satisfy oneself with! Not only are these foods, fast food in particular, high in calories (Table 5), but portions are getting bigger and bigger (Table 6). In fact, the serving size of today's most commonly eaten food products has grown significantly over the last few decades, often under the pretext of giving the hapless consumer more at a lower price. However, studies clearly indicate that the visual appeal of a larger portion short-circuits our internal appetite-regulating mechanisms, pushing us to consume more food than our needs would dictate. It's obvious that the overconsumption of calorie-rich food in oversize packages will have serious repercussions on the size of consumers!

FAST FOOD CALORIE COUNT

Fast-food muffin	500
Large portion of French fries	540
Double hamburger	1,000
Tub of popcorn with butter	1,640

Table 5

ENDLESS HUNGER

Eating this much food is even more perplexing when we consider that the incredible technological advances made in the last century allow us, for the first time in history, to get away with expending very little energy to function. The number of hours spent in front of the television or the computer screen and the shift of the job market toward the service sector combine to ensure that our lifestyle is much more sedentary than ever.

Taking into account our relatively recent sedentary lifestyle, scientists estimate that a daily intake of 2,200 calories is sufficient to satisfy most people's energy requirements. Yet instead of reducing calorie intake to reflect contemporary lifestyle, North Americans are eating more and more: in twenty-five years, from 1981 to 2004, the daily calorie intake of Canadians has risen from 2,294 to 2,674, an increase of 17 per cent!

This avalanche of energy-rich substances is the antithesis of the type of food to which our metabolism has adapted itself over the course of evolution. Whether in prehistoric times, when uncertainties linked to the success of both hunting and gathering could mean a prolonged fast, or after the development of agriculture (subject to bad weather and the presence of crop-destroying pathogens), daily life for humans has always been marked much more by rarity than by the overabundance of food. Our metabolism, the way we assimilate food energy, has had to adapt itself to these feast and famine cycles and develop efficient ways of stocking the energy surplus to save against times when food is scarce. In our current situation of omnipresent food and sedentary lifestyle, these efficient stocking mechanisms perform all too well, especially if little physical effort is required to obtain food: the surplus energy accumulates in the body's fatty tissues. When the accumulation becomes chronic, it leads to overweight and obesity.

OUR EXPANDING UNIVERSE

According to criteria established by the World Health Organization (WHO), people with a body mass index (BMI) between 25 and 30 are overweight; those whose BMI is greater than 30 are obese (Table 7). One *billion* persons around the world are carrying extra weight and 312 million of these, including about 30 million children, are obese.

These statistics become even more impressive when we look at the evolution of this tendency in North America: in barely forty years, the number of obese adults has more than doubled, while the

STANDARDS USED TO DEFINE OVERWEIGHT AND OBESITY *		
BMI (kg/m^2)	Classification (WHO)	Description
<18,5	Insufficient weight	Thin
18,5–24,9	Recommended weight	Ideal weight
25–29,9	Level 1 overweight	Overweight
30–39,9	Level 2 overweight	Obesity
>40	Level 3 overweight	Morbid obesity

Body mass index (BMI) is calculated by dividing weight (in kilograms) by the square of height (in square metres).

*According to the World Health Organization (WHO).

Table 7

WHY EAT SO MUCH ?

The reasons which prod people into always wanting to eat *more*, despite a more and more sedentary lifestyle, are complex. On one hand, the high amounts of energy-rich substances in food agrees with our brain, which has evolved to recognize the importance of these substances for survival in times of food scarcity, which was actually the case for more than 2 million years! The simultaneous presence of elevated quantities of sugar and fats in a food, very rare in nature, is particularly attractive because it induces a feeling of pleasure that encourages repetition. On the other hand, one cannot ignore the impact of advertising on consumption, especially at a time when the number of hours spent in front of the television or the computer screen has never been higher: in 2005, the food industry spent $11 billion on advertising in North America alone, of which $5 billion was spent on television ads.

From a metabolic point of view, the ingestion of huge servings of energy-rich foods produces an excess of blood sugar. The body responds by producing large amounts of insulin to absorb all that sugar . . . paradoxically inducing a hypoglycemic state just a few hours after mealtime! The immediate reflex is to eat again, to re-establish an adequate level of sugar, thus creating a cycle that puts a heavy load on a person's metabolism. Overeating can thus be seen as a kind of dependence, a psychological and physiological "drug" that is strongly pushed on us by an industry that sings the praises of super-sized formats.

number of obese children, boys and girls indiscriminately, has more than *tripled*. It is currently estimated that about 30 per cent of adults and 10 per cent of North American children are obese (Figure 12). Unbelievably, the situation is worsening, as obesity rates continue to grow; obesity and related disorders now threaten countries such as France and China, once thought immune to such phenomena because of their distinct culinary traditions.

Being overweight or obese is often considered a problem of a purely aesthetic nature; people who seek to lose weight often do so with the goal of improving their appearance. However, this is the least of the evils associated with excess weight! Obesity is first and foremost a major medical concern. Not only is it responsible for many skeleton and joint-related complaints, it can also lead to numerous metabolic disorders, such as diabetes, cardiovascular illness, and certain cancers. To fully comprehend the scope of the damage done by obesity, consider the following: studies indicate that in 2003, more Americans died from causes linked to obesity than from smoking and tobacco use.

OBESITY AND CANCER

In addition to being an important risk factor for diabetes and cardiovascular disease, obesity represents a determining factor in the development of certain types of cancers (Figure 13). Obese persons see their risks of developing colon cancer, gall bladder cancer, esophageal cancer, and kidney cancer increase by 200 to 300 per cent, and the figure is 350 per cent higher for cases of endometrial cancer (the endometrium is the inner mucous membrane of the uterus). Obesity alone is responsible for about 30 per cent of all colon cancers in men and about 60 per cent of endometrial cancers in women! Overall, it is estimated that being overweight or obese will cause about 15 per cent of all deaths linked to cancer in the United States; close to 100,000 of these deaths could be avoided each year if the population had a normal body mass index.

Obesity triggers the development of cancer by complex mechanisms that we are only beginning to better understand. Contrary to what is often believed, the function of adipose tissue cells (adipocytes) is not limited to stockpiling surplus energy in the form of fat. These highly active cells act much like glands, secreting different types of

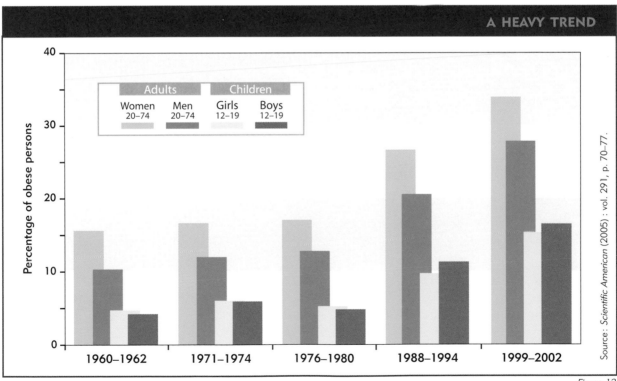

A HEAVY TREND

Source: *Scientific American* (2005) : vol. 291, p. 70–77.

Figure 12

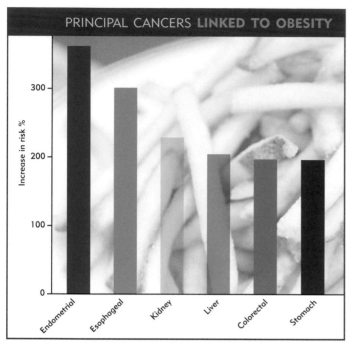

PRINCIPAL CANCERS **LINKED TO OBESITY**

Increase in risk %

300 —

200 —

100 —

0 —

Endometrial Esophageal Kidney Liver Colorectal Stomach

Figure 13

messages destined for surrounding tissue; during an intense athletic workout, for example, adipocytes produce fatty acids that supply muscles with energy. In obese persons, these cells are overloaded with fat, causing them to malfunction (Figure 14).

Adipocytes that secrete too many fatty acids force liver cells and muscles to use these fats instead of sugar to go about their normal tasks. This drop in sugar use has important consequences; blood sugar remains high, despite an increase in the amount of insulin, and "insulin resistance," responsible for the development of type 2 diabetes, sets in. The jump in insulin may also be implicated

in the growth of some tumours; it raises the blood levels of other hormones or growth factors, such as IGF-1, which stimulate the proliferation of cells in surrounding tissue, increasing the risk of cancer. Insulin also triggers the synthesis of inflammatory molecules that support the development of diabetes and provide precancerous cells with conditions that are favourable to their continued growth. All of these harmful effects are amplified because adipocytes use the far-flung blood vessel network present in hypertrophied adipose tissue (a kilogram of fat contains no fewer than 3.5 kilometres of blood vessels!) to transport a host of substances and growth factors that promote further inflammation and angiogenesis.

The obesity "problem" is not just about excess weight: obesity is a complex state that has huge consequences on many bodily functions and that may actively contribute to the development of serious, even fatal, diseases, such as cancer.

As is the case for a diet lacking in fruits and vegetables, overeating is a contributing factor in the high incidence of certain types of cancers. The combination of these two factors is particularly favourable to cancer, and dangerous for us, since an inadequate supply of anti-cancer molecules from diet allows cancer cells to progress without obstacle, their growth stimulated by the inflammatory conditions caused by caloric overload and obesity.

We must call into question this way of feeding ourselves, not only for its excesses, its monotony, and its lack of originality, but also for its very negative impact on health. Benefiting from the

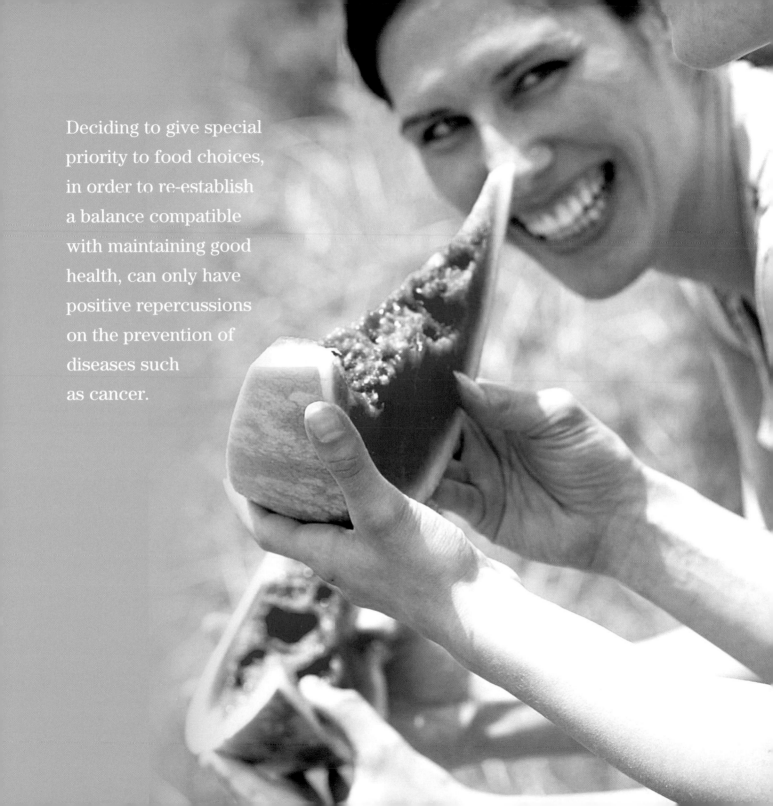

Deciding to give special
priority to food choices,
in order to re-establish
a balance compatible
with maintaining good
health, can only have
positive repercussions
on the prevention of
diseases such
as cancer.

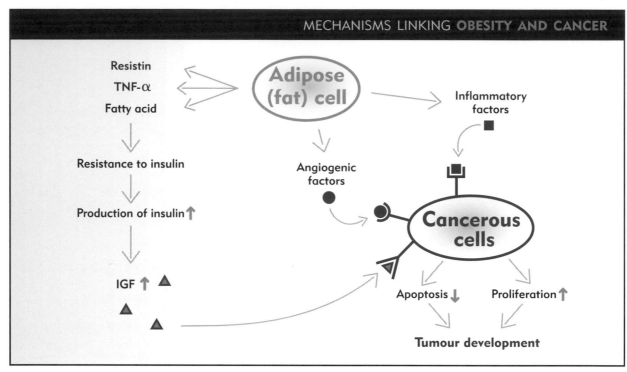

MECHANISMS LINKING **OBESITY AND CANCER**

Figure 14

abundance of food available does not mean that we have to eat more than we need to; it means that we should use these resources available to us to heighten our enjoyment of food, of nourishing ourselves well while simultaneously preventing disease. Food may no longer be a rare commodity, but it is no less precious; it is the best weapon at our disposal today for fighting cancer.

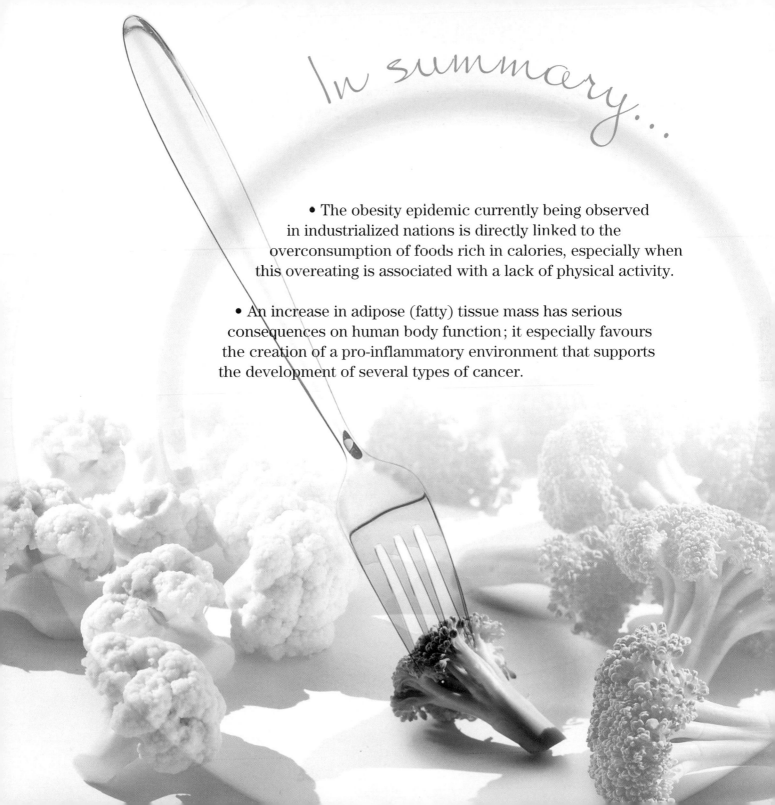

In summary...

- The obesity epidemic currently being observed in industrialized nations is directly linked to the overconsumption of foods rich in calories, especially when this overeating is associated with a lack of physical activity.

- An increase in adipose (fatty) tissue mass has serious consequences on human body function; it especially favours the creation of a pro-inflammatory environment that supports the development of several types of cancer.

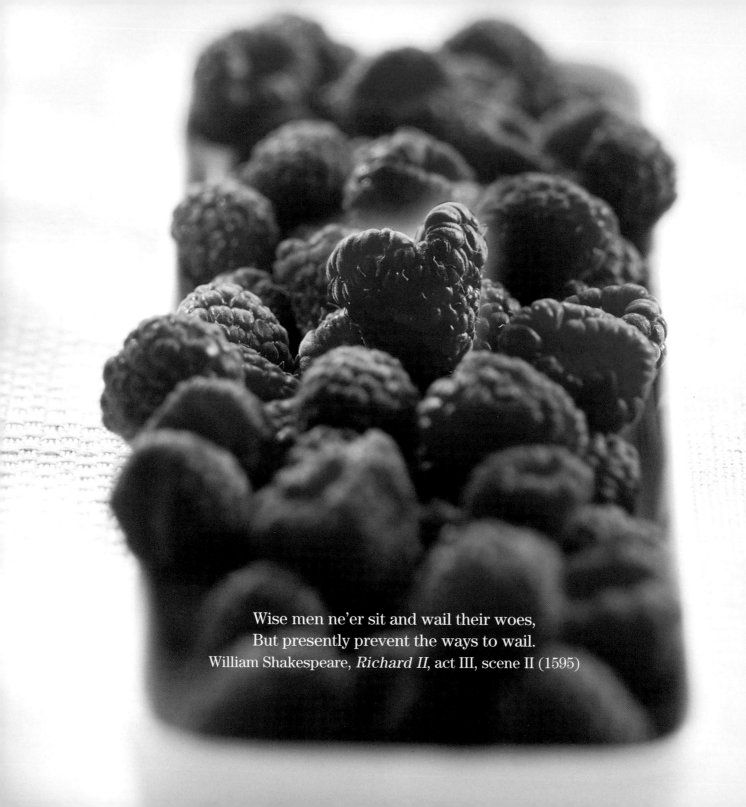

Wise men ne'er sit and wail their woes,
But presently prevent the ways to wail.
William Shakespeare, *Richard II*, act III, scene II (1595)

CHAPTER   4

Diet : At the Heart of Cancer Prevention

There is no doubt that the elevated incidence of many cancers in industrialized countries could be significantly reduced by making profound and long-lasting changes to our diet. Following through with diet and lifestyle changes, however, is not a trivial matter; this is why it is often tempting to choose easier-seeming solutions to our problems. The food industry understands this very well; it offers us an ever-growing number of medicines, dietary supplements, and "natural" extracts, all of which are supposed to solve problems created by a diet poor in quality, without our having to actually ask the hard questions about what we put into our bodies (see inset, page 50). The desire to take medicine, said Sir William Osler, is perhaps the greatest feature which distinguishes man from animals, and one cannot help but agree, considering the astronomical sales of products designed to counteract the harmful consequences of a poor diet.

WHEN MAGIC TRUMPS REALITY

We must be critical of those products that validate our dubious dietary choices and that in practice only encourage them by lulling us into a false sense of security. Addressing the issue of the prevention of diseases as serious as cancer solely by putting faith in the gulping down of a few pills, without changing diet and lifestyle in any way, is, strictly speaking, wishful thinking, and has nothing to do with a truly preventive approach.

A hot-button issue from the time of Hippocrates onward, it seems that the eternal struggle opposing science and magic has not yet been resolved. We are still caught up in the frantic and ongoing pursuit of the elixir of youth and longevity that has garnered huge profits for generations of charlatans and snake-oil salesmen, investing in "universal" remedies made of so-called "natural" ingredients that promise the prevention and cure of any and every disease without undue effort.

THE "DIGESTOL® SYNDROME"

A few years ago, an advertisement vaunting the merits of a certain antacid showed an American homemaker frazzled by the streak of bad health luck her family was experiencing: "My husband has diarrhea, my older daughter is constipated, my son has a stomach ache, and I have gastric reflux. What is the one thing I need for all this? Digestol®." It might seem obvious to the casual observer that, rather than a particular kind of medicine, what this woman really needs is a good cookbook! This ad is the sign of an unhealthy and unfortunately widespread attitude when it comes to diet and health: instead of making healthier or more sensible dietary choices, we have a tendency to look for the "miracle cure" that will allow us to keep doing what we were doing (eating badly) while avoiding the inevitable unpleasantness associated with this lifestyle. Yet the real answer to getting rid of these diseases or discomforts is simple: instituting profound changes in diet and lifestyle instead of banking on pharmaceutical solutions that only temporarily ease the consequences of a diet that is too heavy or too rich in the wrong kind of fats.

The same logic can be applied to many of the dietary supplements that are promoted as supplying the vitamins needed to compensate for a less than healthy diet. The problem of vitamin supplements is that they create a false sense of security and comfort in consumers by implying they can compensate for poor dietary habits, such as insufficient fruits and vegetables. With respect to cancer, this reasoning is outright dangerous: numerous studies conducted in the past twenty years have not succeeded in demonstrating convincingly any real positive impact of vitamin supplements on the incidence of cancer. Quite the opposite, in fact: two studies have indicated an *increase* in the risk of developing certain types of cancer by taking high doses of vitamins A and E. The generous consumption of fruits and vegetables, however, is a well-established protective factor against many cancers; as we have seen, this protection operates by mechanisms in which vitamins play no role. Fruits and vegetables are thus the only foods able to supply us with both essential vitamins and minerals and the phytochemical compounds that may be able to prevent the development of cancer.

A realistic outlook is best: no drug or multivitamin supplement will ever replace the health benefits offered by a diet rich in fruits and vegetables, low in saturated fats, and rich in polyunsaturated omega-3 fatty acids, in which complex sugars from grains and cereals are the principal carbohydrate sources and proteins are obtained from fish, poultry, and legumes as well as from red meat. Last but not least, such a diet is also the source of greater pleasure than a diet based on a regime of pill-taking!

It's important to be clear-headed; it's time to stop our enthusiastic endorsement of miracle "cures" whose promoters profit from our passivity and our reticence to make lifestyle changes. Whether these pills are made from exotic plants, deer antlers, or other "natural sources," the benefits associated with them have nothing to do with health and everything to do with the financial health of their manufacturers. No tablet alone is capable of preventing a disease as complex and as devastating as cancer, or of compensating for the disastrous consequences of a low-quality diet, especially if that diet is poor in fruits and vegetables and rich in sugar, harmful fats, and foods modified to excess.

The same reasoning may be applied to the principles described in this book: these recommendations should not be seen as a miraculous program that absolutely guarantees being spared from cancer. It remains, however, the strategy most likely to reduce the risk of contracting the disease. As we have seen, cancer is an incredibly complex malady, capable of using to its advantage every weakness in the human organism to pursue its own ends (growth), and it is unrealistic to believe that one can completely and definitively arm oneself against its future appearance. We can compare the risk of developing cancer to that undertaken by someone at the wheel of a car in a poor state of repair. If the person happens to be drunk, and decides to drive while passionately discussing the latest sports results on his cellphone without paying too much attention to his driving, his risk of losing control of the vehicle is much greater than that of a person driving the same car, but who is obeying the rules and not engaging in dangerous behaviour. The same is true for cancer: if a person smokes, suffers from obesity, is physically inactive, and eats too many harmful fats (and thus few omega-3 fatty acids) and few fruits and vegetables, then her risk of being stricken with cancer is high. On the other hand, consider a physically active person, a non-smoker who eats five to ten daily servings of fruits and vegetables (especially those containing large amounts of anti-cancer compounds!), as well as foods containing high levels of omega-3s, while eating all foods in moderation. Such a person runs a lower risk of developing cancer.

One cannot completely eliminate the risk of getting cancer. However, taking charge of one's health in order to make significant lifestyle changes, especially with regard to our diet choices, is the approach most likely to reduce the impact of this disease on our lives.

TOWARD A DIET THAT PREVENTS CANCER

Dietary habits testify to a society's quality of life and the ideas or principles that shape it. The culinary extravagances of Apicius speak to the irresistible attraction of the Romans to splendour and hedonism; the many meatless days imposed on the faithful by clerics of the Middle Ages illustrate the difficult conditions of this period, marked by famine and disease; the importance accorded by Asian societies to good diet and the well-being that results is a sign of the value they place on living to a great age.

Our own society is no different. So characteristic of our time, excessive eating is of a piece with

LET'S BE **REALISTIC**

➤ Reduce serving size.

➤ Change dietary habits instead of following ineffective weight-losing diets.

➤ Drink more water.

➤ Increase fibre consumption; fibres will fill you up without adding extra calories.

➤ Miracle foods and miracle diets do not exist.

➤ Eating vegetables does not lead to weight gain.

Table 8

generalized overconsumption, defined by an unprecedented abundance of revolutionary technologies and merchandise both new and irresistible. Without making a value judgment as to the right or wrong represented by this tendency, we need to take it into account if we want to suggest realistic solutions with a real impact on lifestyle and on the risk of developing a disease as serious as cancer. A consumer society, generally speaking, is a society of workers, stressed and overworked people who have little time to think about hunger and diet, perceiving them most often as secondary concerns or needs that can be quickly satisfied by eating exciting new products fairly bursting with energy.

It is possible, however, to change; to adapt our way of feeding ourselves at this frantic pace without falling into all the excesses that we currently observe and that have such disastrous consequences for health. Eating well is not necessarily all that complicated! It means taking back control over daily diet, reconsidering its place in our lives, and learning to see foods not just as items designed to satisfy vital and immediate needs, but also as major contributors to well-being. In this context, we present below some general principles that may well have an extraordinary impact on the food choices we make daily.

HARA HACHI BUN !

We all know that overeating supplies a body with a calorie surplus that causes it to exceed ideal weight; this exaggerated food consumption plays a preponderant role in the obesity epidemic that we are now witnessing. Excess calories cause our food energy absorption mechanisms to overheat; this in turn creates extra free radicals able to damage DNA and accelerate the aging process. We have known for a long time, in fact, that restricting caloric intake in laboratory animals increases their life expectancy. Why not turn to a famous Japanese expression for inspiration? *Hara hachi bun* means that we should stop eating when the stomach is 80 per cent full. This gives the brain the time it needs to detect satiation and allows us to take advantage of the pleasures and benefits afforded by food without overindulging. It is much easier to modify our nutritional habits by reducing the amount of food we eat than it is to lose unwanted kilos by going on one or another of the countless weight-losing diets now in vogue. These diets generally neither promise nor deliver any gourmet pleasure, so the enthusiasm one might experience upon losing several kilos is quickly squashed by the tedium of the diet, which inevitably leads to giving up on the diet . . . and returning to square one. It doesn't do any good to wait for the arrival of some miracle diet: making profound changes in diet so as to reduce caloric intake while favouring increased consumption of fruits and vegetables is the only effective way of controlling one's weight.

LET'S DO LUNCH

The dinner table has always been an auspicious setting for communication and bringing together family and friends, a historic function that takes on even more importance in a time when life is so hectic. Using mealtimes to socialize, discuss, or reinforce ties with people we care about can only add to the delight associated with the food itself; if we happen to be dining alone, meals can become a privileged moment of introspection and inner reflection.

A LITTLE MORE SALAD, HONEY?

It goes without saying (and this is the guiding principle of this book) that improving diet and nutritional habits starts with making profound changes in the very nature of what we eat daily. In this context, the fundamental change consists of getting more plants on the menu: plant products are exceptional foods with many beneficial effects on health. All foods of plant origin play a crucial part in cancer prevention and are doubtless some of the best weapons at our disposal for fighting against all types of this disease, especially cancers of the digestive system. Some plants may even surprise us! The humble potato, for one, essentially

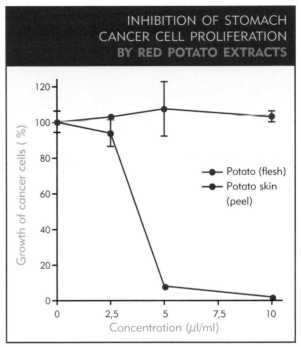

Figure 15

all starch, is often put down as a food with little nutritional value, much less the potential to prevent cancer! We nevertheless studied the ability of this vegetable to interfere with the growth of cancer cells isolated from a stomach tumour. Although the flesh of the potato showed no anti-cancer properties, we noticed that the potato peel exhibited strong inhibitory potential against the growth of the cancer cells (Figure 15). This surprising result illustrates to what extent the presence of anti-cancer molecules is an *intrinsic* characteristic to foods of plant origin; it also underscores the importance of including the greatest possible variety of these foods in our diet to counteract the development of cancer.

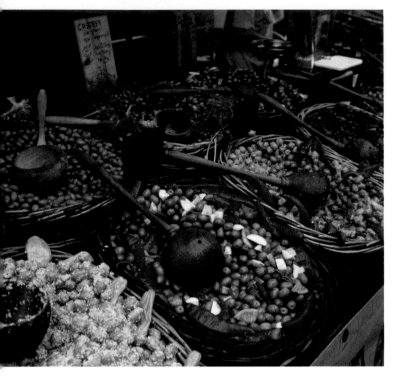

The importance of plants as food is also due to their being excellent sources of fibre, which fills the stomach and gives the eater the impression that he or she has eaten enough, thus reducing caloric intake. This statement may be tested: it is impossible to gain weight by eating vegetables!

ALI, YOUR COUSCOUS IS FANTASTIC!

Seeking health benefits from food does not require giving up the pleasures of the table. On the contrary, this search must derive from the same preventive outlook. This is an important concept because a human being has to experience real satisfaction in eating healthily to feed himself or herself adequately every day. Over the years, we have established an often ambiguous relationship with what we eat. The well-being associated with diet is often a synonym for excess at the dinner table, or for so-called guilty pleasures, which let us "cheat" by eating "forbidden" foods rich in fats and sugar. Conversely, paying close attention to one's diet ("healthy eating") is somehow seen as boring, a kind of bodily deprivation made up of sad, bland meals which give absolutely no pleasure. This perception is a false and insidious one, since eating healthily certainly does not imply banishing all forms of enjoyment associated with food; on the contrary, as you will see in the recipes that follow, dishes that are very rich in anti-cancer compounds are true delicacies! We need to break with this negative attitude toward a healthy diet, and to stop seeing such a diet as evidence for bizarre, Puritan, or countercultural behaviour.

Such a diet must instead be seen as an epicurean call to arms, which is to say an important source of satisfaction, since pleasure does not need to be experienced at the expense of its long-term impact on health. To succeed, one must first consider what one eats as the most important aspect of our day, the act that carries the most influence on our interior environment and must accordingly be finely tuned and controlled. At present, many different actions that are very secondary from a health perspective, such as purchasing a new vehicle or new clothes, are often the result of reflection and careful weighing of the pros and the cons so that the purchaser may fully profit from the benefits associated with the merchandise. In light of what we now know about the consequences of poor diet on the development of diseases as serious and as complex as cancer, it goes without saying that our priorities must change. The very nature of what we eat every day must be foremost in our minds.

To help us change our dietary habits, we have the opportunity and the privilege of accessing millennia of culinary traditions from different parts of the world, and in particular from those regions of the globe where lower rates of cancer are found. It should not be surprising that a large number of recipes included in this book are taken from or inspired by the cuisines of China, Japan, India, the Mediterranean coast, or the Middle East, since it is precisely in these countries that we observe the lowest incidences of several types of cancers (see illustration, pages 56–57). We must get to know better the ingredients unique to the cuisines of these areas, since these ingredients contain many anti-cancer molecules that participate actively in preventing the development of cancer. In the following chapters of this book, we offer you a chance to discover, for instance, the important place that marine algae (seaweed!) occupies in the Japanese diet; to appreciate the diversity and complexity of the world of mushrooms; to explore the multiple health benefits of herbs and spices; to appreciate the virtues associated with flaxseed and fermented milks rich in probiotic bacteria. These foods, combined with those discussed in our previous book, constitute important elements in any diet-based cancer prevention strategy, not only because of their positive impact on health, but also for the incomparable gourmet pleasures they provide.

It is thus with much enthusiasm that we draw on our collaboration with an experienced team of fantastic chefs to present you with a wide selection of easy and economical recipes that will familiarize you with the pleasures to be obtained from a healthy and diverse diet. We are convinced that you will be surprised to discover that preventing cancer can be accomplished by paying special attention to the nature of foods, letting you marry simplicity, ease of preparation, and exceptional flavour with well-being.

Bon appétit!

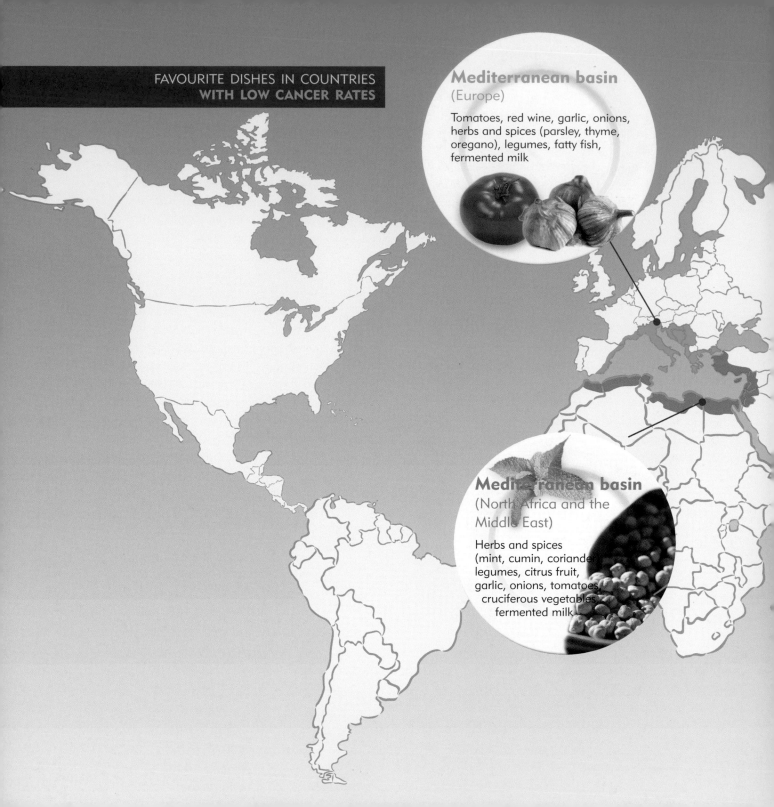

FAVOURITE DISHES IN COUNTRIES
WITH LOW CANCER RATES

Mediterranean basin
(Europe)

Tomatoes, red wine, garlic, onions,
herbs and spices (parsley, thyme,
oregano), legumes, fatty fish,
fermented milk

Mediterranean basin
(North Africa and the
Middle East)

Herbs and spices
(mint, cumin, coriander)
legumes, citrus fruit,
garlic, onions, tomatoes,
cruciferous vegetables,
fermented milk

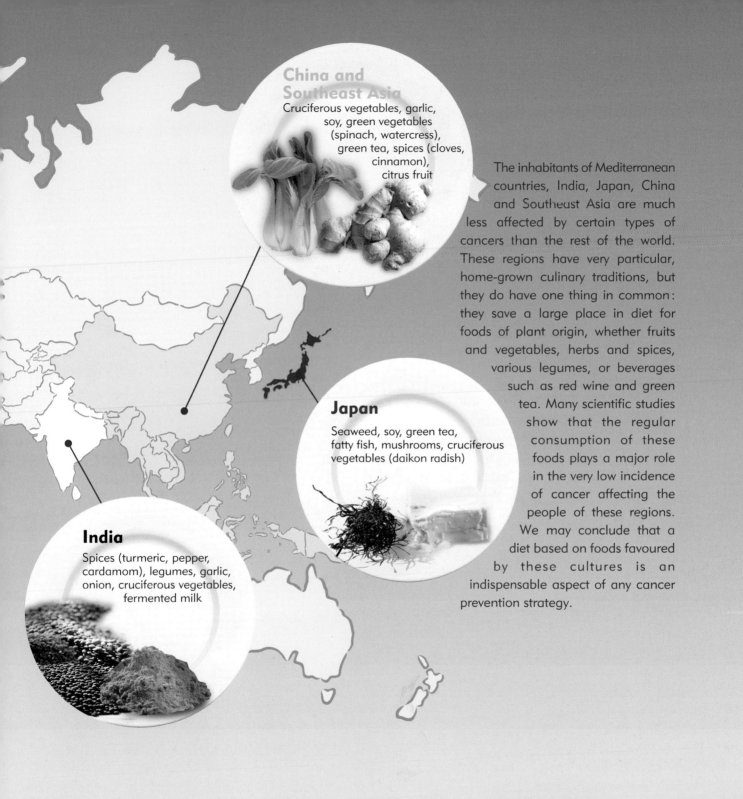

China and Southeast Asia

Cruciferous vegetables, garlic, soy, green vegetables (spinach, watercress), green tea, spices (cloves, cinnamon), citrus fruit

Japan

Seaweed, soy, green tea, fatty fish, mushrooms, cruciferous vegetables (daikon radish)

India

Spices (turmeric, pepper, cardamom), legumes, garlic, onion, cruciferous vegetables, fermented milk

The inhabitants of Mediterranean countries, India, Japan, China and Southeast Asia are much less affected by certain types of cancers than the rest of the world. These regions have very particular, home-grown culinary traditions, but they do have one thing in common: they save a large place in diet for foods of plant origin, whether fruits and vegetables, herbs and spices, various legumes, or beverages such as red wine and green tea. Many scientific studies show that the regular consumption of these foods plays a major role in the very low incidence of cancer affecting the people of these regions. We may conclude that a diet based on foods favoured by these cultures is an indispensable aspect of any cancer prevention strategy.

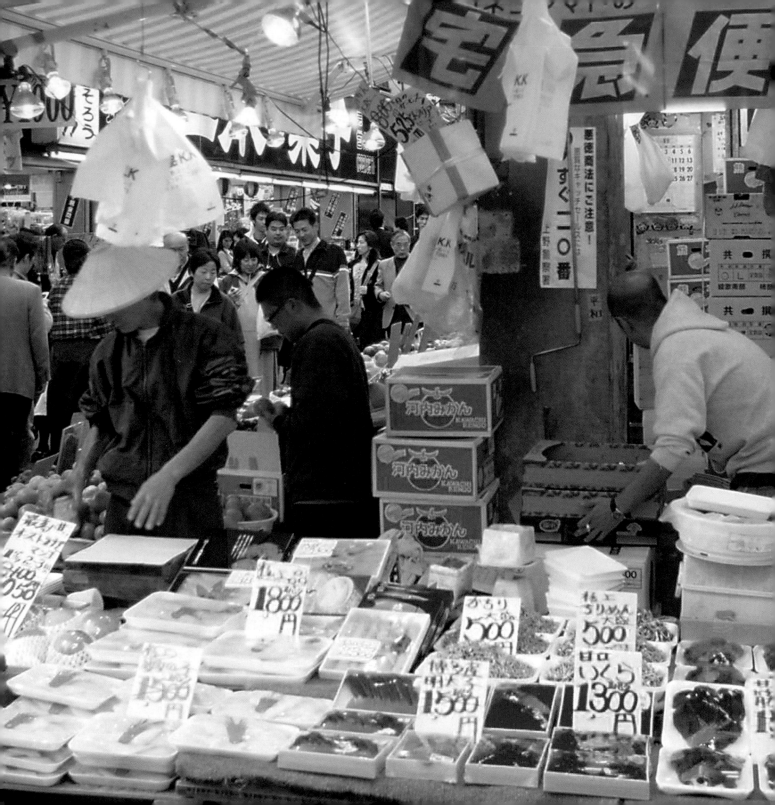

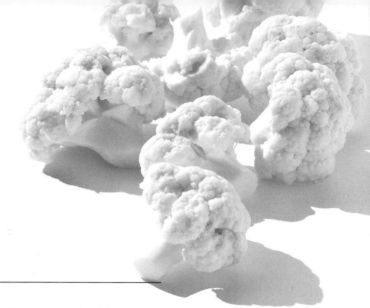

PART *two*

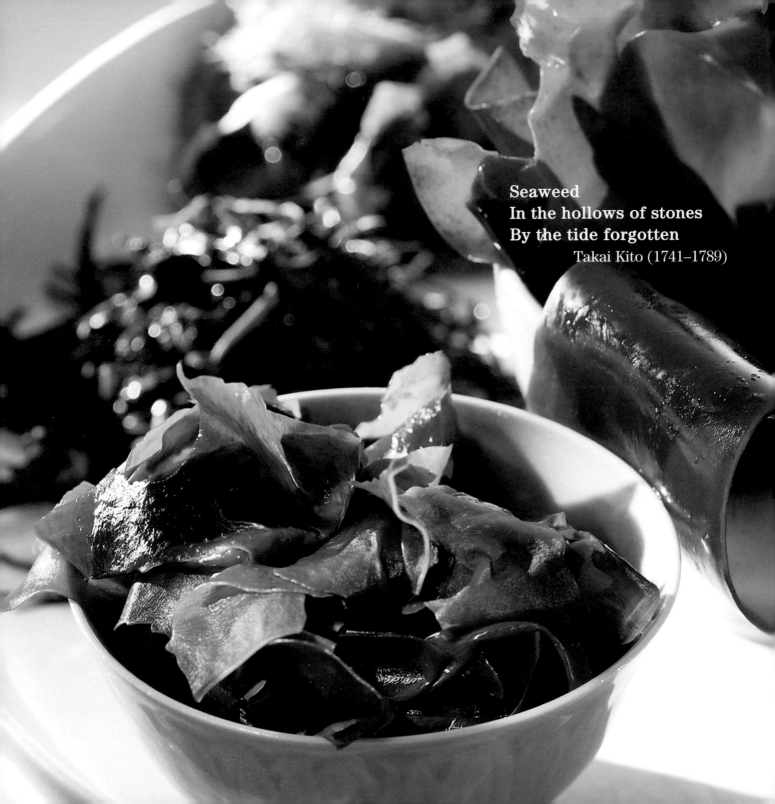

Seaweed
In the hollows of stones
By the tide forgotten
Takai Kito (1741–1789)

CHAPTER 5

Seaweed : Cancer Falls Victim to the Sirens' Song

People living in proximity to the sea have a close and privileged relationship with the vastness of open water. They see in it the only way of satisfying their desire for the exploration of far-off horizons, but they also see it as an almost inexhaustible source of the food essential to their survival. The knowledge gathered over millennia thanks to the symbiosis of human beings and sea has allowed us to identify many delicious fish and shellfish that have become central to diet. Today, the term "seafood" refers to some exceptional delicacies, luxury items often reserved for elaborate and refined feasts.

Not all treasures found in the sea are equally well known. Indeed, some of the foods abundantly present in our oceans and integrated into the diet of certain cultures are today either almost forgotten or neglected by most industrialized societies. This is especially true of marine algae or, more poetically, seaweed.

SEAWEED: MARINE VEGETABLE LIFE

Having made an appearance on Earth about 1.5 billion years ago, marine algae are the ancestors of today's terrestrial plant life. They were the first living species capable of converting the sun's energy into substances necessary to cell function by the process of photosynthesis : an innovation that they have largely benefited from over time, since no fewer than ten thousand species of algae are now spread out over the globe's seashores! These inventors of photosynthesis are responsible for the huge increase in the amount of oxygen on the planet, meaning they played a leading role in the appearance of other kinds of life.

In addition to its starring role in the ecology of the planet, seaweed is the prototype of an ideal health food. It is very rich in essential minerals, especially iodine, potassium, iron, and calcium (some algae contain up to ten times the calcium in cow's milk, and five times the iron found in spinach!), and rich in proteins, all of the essential amino acids, vitamins, and fibre. Seaweed is also

(continued on page 64)

Almost ten thousand varieties of marine algae exist: green (*Chlorophyceae*), red (*Rhodophyceae*), and brown (*Phaeophyceae*), their colour being a function of their content in light-absorbing pigments. Particularly abundant along the coasts of Japan, whose population counts among the most enthusiastic consumers of algae worldwide, most types of seaweed are known today under their Japanese names.

NORI (*Porpyhra spp.*, especially *Porphyra yezoensis*)
Nori means "algae" in Japanese; nori is red or purple in the sea, turning black when dried. It is most often sold in the form of thin dried sheets which have served from the eighteenth century onward in the preparation of certain types of sushi, maki, and termaki sushi. Nori was harvested for centuries in its natural state in the Ariaki Sea, on the island of Kyushu, but it wasn't until 1947 that a British professor, Kathleen Mary Drew, determined its reproductive cycle. Her findings have since allowed fishermen and farmers to practise large-scale cultivation and thus considerably increase nori production, which stands today at 350,000 tons per year: a crop worth US $1 billion. Ten billion sheets of dried nori are now eaten every year, making it by far the world's most popular type of seaweed! Nori contains large amounts of proteins (35 per cent of its dry weight), several vitamins, including vitamin B12, and a whole host of minerals. It is one of the only plant species to contain the long-chain omega-3 fatty acids (specifically EPA, eicosapentaenoic acid) that are crucial to proper brain function, reduce inflammation and diminish the risk of cardiac disease and cancer.

KOMBU (*Laminaria japonica*)
Probably eaten in Japan more than ten thousand years ago, during the Jomon period (14,000–300 B.C.), kombu is a brown algae that is indispensable in Japanese cuisine; starting in the seventh century, it has been the principal ingredient in *dashi*, Japanese cooking's standard soup stock. This algae grows deep within cold waters (the highest-quality kombu comes from the northern Japanese island of Hokkaido) and is a particularly rich source of both iodine and glutamic acid, giving it the nickname of "natural" monosodium glutamate. With a slightly sweet, iodine-like flavour, kombu is thought to promote digestion and shorten the cooking time of different foods, mainly legumes. Kombu has long been considered a luxury item, one reserved for the emperor, as well as a symbol or promise of happiness; it was once part of a gift package sent to the Chinese imperial court. With the colonization and development of the island of Hokkaido during the Edo period (1603–1868), this seaweed became available to all and acquired its status of kitchen ingredient extraordinaire. In Japan, the average per capita consumption of kombu is half a gram per day; it reaches one gram per day in Okinawa, where this algae is particularly appreciated when paired with pork and vegetables, as it is in *kubuirichi*. For the inhabitants of Okinawa, known for their exceptional longevity, kombu is an important component of *ishokudogen*, an expression or belief signifying that every food is a kind of medicine.

WAKAME *(Undaris pinnatifida)*

Very tender, with a lovely dark green colour, wakame is the algae most often added to that great classic of Japanese cuisine, miso soup. This type of seaweed has a pronounced taste of the sea, which may remind the eater of oysters. Other than its astonishingly high calcium content (thirteen times higher than that of milk), wakame, like kombu, also contains appreciable amounts of fucoxanthin and fucoidan, two powerful inhibitors of cancer cell growth. Both wakame and its immature form, mekabu, show strong activity against cells isolated from breast cancer tumours.

ARAME *(Eisenia bicyclis)*

This mild-tasting, almost sweet algae is ideal for initiating oneself into the gourmet delights long associated with seaweed. Arame is traditionally harvested in the Ise region of Japan, where it has served for millennia as an offering in local Shinto shrines, among the most venerated in Japan. Arame closely resembles another algae, *hijiki (Hizikia fusiforme)*, whose consumption, according to legend, is thought to be responsible for the shiny black hair of the Japanese. Contrary to hijiki, which may contain traces of arsenic and must thus be eaten in moderation, arame may be eaten freely, in salads, soups, or as an accompaniment to a great variety of dishes, where its intense black colour adds a vivid touch of contrast that enhances the food's appearance.

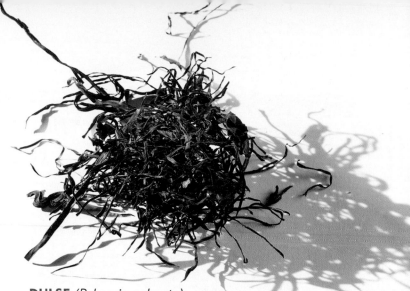

DULSE *(Palmaria palmata)*

Among the algae that are not of Japanese origin, dulse (also known as dillisk or Neptune's Girdle) is one of the most famous. This reddish-purple algae has been eaten for thousands of years in Ireland, Scotland, Wales, and especially in Iceland, where its harvest was already being strictly regulated in the tenth century! In Canada, dulse is found in important amounts around Grand Manan Island, in the Bay of Fundy off the coast of New Brunswick. Featuring a soft texture and a tangy, nutty taste, dulse is very rich in proteins, iron, and various vitamins. A little-known legacy of the British Empire, it is still consumed today in many British and North American coastal communities; dried dulse is a popular snack that often accompanies a pint of beer . . . a tradition that is at least eight hundred years old!

Fucoxanthin

low in fat, and the fat it does contain is mostly omega-3 and omega-6 fatty acids, present in an ideal 1:1 ratio. Some types of red algae, such as nori, even contain long-chain omega-3 fatty acids, which are powerful agents in preventing the development of different diseases; the only other source of these particular acids are fatty fish. Algae are true vegetables of the sea; they constitute a class unto themselves from a nutritional point of view and deserve pride of place in a sensible disease-preventing diet.

This great wealth has been known to Asians for millennia. The Chinese, for example, were already using algae for food and medicinal purposes five thousand years ago, and Chinese manuscripts dating from more than two thousand years before Christ mention that some types of seaweed are "a delicacy reserved for the most distinguished guests and the king himself." It was in Japan that algae found their preferred sea: the geography of the Japanese islands and the rareness of arable land have always motivated the Japanese to seek in the sea a large number of foods of both plant and animal origin. Even today, Japan is one of the very few countries where algae occupy a place of honour in diet (see pages 62-63). Japanese algae

consumption represents up to 10 per cent of daily diet, an amount equal to the ingestion of almost two kilograms of seaweed per person per year!

The systematic Japanese use of algae is diametrically opposed to what is practised in the West. With the possible exception of the Scottish and Irish, Occidentals have always snubbed such humble food; the ancient Greeks used seaweed as cattle feed or fertilizer. Today, algae find relatively little use as food in North American and European countries, except as a source of agar, carrageenan, and alginates, complex polymers with gelling and thickening properties that serve in the manufacture of milk products such as ice cream and yogurt, pastries, prepared meals, animal food, toothpaste, antacids, and lipstick!

Although these differences in regional cuisine nicely illustrate what the French writer Rabelais wrote in *Gargantua and Pantagruel* more than five hundred years ago: "Then I began to think that it is very true which is commonly said, that the one half of the world knoweth not how the other half liveth," it remains that the copious Japanese consumption of seaweed is not just the product of a cultural difference between East and West. In fact, much research conducted over the last few years indicates that algae contain significant quantities of anti-cancer compounds and that their consumption may in part explain the important discrepancy between cancer incidence in Japan and that in Western societies, especially in the case of breast and prostate cancer.

THE ANTI-CANCER PROPERTIES OF ALGAE

The huge discrepancies in the incidence of several types of cancer affecting Asians and people living in the West are in large part linked to important differences in the nature of diet in these countries.

For example, the generous consumption by Asians of soy-based foods is often thought to be responsible for the relatively low incidence of hormone-dependent cancers (breast cancer, endometrial cancer, ovarian cancer, prostate cancer) in the East. This protection is usually ascribed to the exceptionally high phytoestrogen content of soy products (phytoestrogens are molecules able to counteract the harmful effects caused by elevated levels of sex hormones). Indeed, several studies have shown that Japanese women have longer menstrual cycles, and thus lower bloodstream estrogen levels, than Western women: two factors that reduce the potential exposure of tissue targeted by these hormones (breasts, endometrium, and ovaries), and consequently lower the risk of developing cancer. Recent research indicates that marine algae may have the same kind of effect: lab animals who were fed brown algae experienced a 37 per cent lengthening of their menstrual cycles and a significant lowering of blood estrogen levels. These results are representative of the effects of these algae on humans; a study conducted on premenopausal women obtained similar findings, namely a significant prolongation of the menstrual cycle and a drop in blood estrogen levels. Algae thus look to be extremely promising agents in the prevention of hormone-dependent cancers; their anti-estrogenic activity certainly contributes to the low incidence of these cancers in women who regularly consume algae as food, especially Japanese women.

The *Codex Ebers*, or Ebers papyrus, a 3,500-year-old Egyptian medical treatise, mentions the use of algae in the treatment of women suffering from breast cancer. This intuition is not far from reality; according to recent research, algae may not only interfere with estrogen levels, but also with the development of cancer itself, by acting directly on cancer cells. In fact, adding algae extracts to the diet of lab animals significantly reduces the progression of breast, colon, and skin cancers induced by carcinogenic substances. Even though the mechanisms responsible for these anti-cancer properties are not well understood, there is no doubt they are in large part linked to the elevated fucoxanthin and fucoidan content of algae. These two compounds disrupt several processes vital to the growth of cancer cells.

Fucoidan, a complex polysaccharide that is found abundantly in many types of seaweed, especially kombu and wakame, prevents the growth of a large variety of cancer cell lines cultivated in the lab, often causing cell death by apoptosis. In addition to this cytotoxic activity, it seems that fucoidan may also have a positive impact on immune function: it increases the activity of cells involved in defence against pathogens, which may contribute to creating an environment more hostile to microtumours and thus slowing down their development.

Fucoxanthin is a yellow pigment that, depending on its concentration, imparts an olive-green to purplish-brown colour to plants. A close relative of other pigments in the carotenoid family (β-carotene, lycopene, etc.), fucoxanthin is found abundantly in nature, mostly in marine plant life, where it participates in photosynthesis by way of its unique ability to absorb sunlight through deep waters. Of all the dietary carotenoids tested, fucoxanthin shows some of the most important anti-cancer

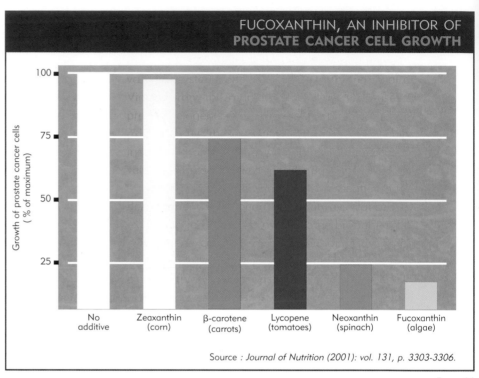

Figure 16

activity, in lab animals and in cancer cells isolated from human tumours. For example, as seen in Figure 16, the addition of fucoxanthin to prostate tumour cells significantly slows down the growth of these cells. Amazingly, this inhibitory effect is much more pronounced than that of lycopene, a carotenoid found mainly in tomatoes and which has long been theorized as playing a preventive role in the development of prostate cancer. Only neoxanthin, a carotenoid present in green vegetables such as spinach, possesses an activity as powerful as fucoxanthin's: the inhibiting effect of these two molecules is associated with their ability

to destroy prostate cancer cells by apoptosis. Because algae are the only dietary source of fucoxanthin, they should become a part of any cancer prevention strategy linked to diet, especially for breast cancer and prostate cancer.

To conclude: marine algae should be considered not just culinary curiosities, but valuable allies, with powerful protective effects, in the fight against several types of cancer. They are capable of counteracting the progression of latent microtumours in two ways: by acting directly on their growth, and by exercising a measurably positive influence on the immune system and on inflammatory processes.

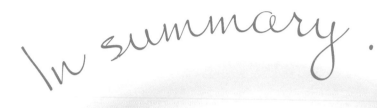

In summary . . .

• To take full advantage of the health benefits offered by algae, use dried seaweed that you can rehydrate and then add to soups or main dishes. Dietary supplements containing marine algae extracts are not recommended, as they contain large amounts of iodine as well as traces of several heavy metals.

• The taste of algae goes well with other kinds of seafood : why not make seaweed a regular side dish to a meal created around fish?

• Many supermarkets offer scaweed salad samples for tasting. Discover them! Enjoy them!

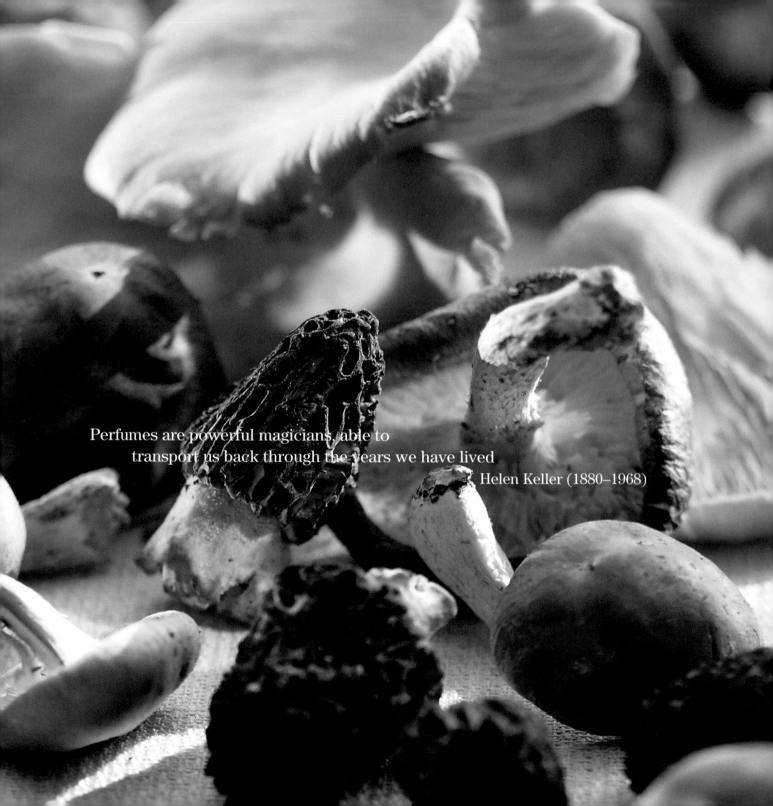

Perfumes are powerful magicians, able to
transport us back through the years we have lived

Helen Keller (1880–1968)

CHAPTER 6

The Magic of Mushrooms

Being initiated into the mysteries of mushrooms is like entering into a strange realm, full of secrets and legends: a unique world, both diverse and complex, where the most sought-after gourmet pleasures are close cousins to fabled, fatal poisons. Faithful reflections of the human soul, mushrooms are truly extraordinary foods, capable of the best – attaining heights of subtlety and exquisite flavour, as well as the worst – able to cause serious, often irreparable harm to health. Beyond their mythic and magical character, however, mushrooms are first and foremost foods that cannot be dissociated from the history of human diet, as much for their exceptional taste as for their very real health benefits.

"PLANTS" THAT ARE NOT LIKE THE OTHERS!

Unique from a biological point of view, mushrooms are not plants, but fungi; they have neither leaves nor roots, and they contain no chlorophyll, which means they cannot use sunlight to produce the nutrients essential to a plant's survival. Mushrooms are thus reduced to scavenging for nutrients in their immediate environment by means of their mycelium, an underground network of slender filaments. What we call a mushroom is the very small, visible portion of this vast network of filaments (1 cubic centimetre of fertile soil may contain up to 100 metres of mycelium!), the part that serves as a reproductive organ. This organ, known as a carpophore (from the Greek *karpos*, "fruit," and *phora*, "to bear"), contains the mushroom's genetic material in the form of tiny spores that are destined to be scattered widely by the wind. When conditions are favourable, a carpophore is literally able to "spring up like mushrooms after rain," growing with incredible speed: certain species can go from the size of the head of a needle to maturity in a scant few hours!

Mushrooms constitute a distinct and extremely diverse life form; of its 100,000 species, at least 2,000 are edible, and 500 are known for

(continued on p. 72)

BUTTON MUSHROOMS *(Agaricus bisporus)*

Button mushrooms, more elegantly known as *champignons de Paris*, or Parisian mushrooms, in French, are rare in the wild, but remain the most cultivated mushrooms in the world. Introduced into Western diet by Jean-Baptiste de La Quintinie (1624–1691), gardener to Louis XIV, this mushroom literally took off in the time of the First Empire, under Napoleon in 1810, thanks to the efforts of a certain Monsieur Chambry, an agronomist who discovered by sheer accident that the abandoned quarries around Paris provided ideal growing conditions for fungi, due to optimal temperature (10–15 °C) and humidity. Despite its Gallic antecedents, this "Parisian" mushroom is now mostly cultivated in the United States, especially in Pennsylvania, in China, the Netherlands, and the Anjou region of France. Boasting a relatively subdued flavour, it is popular mostly in the West, where its consumption can reach one kilogram per person per year. A slightly different variety of the button mushroom, the cremini ("coffee") mushroom, dark brown in colour and with a firmer texture, is widely available and particularly appreciated in its mature form, the famous Portobello mushroom. Although button mushrooms have less of a reputation for medicinal use than do their Asian cousins, they contain lectins, proteins similar to those present in certain legumes, which under laboratory conditions impede the growth of some cancer cells.

SHIITAKE *(Lentinus edodes)*

As common in Asia as button mushrooms are in the West, the shiitake is a mushroom (*take*, in Japanese) that grows wild on the *shii* (*Castanopsis cuspidata*), an evergreen related to the beech and oak trees and indigenous to Southeast Asia. For several millennia, the peoples of this region used shiitake both as food and medicine. The cultivation of shiitake probably began in China, in the area of Qingyuan, about two thousand years ago, and was refined over the centuries, particularly in Japan. Today, the shiitake is the second most widely cultivated mushroom in the world, after the button mushroom: Asian eaters account for 790,000 tons of the 800,000 tons produced and eaten yearly! Known as the "elixir of life" in Asia, the shiitake enjoys an ever-growing reputation among those seeking longevity, sexual vigour, and physical endurance. Although this mushroom is now being cultivated in America and Europe (mostly in the Netherlands and in the Brittany region of France), where it can be found fresh on supermarket shelves, the lion's share of production still occurs in Asia. The shiitake is most often sold in dried form. The drying process does not degrade the unique taste; many Asian connoisseurs prefer the dried mushrooms over fresh shiitake because of their more

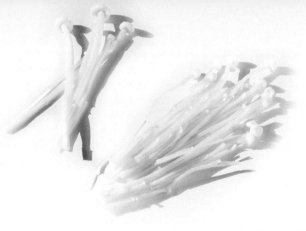

pronounced flavour. Lastly, the popularity of shiitake is due to its exceptional culinary potential, yes, but also to its medicinal virtues: this mushroom is particularly rich in lentinan, a complex sugar that possesses powerful anti-cancer activity.

OYSTER MUSHROOMS (PLEUROTUS)

(Pleurotus ostreatus)

Very common in Europe and North America, oyster mushrooms, or pleurotus (from the Greek *pleura*, meaning "side," and *otos*, "ear") grow in compact bunches resembling store displays of oysters, hence their common English name. With their firm texture and a delicate flavour reminiscent of wild mushrooms, oyster mushrooms are the perfect accompaniment to meat and poultry. Both the common oyster mushroom and its cousin from the south of France, the king oyster mushroom (*Pleurotus eryngii*), are among the mushrooms exhibiting the strongest anti-cancer activity against isolated tumour cells (see Figure 17).

ENOKITAKE *(Flammulina velutipes)*

Also known as velvet foot collybia, this mushroom often grows in the wild on the stumps of Japanese enoki trees (*Celtis sinensis*), relatives of the elm, from which it takes its Japanese name. Nurtured to maturity in dark, narrow jars, the cultivated enokitake is formed of several thin, white stems collected in a bouquet shape, and does not at all resemble the wild form of the mushroom. Delicate-tasting, with a pleasing appearance, it is often eaten raw in salads or added at the last minute to soups and stir-fries. From a medicinal point of view, the enokitake, like most mushrooms, contains polymers of complex sugars that stimulate immune system function.

MAITAKE *(Grifola frondosa)*

Originally from northeastern Japan, this small brown gilled mushroom grows in bunches that may reach impressive dimensions. Maitake means "dancing mushroom"; it may have received this name because of its innumerable superimposed tiny leaves, which look like butterflies in flight. (A Japanese legend attributes the "dancing" to the joy of peasants who discovered the mushroom and exchanged it for its weight in silver, its unique taste making it much prized among gourmets.) It wasn't until much later, in the 1980s, that the cultivation of maitake really took off, allowing greater numbers of mushroom fans to benefit from its properties. In fact, the maitake was long used in both Chinese and Japanese medicine, which consider it an essential ingredient for good health and longevity. Interestingly, recent research indicates that the maitake among all mushrooms is the one that most strongly stimulates the immune system.

The Magic of Mushrooms | Chapter 6

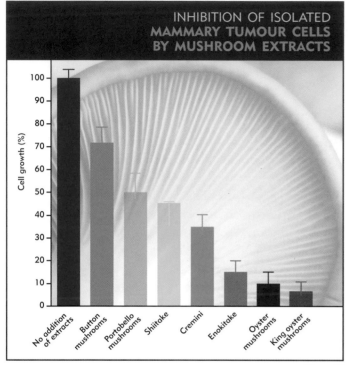

INHIBITION OF ISOLATED
MAMMARY TUMOUR CELLS
BY MUSHROOM EXTRACTS

Figure 17

source. Mushrooms have always occupied a place of privilege in most of the great culinary traditions, often attaining the status of a "superior" food, a symbol of wealth and taste. Egyptian pharaohs, for example, reserved mushrooms for their own personal use; in ancient Greece and Rome, the ruling class had a special fondness for the truffle (another type of fungus) and the royal amanita (Caesar's amanita). Fortunately for humbler gourmets, enjoying these delicious mushrooms is no longer the privilege of kings, and the domestication of many species has contributed greatly to making them available year-round (see pages 70-71).

Beyond their value in the kitchen, mushrooms have always been an important component of traditional medicine in Asia, Russia, and Africa, among the Yoruba of Nigeria, for example. Scientific findings over the last few years tend to demonstrate that these fungi do indeed possess properties beneficial to health, especially when it comes to cancer prevention.

THE ANTI-CANCER PROPERTIES OF MUSHROOMS

Several epidemiological studies have examined the relationship between mushroom consumption and a decrease in the risk of developing cancer, with encouraging results. A Japanese study, for example, found that farmers whose principal occupation was enokitake cultivation (and who were thus likely to eat this mushroom on a regular basis) had a much lower cancer mortality rate than the general population. Similarly, another study conducted in the Japanese city of Chiba showed that the regular

having in varying degree some influence on human body function. This total does not take into account numerous microscopic fungi, such as yeast and moulds, long used and appreciated for their indispensable role in the making of bread, wine, cheese, and soy sauce, among other products. Mushrooms are the keepers of many secrets. . . .

What we know about the nutritional, toxic, and hallucinogenic properties of mushrooms (see pages 74-75) is the sum total of much human trial and error; the abundance of these fungi in the immediate environment of the experimenters must have made them a non-negligible nutritional consumption of *Hypsizygus marmoreus* (buna-shimeji) and *Pholiota nameko* (nameko), two locally popular mushrooms, was associated with a 50 per cent decrease in the risk of stomach cancer; these preventive effects were also observed in lab animals exposed to methylcholanthene, a powerful carcinogenic substance. In accordance with these observations, we have recently noted that the addition of mushroom extracts to isolated mammary tumour cells blocked the growth of these cells. This inhibitory effect was particularly strong for enokitake and oyster mushrooms (Figure 17).

A certain number of polysaccharides, complex polymers made up of multiple units of specific sugars, are responsible for the anti-cancer effects observed with different mushrooms. Of variable structure and composition, these polymers are present in large quantities in many mushrooms of Asian origin, and especially in shiitake, enokitake, and maitake, as well as in kawaratake (*Coriolus versicolor*), a species of inedible mushroom that is nevertheless extremely rich in polysaccharides.

Lentinan, a compound present in shiitake mushrooms, is a polysaccharide whose anti-tumour activity is relatively well documented. In patients suffering from stomach or colon cancers, adding lentinan to a course of chemotherapy causes a significant, life-prolonging regression in tumour size, compared to chemotherapy undertaken without supplemental lentinan, suggesting that this polysaccharide possesses in itself anti-cancer activity. The administration of PSK, a preparation similar to lentinan, is currently used in Japan in conjunction with chemotherapy to treat several

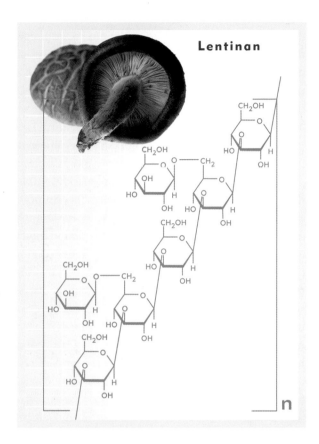

Lentinan

types of cancers; particularly in colon cancer cases, the addition of this extract to treatment actually improves the quality of life and the odds for long-term survival for patients in remission.

The mechanisms responsible for the anti-cancer activity of the polysaccharides contained in mushrooms are very complex, but it is now acknowledged that these compounds stimulate immune system activity. Numerous studies have shown that the lentinan in shiitake mushrooms, as well as a polysaccharide isolated from maitake,

(continued on page 76)

The Magic of Mushrooms | Chapter 6

Whether because of their honoured place in royal feasts, their use in violently accelerating the course of history, or their ability to enhance communication with the divine, mushrooms have always exercised a certain fascination on human beings.

From the gourmet's perspective, the truffle is probably the best example of the mushroom phenomenon. Considered a food of incomparable delicacy in the reign of the pharaoh Cheops, more than four thousand years ago, celebrated in Greek and Roman civilization, this mysterious fungus matures underground and its finding, then and now, has necessitated an animal's intervention, usually that of a dog or a pig. Fully deserving its "black diamond" moniker, the truffle remains above all a food prized for its exceptional culinary qualities: one kilogram of the best truffles currently fetches a market price of more than two thousand dollars!

Mushrooms have not always been pursued for their value as a pleasant side dish! Some well-known fungi are prized for their powerful hallucinogenic properties. Aztec *pahini*, or shamans, in particular, regularly consumed *teonanacatl* (literally, "the flesh of God") as a path to communing with the gods during sacred religious ceremonies: "With the help of mushrooms, these ancient priests had visions in which the future was revealed to them, as the devil spoke to them while they were in a state of intoxication" (Diego Durán, *Historia de los Indios de Nueva España*, 1581). It is believed that this particular mushroom was the *Psilocybe caerulescens*, whose principal active ingredients, psilocybin and psilocin, are powerful hallucinogens with effects similar to those of LSD. The fly agaric (*Amanita muscaria*), another hallucinogenic mushroom, is easily recognized by its orange cap spotted with white warts. The sensory distortions and euphoria associated with the consumption of this mushroom are due to muscimol, a substance that is not transformed in the body, but excreted as is in urine; enthusiasts can reabsorb the substance by drinking their own urine or someone else's! A cautionary note: ingesting large quantities of *Amanita muscaria* is dangerous, not to mention illegal, as it also contains a high percentage of muscarine, a compound that is lethal in high doses.

Other types of mushrooms leave no ambiguity as to the fate of the person who ate them: the Roman emperor Claudius (Tiberius Claudius Drusus Nero Germanicus) in 54 A.D., Pope Clement VII in 1534, and the Holy Roman Emperor Charles VI in 1740 are all among the celebrities famous for succumbing to the toxic effects of fungi. The best-documented case of death by mushroom poisoning is that of Claudius. The emperor fell ill on October 13, 54 A.D. after eating a generous helping of royal amanitas (Caesar's amanitas); he died in wracking pain shortly afterward. History suspects Agrippina, his niece and second wife, of having introduced a few death cap mushrooms (*Amanita phalloïdes*) into the emperor's plate; the idea was that her own son Nero succeed Claudius, thereby preventing the other heir, Britannicus, from ascending the imperial throne. Today, the death cap is still responsible for the majority of fatal poisonings linked to mushroom eating; it contains very powerful toxins, amatoxins,

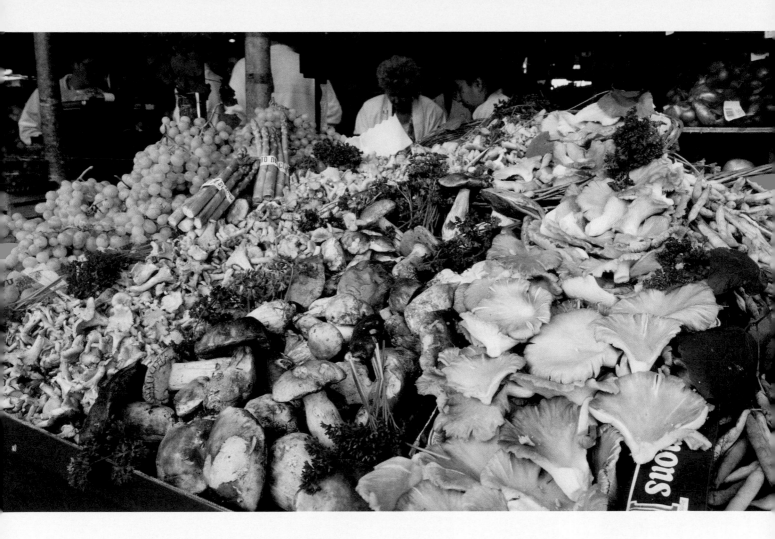

which cause irreversible damage to the liver. About twelve hours after ingestion, the patient falls very ill, but may feel a little better after a certain time. This respite is, however, both temporary and misleading; the toxins continue to attack the liver and the patient rapidly deteriorates, soon reaching the stage where only a liver transplant can save his or her life.

Common in Europe but rare in North America, except perhaps on the American west coast, the death cap has a close New World cousin that must be taken seriously: the death angel (*Amanita virosa*), a widespread mushroom that possesses sufficient quantities of toxins to kill the careless mushroom gatherer.

The Magic of Mushrooms | Chapter 6

cause a strong increase in both white blood cell count and white blood cell activity, thus improving the effectiveness of the accompanying chemotherapy. It seems that the immune system stimulation by the active compounds in these mushrooms increases our chances of controlling early-stage tumours, thus preventing them from reaching a later, more advanced stage.

The anti-cancer and immuno-stimulating activity exhibited by edible mushrooms does not seem to be restricted to species of Asian origin. Boletes and button mushrooms, for example, also contain molecules that look effective in impeding the development of certain cancers, especially colon cancer, by directly attacking cancerous cells and causing their death by apoptosis.

To summarize, research conducted on the anti-cancer properties of mushrooms has mostly focused on the use of polysaccharides isolated from fungi as immunoregulators destined to improve the effectiveness of chemotherapy and the general well-being of patients. The positive results obtained are extremely encouraging, especially if we consider the seriousness of certain cases and the comparative difficulty of treating them. In light of these findings, there is no doubt that mushrooms may play an

---

MUSHROOM TIP

Dried mushrooms may be substituted for fresh mushrooms in many recipes. Many supermarkets now regularly stock mixtures of various dried mushrooms : morel mushrooms, boletes, shiitake, chanterelles, porcini . . . To rehydrate dried mushrooms, place them in a bowl and cover with boiling water. Leave them to soak for about half an hour, and then squeeze out the remaining liquid. They may then be sliced and used in the same manner as fresh mushrooms. Always keep the soaking water if making broth or for water for cooking, as it is both delicious and nutritious.

---

important part in cancer prevention : by stimulating the immune system in a positive manner, they improve the effectiveness of the immune response in the face of the aggression represented by the cancer cell seeking to reproduce.

Learning about these marvellous foods, rich in subtle perfumes and flavours, allows us to add a whole other dimension to our cooking; it also motivates us to include in our daily diet new allies that help prevent the development of cancer.

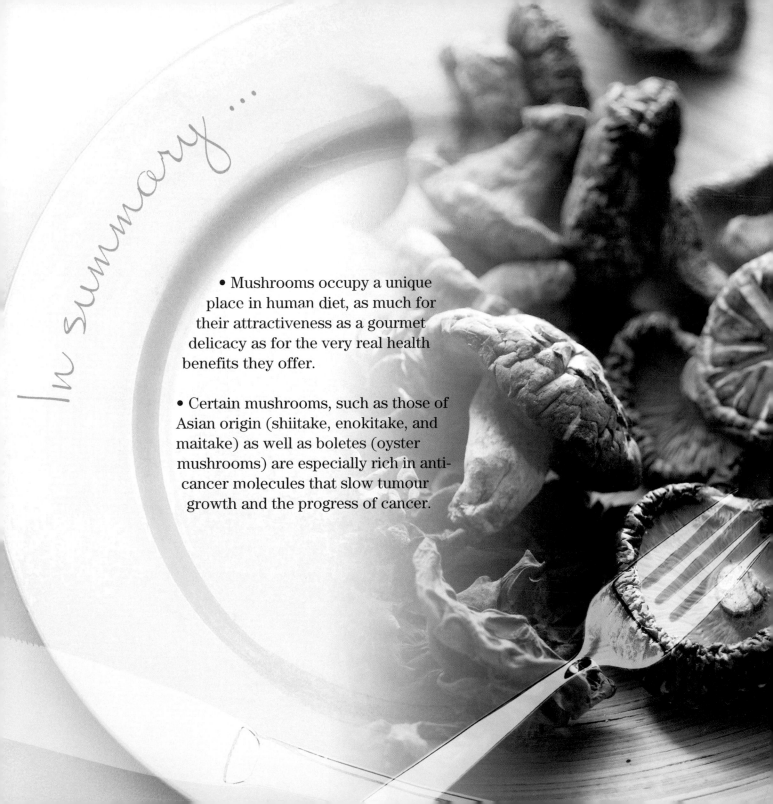

In summary ...

• Mushrooms occupy a unique place in human diet, as much for their attractiveness as a gourmet delicacy as for the very real health benefits they offer.

• Certain mushrooms, such as those of Asian origin (shiitake, enokitake, and maitake) as well as boletes (oyster mushrooms) are especially rich in anti-cancer molecules that slow tumour growth and the progress of cancer.

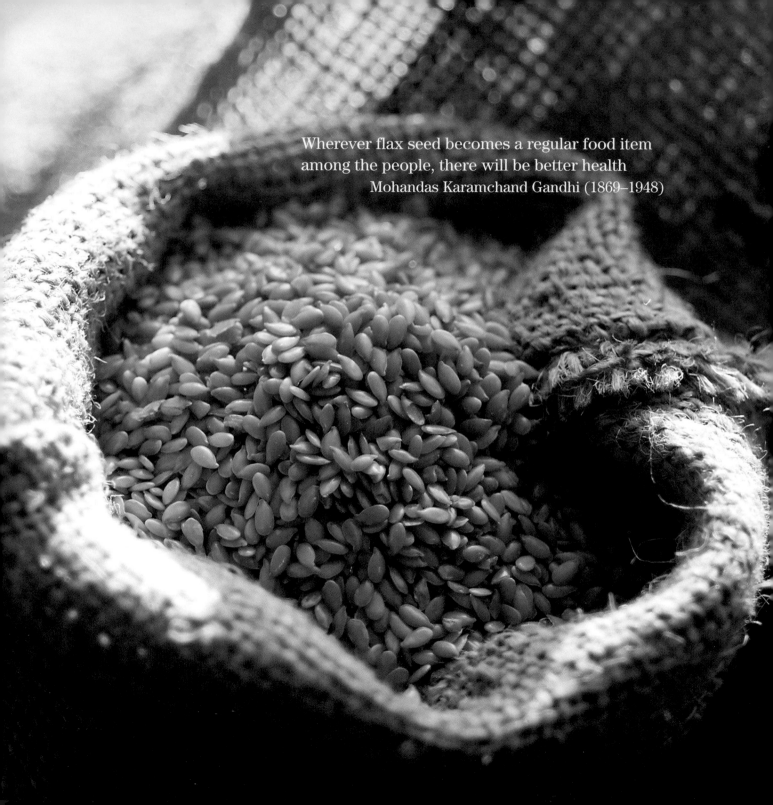

Wherever flax seed becomes a regular food item
among the people, there will be better health
Mohandas Karamchand Gandhi (1869–1948)

CHAPTER 7

Flaxseed : Weaving Better Protection Against Cancer

Flax (*Linum usitatissimum*) was one of the first plant species to be domesticated and cultivated on a large scale. Particularly appreciated for its textile properties (linen is woven from flax), flax was already used by the Egyptians at least ten thousand years ago to make clothing, as well as the linen burial wrappings needed for mummification rites. Phoenician merchants subsequently played an important role in spreading flax throughout Europe, where the popularity of linen as a light fabric, ideal as protection against the heat, has grown over the centuries. Weavers' enthusiasm has led to the development of new fabrics made from linen, such as crinoline, a type of cheesecloth, in which linen is woven together with bristle (*crin*, in French).

MORE THAN JUST FABRIC!

Eating flaxseed for both food and medicinal purposes is probably as old as the cultivation of flax itself. Recognized as a source of high-quality nutrients, flaxseed appeared on the daily menu of the Pharaohs, and flaxseed meal was used in the preparation of many Ethiopian, Indian, and Chinese dishes. It is said that in the eighth century, Charlemagne, king of the Franks, was so impressed by the multiple qualities of flax that he imposed the eating of flax seeds by decree! It turns out Charlemagne was right; research carried out over the last few years shows that humble flaxseed contains many substances that are beneficial to health, even playing an important role in the prevention of cancer.

FILLING UP WITH OMEGA-3S

As mentioned previously (see chapter 2, page 35), our modern-day diet suffers from a serious lack of omega-3 fatty acids. This phenomenon, associated with excessive consumption of omega-6 fatty acids, favours the creation of an inflammatory environment that is conducive to the development of cancer. Re-establishing the proper balance between levels of these two essential fatty acids can only be of help in fighting this disease.

Flaxseed is by far the best plant source of linolenic acid, an omega-3 fatty acid used by cells to make EPA (eicosapentaenoic acid) and DHA (docosahexaenoic acid), two anti-inflammatory substances. For example, only two tablespoons of flaxseed supply more than 140 per cent of the recommended daily allowance of omega-3s! However, in order to optimize the benefits associated with the omega-3s present in flaxseed, we should remember that the conversion of linolenic acid to EPA and DHA is a relatively inefficient process if the corresponding intake of omega-6s is too high. This is why any increase in the consumption of omega-3s must be accompanied by a marked lowering in that of omega-6s, so that a better equilibrium of omega-6/omega-3 is reached and inflammation prevented.

This equilibrium is all the more important when one considers that an "improvement" in the omega-6/omega-3 ratio plays a crucial role in cancer prevention (Table 9). A recent study suggests that approximately equal amounts of omega-3 and omega-6 fatty acids in adipose (fatty)

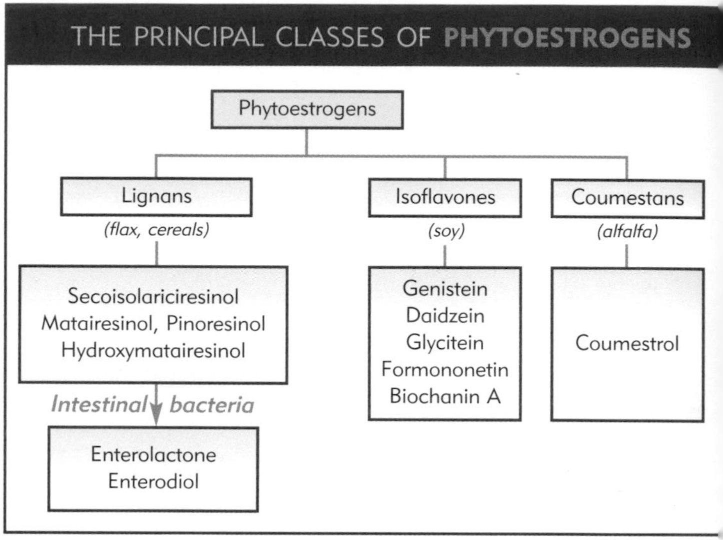

THE PRINCIPAL CLASSES OF **PHYTOESTROGENS**

Figure 18

tissues, combined with increased levels of monounsaturated fatty acids such as those found in olive oil, are associated with a definite decrease in the risk of developing breast cancer. The omega-6/omega-3 equilibrium also seems to have such an effect on prostate cancer (we now know that a surplus of omega-6s promotes the development of this disease), as well as on the bone metastases linked to prostate cancer: two phenomena, incidentally, that are inhibited by omega-3s.

There is no doubt that flaxseed may have a highly positive and valuable impact on a diet designed to stave off cancer; it supplies a significant amount of the omega-3 fatty acids needed for the synthesis of powerful anti-inflammatory molecules that impede the creation of a context favourable to tumour growth.

OMEGA-3 FATTY ACIDS AND
CANCER PREVENTION

➤ Omega-3 fatty acids lower the risk of contracting breast, colon, and prostate cancer.

➤ Omega-3s inhibit the metastatic potential of cancer cells; this is the principal factor affecting the immediate prognosis and long-term survival of cancer patients.

Table 9

LIGNANS: A CLASS OF ANTI-CANCER PHYTOESTROGENS

In addition to omega-3 fatty acids, flaxseed contains exceptional quantities of phytoestrogens, molecules whose structure resembles that of estrogens and which are thus able to attenuate the harmful effects caused by excessively high levels of these hormones. Although the isoflavones present in soy are the phytoestrogens having received the most attention from the medical and scientific communities, other classes of phytoestrogens exist

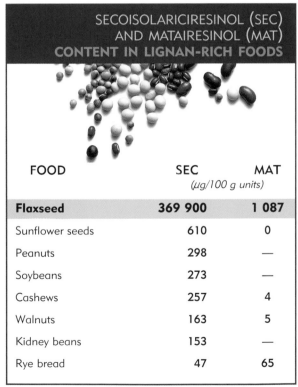

SECOISOLARICIRESINOL (SEC) AND MATAIRESINOL (MAT) CONTENT IN LIGNAN-RICH FOODS		
FOOD	**SEC**	**MAT**
	(μg/100 g units)	
Flaxseed	**369 900**	**1 087**
Sunflower seeds	610	0
Peanuts	298	—
Soybeans	273	—
Cashews	257	4
Walnuts	163	5
Kidney beans	153	—
Rye bread	47	65

Figure 19

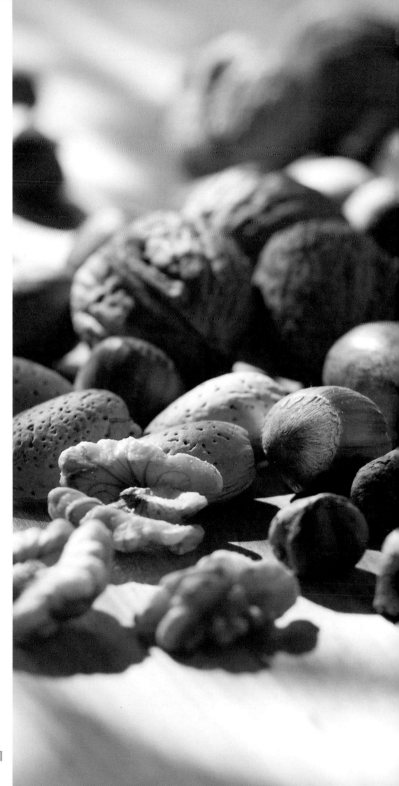

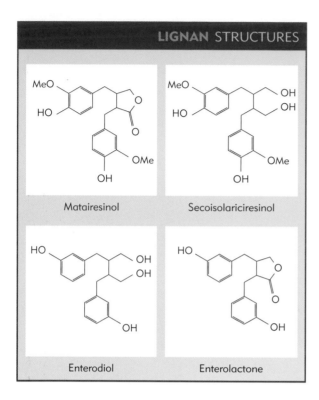

LIGNAN STRUCTURES

Mataïresinol

Secoisolariciresinol

Enterodiol

Enterolactone

in nature and may also participate in the prevention of breast cancer (Figure 18). This is notably the case of lignans.

Lignans are complex compounds present in many plants, although flaxseed is by far the best dietary source of these molecules (Figure 19). Flaxseed contains very high levels of secoisolariciresinol and its close relative mataïresinol. These compounds are important in the prevention of cancers whose growth depends on estrogens, because intestinal bacteria are able to convert them into enterolactone and enterodiol, two molecules that interfere with the bonding of estrogens to breast cells.

Epidemiological studies focusing on the possible role of lignans in the breast cancer prevention have produced extremely encouraging results. In most cases, an increase in enterolactone blood levels (enterolactone being produced by the conversion of secoisolariciresinol) is linked to a decrease in breast cancer risk, especially in premenopausal women, whose estrogen levels are higher. These findings agree with the results of several studies carried out on laboratory animals grafted with breast tumours. Researchers observed that the addition of lignans to diet blocked the growth of tumours implanted in these animals. Contrary to soy isoflavone supplements, which in elevated doses, it is now known, *promote* the growth of mammary tumours in lab animals, lignans typically induce tumour regression. The phytoestrogens present in flaxseed thus represent a valuable dietary alternative to those present in soy, and may become a very interesting addition to the diet of women already affected by breast cancer, who are strongly discouraged from eating soy.

Flaxseed is a very useful, multifunctional anti-cancer food, capable of interfering with the development of cancer by reducing chronic inflammation, and thus preventing precancerous cells from benefiting from a milieu that favours their further growth. The high lignan content of flaxseed makes this substance a natural and efficient rampart against breast cancer.

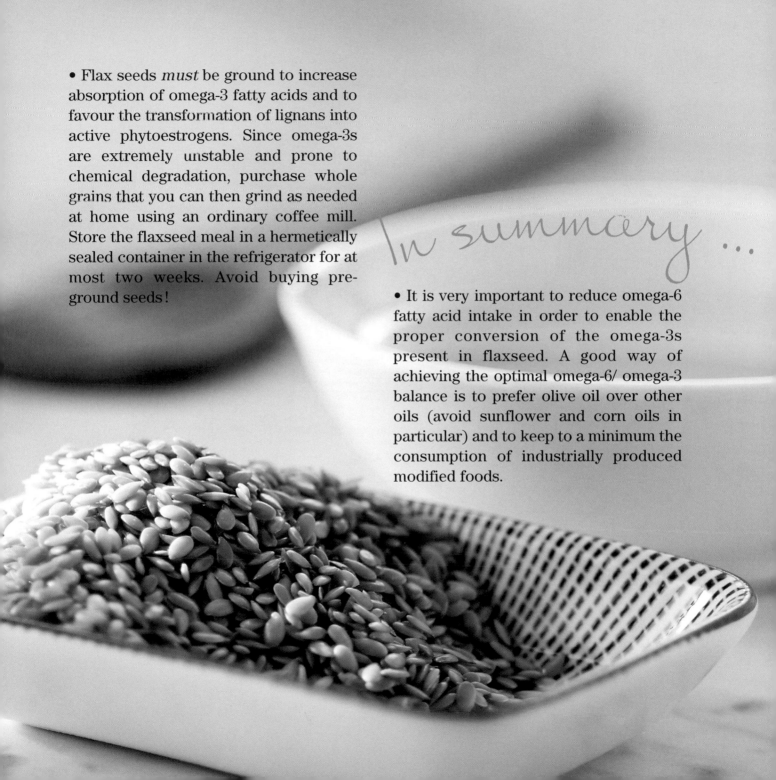

• Flax seeds *must* be ground to increase absorption of omega-3 fatty acids and to favour the transformation of lignans into active phytoestrogens. Since omega-3s are extremely unstable and prone to chemical degradation, purchase whole grains that you can then grind as needed at home using an ordinary coffee mill. Store the flaxseed meal in a hermetically sealed container in the refrigerator for at most two weeks. Avoid buying pre-ground seeds!

In summary ...

• It is very important to reduce omega-6 fatty acid intake in order to enable the proper conversion of the omega-3s present in flaxseed. A good way of achieving the optimal omega-6/ omega-3 balance is to prefer olive oil over other oils (avoid sunflower and corn oils in particular) and to keep to a minimum the consumption of industrially produced modified foods.

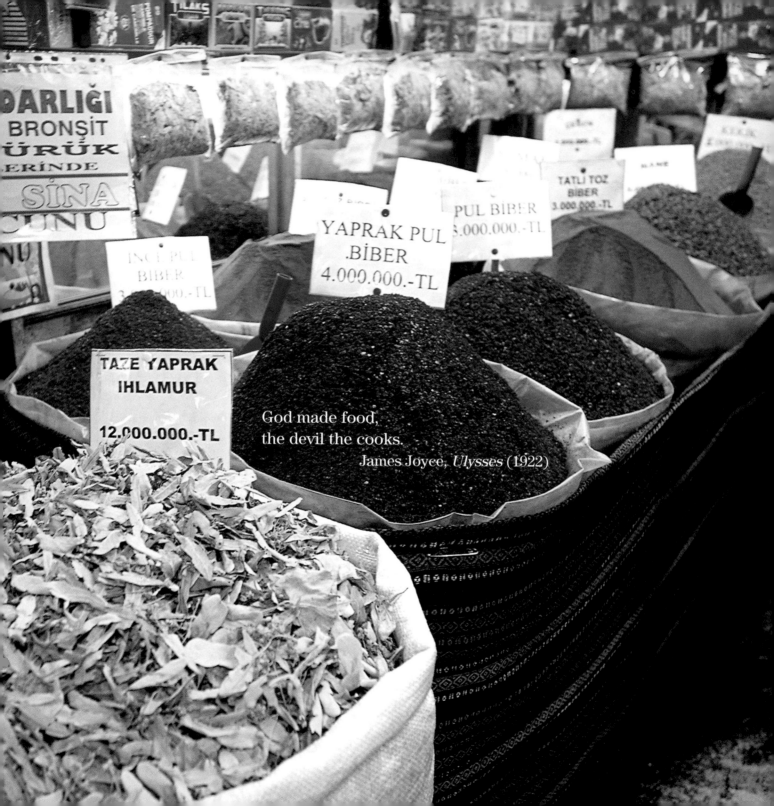

God made food,
the devil the cooks.

James Joyce, *Ulysses* (1922)

CHAPTER 8

Herbs and Spices :
A Taste of Cancer Prevention

The systematic use of herbs and spices in the world's great culinary traditions is one of the best examples of a sense of pleasure becoming an inseparable dimension of daily diet. Throughout history, these ingredients were considered precious luxury items, often reserved for wealthy and powerful people, their value in palace kitchens and dining halls easily equal to their political and economic value (see inset, page 87). Now readily available, spices are essential in today's kitchens; they are a matchless source of flavours and aromas without which most food would turn out pretty bland indeed.

Although the place of spices in cookery is first and foremost a question of taste, spices are recognized today for their medicinal properties; over the centuries, apothecaries, the forerunners of today's pharmacists, exercised strict control over the use of spices to treat afflictions ranging from hiccups to rather more serious digestive diseases. If some of these uses now make us smile, recent

research into the spice cabinet suggests that many herbs and spices may serve effectively as weapons in disease prevention, and especially cancer prevention.

HERBS IN THE FIGHT AGAINST CANCER
It is fascinating to note that many herbs and spices commonly used in modern cooking contain molecules that may influence the processes associated with the development of cancer (Figure 20). One remarkable characteristic is their high content in anti-inflammatory molecules, molecules able to reduce inflammation of the cell environment in which precancerous tumours are found, thus preventing these microtumours from benefiting from a climate favouring their growth, as explained earlier. Precancerous cells definitely do not appreciate a well-seasoned meal !

Among the most thoroughly studied spices, three families stand out because of their rich anti-cancer and anti-inflammatory molecule content,

(continued on page 88)

SPICING UP THE FIGHT AGAINST CANCER

Spice	Active Molecule	Biological Activity		
		Anti-inflammatory	Anti-cancer	Antimicrobial
Turmeric	Curcumin	■	■	■
Ginger	Gingerol	■	■	■
Chili pepper	Capsaicin	■	■	■
Clove	Eugenol	■		■
Lamiaceae Family				
Mint, thyme, marjoram, oregano, basil, rosemary	Ursolic acid	■	■	■
	Perillic acid		■	
	d-Limonene	■	■	
	Carvacrol		■	■
	Thymol		■	■
	Carnosol		■	
	Luteolin	■	■	
Apiaceae Family				
Parsley, coriander, cumin, fennel, anise, chervil	Anethol	■		■
	Apigenin	■	■	
	Polyacetylenes	■		■

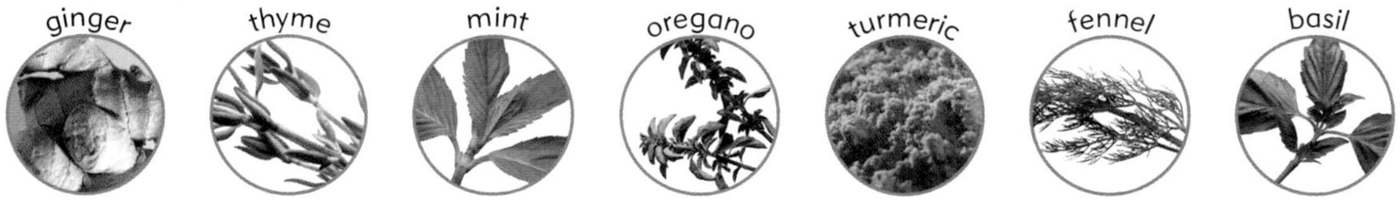

ginger thyme mint oregano turmeric fennel basil

Figure 20

ON A SPICY NOTE !

The Romans were the first to introduce spices in abundance into Western cuisine, the most celebrated example of their prowess being Marcus Gavius Apicius (25 B.C.–37 A.D.). Apicius, a food-lover renowned for his prodigious tastes and appetites, himself created many recipes containing incredible amounts of spices! The fall of the Roman Empire, unfortunately, led to the quasi-disappearance of spices in the West. It was not until the Middle Ages that infatuation with spices resurfaced, stimulated in part by Marco Polo's sumptuous, sometimes exaggerated descriptions of his travels in *The Description of the World* (or *The Book of Marvels*), first published in 1298. Spices were a great draw in the kitchen; beyond that, the desire to control the spice market, as well as the famed "spice routes" that fed this market, grew because of the considerable sums involved: the long road travelled by spices from Asia to Europe made them that much more expensive. Common pepper, for example, long considered the "queen of spices," was found only on the tables of the nobility because a handful cost as much as a bull or a sheep! The exorbitant prices reflected the time spent in transit: it took one to two years for pepper and ginger to arrive from India, or cinnamon and nutmeg from Indonesia. Different monopolies en route also succeeded in driving up the price. Arab merchants served as intermediaries between Indian

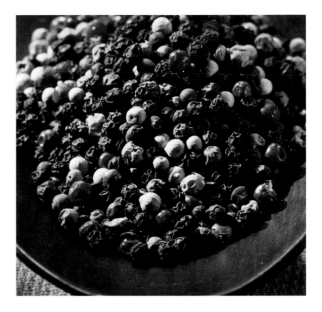

merchants and Venetian navigators (who owed their monopoly to their participation in the Second Crusade), each group drawing considerable benefits from its situation. Fortunately for continental spice-lovers, new routes leading to the sources of these spices, India and Indonesia in particular, were discovered by Portuguese and Dutch sailors. These routes allowed traders to circumvent the established monopolies and made the precious spice cargo available to an ever growing number of people. Certain spices are still apparently worth extraordinary sums, judging by the price of saffron, which can fetch up to $10,000 per kilogram! That quantity, incidentally, would require collecting about three hundred thousand *Crocus sativus* (saffron crocus) flowers.

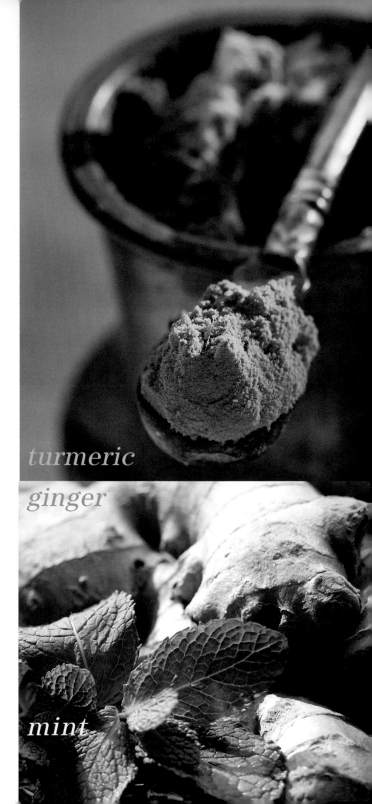

turmeric

ginger

mint

> **TURMERIC** TIP
>
> Turmeric needs to be stabilized in oil before it can be absorbed by the body. Add turmeric to soup by first sautéing onions and garlic in oil, adding the turmeric, and then adding the mixture to the broth. Always add black pepper to a recipe containing turmeric : the pepper dramatically increases the absorption of turmeric. Turmeric may also be added to salad dressing (be sure to add the spice to the oil before adding vinegar or lemon juice), or used to give a special zest to tomato or other vegetable juices : mix in one teaspoon of olive oil into which some turmeric has been dissolved. Sprinkle in liberal amounts of pepper, and serve.

giving them high potential to interfere with the development of cancer.

THE ZINGIBERACEAE FAMILY

A family whose members include ginger (*Zingiber officinale*) and turmeric (*Curcuma longa*), the Zingiberaceae come from Southeast Asia, particularly China and India, where they have been cultivated and used for food and medicine for more than five thousand years. Although these roots are very different from one another in appearance and taste, they both contain important quantities of molecules with very powerful anti-inflammatory effects: curcumin, in turmeric, and gingerol, in ginger. The addition of curcumin or ginger to lab-grown cancer cells, for example, efficiently blocks the production of COX-2, the principal enzyme used by these cells to cause inflammation (see page 33). This anti-inflammatory effect also manifests itself in the human body: the daily consumption of turmeric lowers the amounts of pro-inflammatory molecules in the bloodstream. Studies have shown that a daily dose of ginger in patients suffering from rheumatoid arthritis (a disease where the preponderant role played by inflammation is well-documented), leads to a lessening of symptoms. This effect supposes a decrease in the number of inflammatory molecules present (molecules whose formation was catalyzed by COX-2). Since inflammation plays an important part in the development of cancer, the anti-inflammatory activity of ginger and turmeric suggests interesting avenues for cancer prevention. Curcumin and gingerol also possess the ability to interfere with other processes implicated in the spread of cancer; they may act by directly targeting different types of cancer cells, thus forcing these cells to self-destruct by apoptosis, or they may prevent the formation of the new network of blood vessels that is needed by the tumour for growth. Other studies have shown that turmeric and ginger administered to laboratory animals block the development of different kinds of cancers, especially colon cancer, that were induced by carcinogenic substances. Turmeric and

ginger may thus be considered multifunctional preventive agents, capable of interfering with the growth of cancer cells as much by their direct action on microtumours as by indirect effects, for example, by reducing the chronic inflammation that is essential to tumour progression.

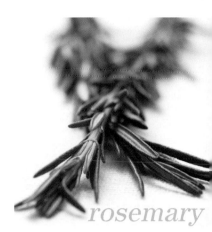

rosemary

THE LAMIACEAE FAMILY

Most lamiaceae used in cooking today (mint, thyme, marjoram, oregano, basil, rosemary) come from the shores of the Mediterranean, where they have played a fundamental role in creating the traditional cuisine of the region. Plants belonging to this family all have very fragrant leaves, due to their high content

Gingerol

Curcumin

in essential oils containing odorous molecules from the terpene family.

Terpenes interfere with the development of cancer by blocking the function of many oncogenes involved in cancer cell growth. Adding terpenes (carvacrol, thymol, perillyl alcohol) to cancer cells derived from a large variety of tumours considerably reduces their proliferation and, in certain cases, leads to their death. Another study showed that the addition of carnosol (a terpene that is particularly abundant in rosemary) to the diet of mice genetically predisposed to suffer from colon cancer prevented the development of this cancer by repairing the intestinal cell defects that cause the disease. It should also be noted that the plants of this family contain ursolic acid, an anti-cancer molecule whose multiple functions include its ability to directly attack cancer cells, to prevent angiogenesis from occurring, and to block COX-2 production, thus reducing inflammation.

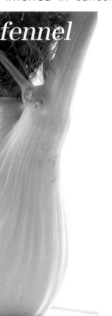
fennel

This anti-cancer activity is not, however, restricted to the terpenes contained in these plants, since luteolin, a polyphenol that is particularly abundant in thyme and mint, also exhibits multiple anti-cancer activity. We have recently observed that luteolin is a potentially strong inhibitor of angiogenesis, by way of its ability to prevent the recruitment of cells essential to the functioning of the blood vessel network used by tumours as supply routes for growth. This inhibitory effect becomes even more interesting when one considers that it occurs at relatively weak luteolin concentrations, similar to those of synthetic molecules derived from pharmaceutical research (see Figure 6, page 25).

THE APIACEAE FAMILY

Also known as the Umbelliferae family, the Apiaceae form a diverse family of plants that includes savoury herbs such as parsley, coriander, chervil, fennel, and cumin, as well as vegetables such as carrots, parsnips, and celery. Of historic importance to Mediterranean regions, the Apiaceae family occupies pride of place in the *Capitulare de villis vel curtis imperii*, an edict written during the reign of Charlemagne (742–814 A.D.), which describes plants needed for medicinal, aromatic, and culinary purposes that were to be cultivated in monasteries.

In a cancer prevention context, the interest of some of these plants, especially parsley and celery, lies in their high content in apigenin, a polyphenol possessing extremely powerful anti-cancer activity. In the laboratory, this molecule inhibited the growth of an impressive number of cancer cells, many derived from the principal cancers that afflict Western societies: breast cancer, colon cancer, lung cancer, and prostate cancer. Although apigenin is a very different molecule from those found in other herbs and spices, the mechanisms involved are in many ways similar: apigenin acts both directly, on cancer cells and angiogenesis, and indirectly, by decreasing inflammatory processes. Even though we are only beginning to characterize the anti-cancer effects of apigenin, its multiple modes of activity and its unusual power mark it as a fascinating future subject of research into cancer prevention.

In summary, recent research indicates that the anti-cancer properties exhibited by herbs and spices are directly linked to their ability to block inflammation. Turmeric, ginger, chili peppers, cloves, and fennel; mint, thyme, and basil : all of these herbs and spices contain molecules that block the activation of NFκB, thus reducing the production of COX-2 and the onset of inflammation. Given that many of these molecules also exert direct anti-cancer activity on precancerous cells, herbs and spices should be considered important sources of anti-cancer molecules that may actively contribute to preventing the development of the disease. In other words, cancer prevention may also be, among other things, a question of good taste !

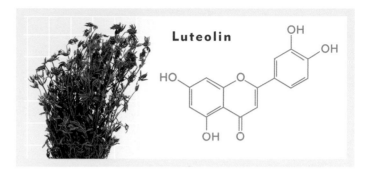

Luteolin

In summary ...

• Herbs and spices contain anti-inflammatory molecules that contribute to slowing down the development of cancer. They act by preventing tumours from taking advantage of nearby favourable conditions for growth.

• The anti-inflammatory property of spices, especially turmeric and ginger, seems to play an important role in the prevention of several types of cancer, particularly colon cancer.

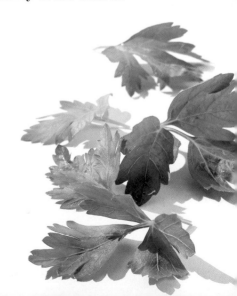

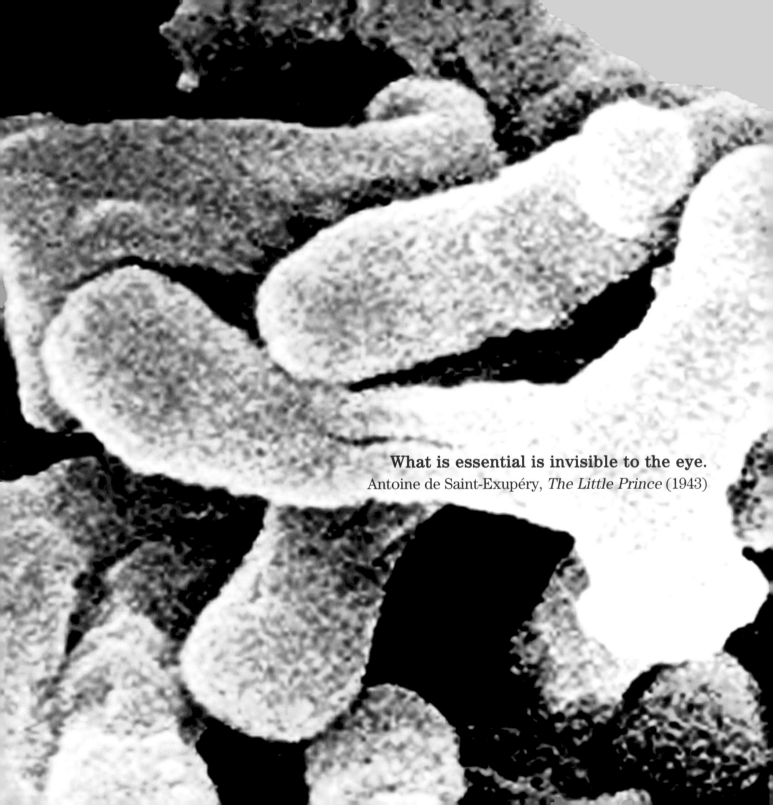

What is essential is invisible to the eye.
Antoine de Saint-Exupéry, *The Little Prince* (1943)

CHAPTER 9

Probiotics : Bacteria
That Want What's Good for You

If we were to use a microscope to examine the world around us, we would be astonished to discover the presence of a universe parallel to our own: a world invisible to the naked eye, an incredibly complex world containing millions of species of bacteria living in direct contact with us! Some bacteria are a threat to human beings and must be eliminated, but others are essential to the healthy functioning of the human body, especially that of the digestive system.

The human digestive tract, stretching about five metres from the mouth to the anus and boasting a surface area of three hundred square metres, or the equivalent of two tennis courts, is the part of the body that has the most direct contact with the outside world and is the most susceptible to colonization by bacteria (Figure 21). The initial colonization takes place early in life: just hours after birth, the intestine already contains important numbers of bifidobacteria (Table 10), bacterial "armies" that predominate all through the nursing

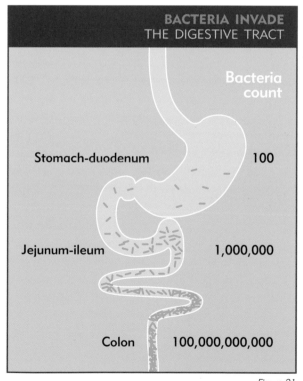

BACTERIA INVADE
THE DIGESTIVE TRACT

Bacteria count

Stomach-duodenum   100

Jejunum-ileum   1,000,000

Colon   100,000,000,000

Figure 21

BIFIDOBACTERIA . . .
➤ 100 million to 100 billion bacteria per gram of human stool
➤ 10 per cent of all intestinal flora
➤ Fourth in importance among all species of bacteria present in the body
➤ Optimal at birth, their number decreases with age: • 95 per cent of bacteria present in breast-fed newborn

Table 10

period, but which are in turn joined by some four hundred other species, forming a very diverse bacterial flora. Rare in the upper sections of the digestive tract, because of the stomach's extreme acidity and the presence of bile salts, bacteria congregate in astronomical numbers in the most far-off regions of the intestine. The colon, for example, contains on average 1,000 billion (1 trillion) bacteria per millilitre (10^{12}/ml), making it the planet's mostly densely populated microbial habitat! For some idea of how huge this bacterial presence is, consider that an adult's body is estimated to be 90 per cent bacteria cells; this means that it contains ten times more bacteria than it does actual human cells, and that the one hundred thousand billion bacteria living in it make up about two kilograms of its weight! Bacteria play a very important part in the life of the body, and it is vital to learn more about their secrets.

IMPORTANT FUNCTIONS OF INTESTINAL BACTERIA

The bacteria present in the digestive system interact closely with the immune system and the cells of the intestinal lining, forming a kind of "ménage à trois" that is essential to the proper functioning of the intestine, as well as that of health in general (Figure 22). Friendly bacteria have an essential role to play in the development of our immune system: they defend the body against outside aggressors, allowing us to survive in spite of the massive number of pathogenic agents surrounding and penetrating us!

An example: mice placed in a sterile (microbe-free) environment at birth subsequently suffer from a gravely compromised immune system. Their immune system can, however, be restored to normal in a few weeks if they cohabit with mice having normal intestinal flora; this corresponds roughly to what happens to us at birth. Because the intestinal mucus is the part of the body that is most vulnerable to outside attack, close to 75 per cent of the body's immune cells are concentrated in the digestive tract. Ideally located to influence the function of this immune defence, intestinal bacteria work either by stimulating the immune response to bolster up defences against pathogenic bacteria or viruses, or by selectively suppressing the immune response, so as to tolerate the presence of certain substances in the outside environment that do not pose any threat: this limits the harmful effects of autoimmune diseases. Intestinal bacteria are the true maestros of the immune system; they play a key role in maintaining and optimizing our ability to

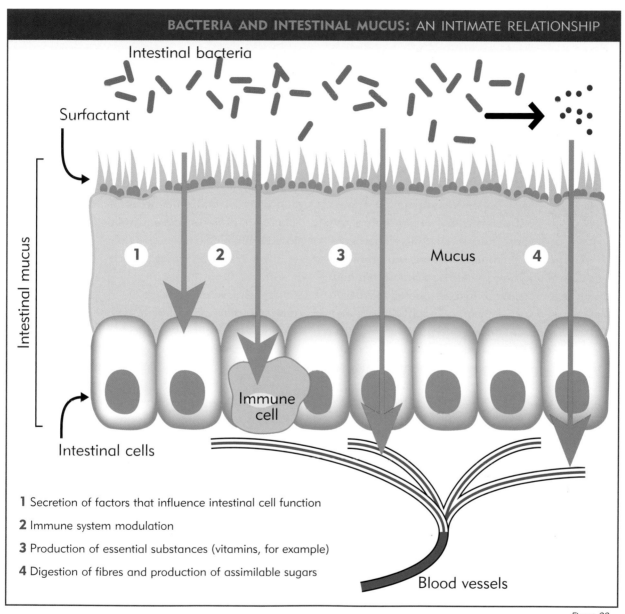

BACTERIA AND INTESTINAL MUCUS: AN INTIMATE RELATIONSHIP

Intestinal bacteria

Surfactant

Intestinal mucus

Intestinal cells

1

2

Immune cell

3

Mucus

4

Blood vessels

1 Secretion of factors that influence intestinal cell function

2 Immune system modulation

3 Production of essential substances (vitamins, for example)

4 Digestion of fibres and production of assimilable sugars

Figure 22

THE SECRET LIES IN FERMENTATION

Fermentation is a reaction used by different micro-organisms in the absence of oxygen to produce energy from sugar. Occurring in the colon, lactic fermentation is analogous to a process known from ancient times; indeed, the first humans to raise cattle must have observed that milk produced by their animals had a definite and short conservation time. If the milk were placed in a hermetically sealed container, however, it curdled, and its conservation time increased significantly. Without knowing the science involved, people discovered the virtues of lactic fermentation, or "life in the absence of air," as Louis Pasteur put it: milk sugars are transformed into lactic acid, which acidifies the environment and prevents the proliferation of undesirable or pathogenic micro-organisms, such as moulds. Although it is generally held that the

discovery and later refinement of these processes took place in the Middle East and the Balkans, almost every culinary tradition has its own version of products made from fermented milk: *skyr*, *langfil*, *viili*, and *ymer* are Scandinavian favourites; *amasi*, *irgo*, and *nono* are well known in Africa; buttermilk and yogurt are popular throughout Europe, while kefir and koumiss are enjoyed in Eastern Europe and Central Asia. All of these foods testify to the importance that human beings accord to fermented milk.

Other than the more convenient expiry date, fermented milk products have several other advantages over ordinary milk: 1) increased digestibility, because the milk sugar lactose has been transformed into lactic acid; 2) higher amounts of essential nutrients such as proteins, amino acids, fatty acids, and vitamins from bacteria (Table 11); and 3) a greater food diversity, thanks to the different aromas, flavours, and textures created by the fermentation process.

Lactic fermentation is not restricted to milk products! It also plays a key role in the preparation of certain vegetable dishes such as sauerkraut (pickled cabbage) and in various types of sourdough breads.

FOLIC ACID CONTENT OF NON-FERMENTED MILK AND OTHER MILK PRODUCTS

Milk product	Folic acid (µg / 100 g)
Milk	0.42
Cheddar cheese	4.2
Yogurt	3.9
Cottage cheese	3.5

Table 11

interact efficiently and safely with our surroundings.

Intestinal bacteria also participate in the good working order of the body by degrading several substances that cannot be digested by the stomach, especially plant fibres (those found in fruits, vegetables, cereals, etc.). The degradation of those fibres frees up the sugars they contain, which are then used as an energy source by the body. The metabolic activity of intestinal bacteria leads to the formation of different molecules, such as vitamins (K1, B, folic acid) and some fatty acids. Finally, as we have seen in chapter 7, this metabolic activity is essential to the production of certain anti-cancer molecules from different foods, especially oleaginous grains and cereals.

Intestinal bacterial flora is an essential component of our bodies, an environment necessary for maintaining good health with which we need to cohabit. In this context, any disturbance that negatively affects the composition and the activity of microbial flora, whether induced by environmental, physiological, or pharmacological factors, facilitates the development of different diseases, ranging from such minor but unpleasant annoyances as the famed *turista* (enteritis) to serious gastrointestinal disorders, including infectious diarrhea, inflammatory diseases such as ulcerative colitis and Crohn's disease, and even cancer.

OUR GOOD FRIENDS: LACTIC BACTERIA

To adequately fulfill its function, intestinal flora must be principally made up of beneficial ("good") bacteria occupying the maximum possible available area to prevent potential harm brought on by pathogenic bacteria strains. Among these friendly bacteria, bifidobacteria and other species of lactobacilli are considered those with the most positive possible effect on the composition and function of intestinal flora. In the absence of oxygen, as is the case in the colon, these bacteria are capable of transforming substances rich in fibres into lactic acid, through the process known as lactic fermentation (see inset, page 96).

The production of lactic acid acidifies the intestine and slows the proliferation of several pathogenic micro-organisms that prefer more temperate conditions for growth. In other words, the presence of lactic bacteria in the colon has an extremely positive impact on intestinal equilibrium, and by extension, on the immune system and on overall health.

PROBIOTICS

The Russian biologist Elie Metchnikoff (1845–1916), a Nobel Prize winner in physiology and medicine who is considered the founding father of immunology, is the person most responsible for today's interest in the beneficial effects of lactic bacteria. Starting from his observations on the unusually long lifespans of Bulgarian mountain-dwellers, Metchnikoff hypothesized that the observed longevity was linked to the consumption of *yahourth*, a fermented milk drink containing large numbers of lactic bacteria. According to him, the acidity produced by these "friendly" bacteria created an inhospitable environment for the toxin-producing bacteria present in the intestine, thus neutralizing the auto-intoxication process and

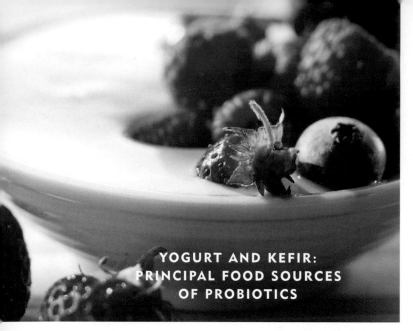

YOGURT AND KEFIR: PRINCIPAL FOOD SOURCES OF PROBIOTICS

YOGURT

Of probable Bulgarian origin, this "divine essence," as Pliny the Elder (20–79 A.D.) called it, is still made today by the combined action of *Lactobacillus bulgaricus* and *Streptococcus thermophilus*. These bacilli cooperate to rapidly transform lactose (a milk sugar) into lactic acid, inducing a slightly sour taste and a modification of the structure of milk proteins that leads to its coagulation. Yogurt had long been consumed in Central Europe and Asia Minor, but once it began to appear on supermarket shelves in the 1950s, and new fruit-flavour varieties became available, its consumption and popularity began to rise steadily. In Canada, for example, annual yogurt consumption grew from 0.1 kilogram to 6 kilograms per capita from 1968 to 2004; this is still, however, significantly lower than the average in certain European countries, 20 kilograms. To have a beneficial effect on the intestine, yogurt must be fortified with lactic bacteria, usually bifidobacteria

and lactobacilli. Very popular throughout Japan and Europe, milk products containing large amounts of bifidobacteria and/or lactobacilli are gradually starting to assert themselves on the North American palate.

KEFIR

Eaten mostly in Russia and other East European countries, where it represents up to 15 per cent of all milk products sold, kefir (from the Turkish word *keif*, or "well-being") is a particular type of fermented milk resulting from the combined action of hundreds of different bacteria and yeasts that are added to cow's milk in the form of gelatinous "grains" that resemble cauliflower heads. The bacteria produce lactic acid which imparts a sour taste resembling that of yogurt, while the yeasts transform part of the lactose into carbon dioxide and alcohol. The thick, fizzy liquid that results has a slight alcohol content (0.5 per cent) . . . and may just prove an unforgettable experience for seekers of strong gourmet sensations! The "Champagne of yogurts" contains more bacteria than yogurt, mostly different types of lactobacilli, as well as kefiran, a complex polysaccharide, which seems to have decided positive effects on the immune system. In fact, kefir has long been used in Russia to promote overall good health, as well as for treating various diseases ranging from stomach ulcers to pneumonia. Koumiss, a fermented product similar to kefir, is prepared from mare, camel, or donkey milk; it is a drink of choice in Central Asia, especially Siberia, where it is very much a part of the daily diet.

HEALTH BENEFITS AND THERAPEUTIC ACTIVITY OF PROBIOTIC BACTERIA IN HUMANS

Health Benefits

➤ Maintenance of healthy intestinal flora

➤ Immune system reinforcement

➤ Decrease in lactose intolerance

➤ Decrease in cholesterol levels

➤ Anti-cancer activity

➤ Improved nutritional value of certain foods

Therapeutic Activity

➤ Prevention of urogenital infections

➤ Decrease in constipation

➤ Protection against *turista*

➤ Prevention of infantile diarrhea

➤ Decrease in diarrhea caused by antibiotics

➤ Prevention of hypercholesterolemia

➤ Prevention of colon and bladder cancer

➤ Prevention of osteoporosis

Table 12

slowing down premature aging. Metchnikoff's observations, coupled with the discovery of bifidobacteria by Henri Tissier at about the same time, influenced the development of a whole new class of foods enriched with these beneficial bacteria: foods we now know as probiotics.

Probiotics (from the Greek "for life") are defined as "living micro-organisms that when administered in adequate amounts produce benefit for the life of the host." Today, to earn "probiotic" status, a product or food must contain bacteria that are able to tough out their passage down the gastrointestinal system and find their way to the colon, where they can exert a certain influence on the composition and activity of the resident bacterial flora. According to this newer, operational definition, ordinary yogurt, even though it may contain up to 500 million living bacteria per gram, cannot be considered a real probiotic, because the bacterial strains used in its fabrication do not survive the encounter with either stomach acid or bile, and are thus not able to reach the colon. It is possible, however, to confer probiotic character upon yogurt by adding bacterial strains that resist the trip down the digestive tract. Since about 30 per cent of certain bifidobacteria strains and 5 per cent of lactobacilli strains do manage to reach the colon after ingestion, these bacteria have, over the years, become the go-to bacterial cultures for use in preparing fermented milk products (see page 98).

THE ANTI-CANCER PROPERTIES OF PROBIOTICS

Many health benefits and positive therapeutic results have been attributed to probiotics (Table 12). The best-documented effect of these bacteria is their positive impact on the prevention and treatment of many types of diarrhea, especially those caused by rotavirus infection. This property may prove extremely useful, if we consider that somewhere in the world, a child dies every fifteen seconds of the consequences of this type of diarrhea.

What of probiotics and cancer? Although no long-term epidemiological study has yet evaluated the impact of the regular consumption of foods rich in probiotics on the risk of developing colon cancer, preliminary findings are encouraging. For example, the daily intake of three hundred grams of probiotic-containing yogurt by volunteers in good health caused a marked lowering of the ability of carcinogenic substances present in stool to induce damage in cell DNA: a key phase in the development of cancer. Patients suffering from colon adenomas who were given lactobacilli and bifidobacteria over a three-month period experienced an acidification of stools as well as a notable decrease in the excessive proliferation that is characteristic of the cells of these tumours. It seems, therefore, that probiotics may have very positive effects on some phases in the development of colon cancer.

In many respects, these observations agree with studies carried out on laboratory animals suggesting that the preference of probiotic lactic bacteria for ending up in the colon may reduce the development of cancer in that organ. For example, the administration of probiotics to these animals prevents the appearance of precancerous cells as well as the development of colorectal tumours induced by azoxymethane or dimethylhydrazine, two powerfully carcinogenic substances. This protective effect of probiotics needs to be better understood, but it seems that a higher concentration of lactic bacteria in the colon does prevent the damage done to DNA by carcinogens, thus reducing the risk of mutations that speed the progress of cancer. The decrease in carcinogenic potential may be linked in large part to a decrease in the number and activity of harmful bacteria that generate carcinogenic substances. In fact, certain bacteria (bacteroids, clostridium, enterobacteria) transform compounds that are excreted by the bile into carcinogenic substances: a mechanism that may be responsible for the impact of these "unfriendly" bacteria on the incidence and growth of colon tumours in lab animals. Such transformations are particularly important in the context of a "Western" diet rich in meats and fats, since this type of diet promotes the growth of harmful bacteria while increasing the production of compounds that may cause mutations. It is interesting to note that some studies on the bacterial content of human feces have observed a higher risk of colon cancer associated with the presence of such bacteria as *Bacteroides vulgatus* and *Bacteroides stercoris*, while a lower risk was associated with the presence of other species, *Lactobacillus acidophilus*, for example.

Another facet of the activity mechanism of probiotics which could certainly contribute to their anti-cancer effects is their capacity to modulate immune system activity. Probiotics stimulate the activity of foreigner-destroying immune cells, and seem to reduce inflammation, an essential condition for the progression of tumours. The impact of this immune system regulation on the development of cancer by probiotic bacteria seems important, but needs to be more fully explored and understood. Adding kefir to the diet of mice grafted with human tumours caused a 70 per cent decrease in tumour growth, a phenomenon that correlates with a stimulation of the immune system in the intestines of these lab animals.

In summary, many sets of data suggest that probiotics actively participate in maintaining good health by exerting a positive regulatory influence on immune system activity, as well as by modifying the composition of intestinal flora. By way of the same mechanisms, probiotics slow the growth of bacteria that activate certain carcinogenic substances present in diet and that increase the risk of damage to intestinal cell DNA. It should be noted, however, that all studies carried out to date indicate that these bacteria stay in the colon for a relatively short time, and that regular probiotic intake is required to renew the friendly bacterial populations and thus fully benefit from their presence. Researchers have also determined that the simultaneous administration of indigestible carbohydrates may encourage the probiotic colonization of the colon and the growth of probiotic bacteria there. These indigestible substances, called prebiotics, are fructose polymers naturally present in a great many foods, including onions, garlic, tomatoes, asparagus, bananas, and wheat. The potent combination of probiotics and prebiotics has proven superior in causing the elimination of cancer cells in animals, especially in tandem with bifidobacteria.

In summary ...

• Intestinal bacteria play an essential role in balancing bodily functions, as much by their metabolic activity as by their impact on the immune system.

• Lactic bacteria such as lactobacilli and bifidobacteria fulfill particularly important functions by preventing the excessive proliferation of harmful bacteria as well as by positively regulating the immune system.

• The daily consumption of foods fortified with probiotics is a simple and efficient way of maintaining high levels of lactic bacteria in the colon and thus preventing the development of cancer.

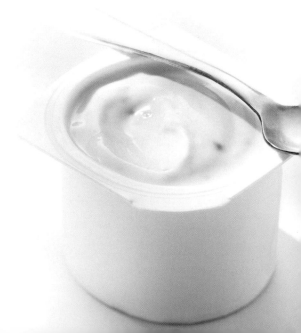

CHAPTER 10

Of Cabbages . . . and Cancer

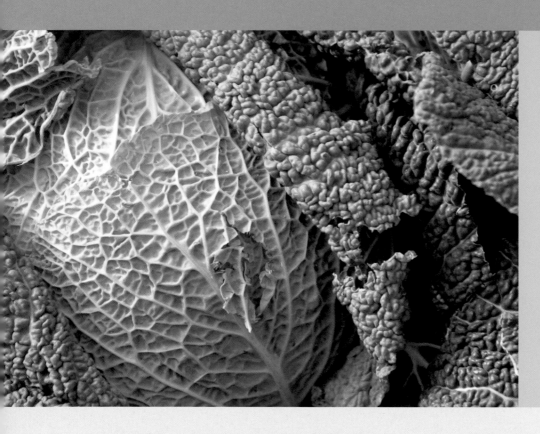

Indole-3-carbinol

Crucifers are vegetables belonging to the cabbage family; they get their name from their distinctive four-petalled flowers that form a cross (*cruci* in Latin). Cabbage is doubtless one of the first vegetables to have been cultivated by humans. It became over time very important in both culinary and medical traditions; starting from the humble wild cabbage, the first cultivators were able to produce a large number of varieties that we still enjoy today. Indeed, broccoli, cauliflower, kale, curly kale, and Brussels sprouts all boast a common ancestor. Each owes its distinct taste and appearance to the selective crop breeding practised by Greek and Roman farmers.

Cruciferous vegetables are extremely important in the prevention of cancer due to their high gluco-sinolate content; glucosinolates are powerful anti-cancer molecules found exclusively in crucifers. Studies carried out over the last few years show that regular crucifer consumption significantly lowers the risk of developing a whole host of cancers, especially lung cancer, bladder cancer, breast cancer, and cancers of the gastrointestinal system (stomach and colon cancers). This protective effect of crucifers derives mostly from their ability to block the carcino-genic potential of a large number of particularly dangerous substances that can alter the cell's DNA, thereby causing damage that leads to the growth of tumours. The glucosinolates present in crucifers prevent this phenomenon from occurring. Glucosinolates stimulate the natural activity of our defence mechanisms, accelerating the elimination of these substances; depriving them of a longer, noxious stay in the body reduces their carcinogenic potential. This property is crucial, since many cancers are directly imputable to deficiencies in these important detox systems. Eating crucifers regularly, on the other hand, improves the performance of these systems. By way of example, a recent study shows that some individuals are more susceptible to developing lung cancer because their immune system falters when confronted with carcinogenic substances. A diet rich in cruciferous vegetables, however, was able to reverse this tendency to develop cancer. Cruciferous vegetables should thus be considered as front-line defence weapons in the fight against cancer. They prevent carcinogenic substances from causing the genetic damage that may over time result in the onset of cancer and the growth of tumours.

As is the case with other cancer-fighting foods, it is essential to eat regular portions of cruciferous vegetables to maximize their health benefits and the protection against cancer they may afford. Fortunately, the very large variety of vegetables now available lets us take full advantage of their healthful properties without them becoming monotonous, predictable, or just plain boring eating. Whether in soups, whether stir-fried or steamed, a minimum of three weekly servings of cruciferous vegetables represents one change in dietary habits that will have the most impact on the risk of being touched by cancer.

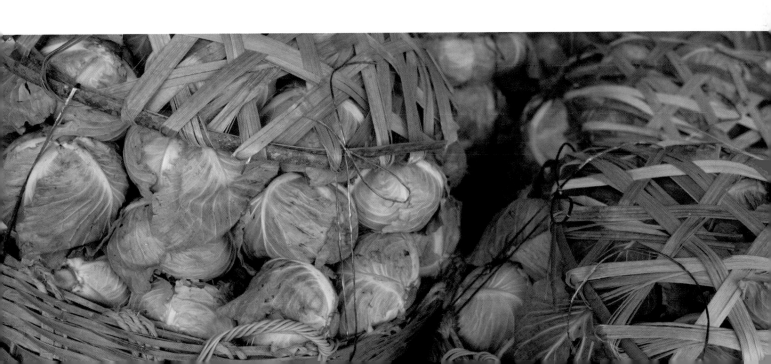

CHAPTER 11

The Garlic Family : Keeping Cancer Far Away

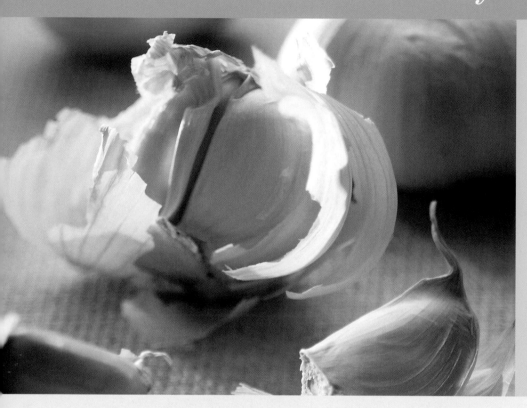

Diallyl sulfide

Crushing a clove of garlic or chopping an onion is hardly, on first glance, a revolutionary act; done mechanically, without much thought, it occurs every day in thousands of kitchens. This routine gesture, however, disguises a process of great importance in the prevention of cancer. Crushing a garlic clove causes important modifications in the vegetable's chemical composition : alliin, a molecule abundantly present in garlic, is transformed by enzyme action into allicin, a very unstable molecule that immediately decomposes into about thirty other compounds. These newly formed molecules have the particularity not only of being extremely unsubtle (in an olfactory sense) but also, much more importantly, of possessing uncommon anti-cancer activity that makes garlic and its cousins important players in cancer prevention.

Studies show that people who regularly consume vegetables from the garlic family have a lowered risk of developing specific types of cancers, in particular those of the digestive system (esophagus, stomach, and colon cancer). Recent research has allowed scientists to identify at least two overall mechanisms by which vegetables from the

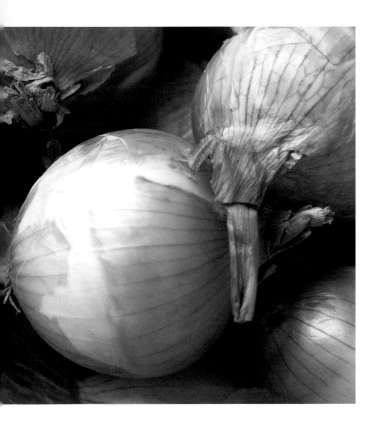

The anti-cancer compounds found in garlic are thus useful as protective shields, but they also have the power to fight the microtumours lying dormant within the body. Certain compounds that form when a garlic family vegetable is chopped up have the ability to stop the growth of cancer cells and, in certain cases, to force them to commit suicide (cell death). Cancer cells have good reason to stay away from garlic!

garlic family play this protective role. In probably the more important model, the odoriferous molecules freed when these vegetables are crushed are able to accelerate the elimination from the body of toxic carcinogenic substances. This accelerated "flushing" lowers the risk of these substances attacking our genetic material (DNA) and causing the multiple mutations that lead to tumour formation. A front-line defence system, like the crucifers, garlic and its relatives may be thought of as border patrols that work to limit the harm wreaked by the different toxic aggressors we face on a daily basis.

GARLIC TIP

To maximize the health benefits found in garlic, try crushing the whole cloves with the flat of a large knife, and then waiting ten minutes before chopping them or putting them through the garlic press. In this way, the molecules that occupy different compartments in the clove come into contact with one another and become active. When you need to chop garlic and other vegetables for a recipe, start by crushing the garlic; prepare the other vegetables during the ten-minute waiting period. The cloves don't need to be peeled before they are crushed; they will be easier to peel afterward.

CHAPTER 12

Soy : A Unique Source of Anti-cancer Phytoestrogens

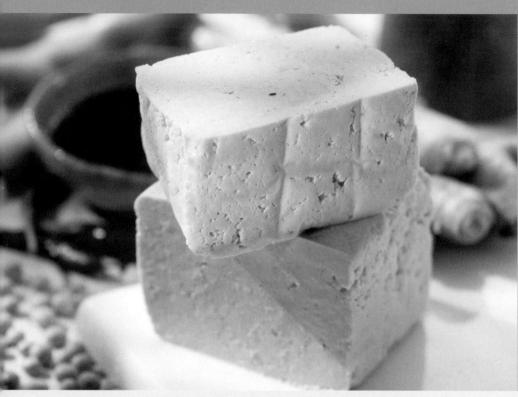

Genistein

Phytoestrogens are molecules derived from plants (phyto-) that are very similar to estrogens, the female sex hormones. Estrogens play a central role in the onset of breast cancer : when the level of these hormones is too high, excessive stimulation of the mammary gland occurs, leading to an increase in cancer risk. Because phytoestrogens so closely resemble estrogens, they get in the way : they are able to prevent estrogens from interacting with breast cells, thus contributing to a lessening of cancer risk.

Phytoestrogens that exist in nature are found only in certain very specific foods. Isoflavones are present exclusively in soy, a legume eaten in large amounts in Asia. Many studies have suggested that the regular consumption of soy-based foods, such as the beans themselves (*edamame*), the bean curd, or tofu, roasted beans, and miso soup, significantly lowers the risk of being affected by breast cancer, and that this preventive effect is amplified if regular soy consumption begins at a young age, before the jump in hormones that accompanies the onset of puberty. On the other hand, the isoflavones in soy may not have the same beneficial effects on women who have a history of breast cancer : these women

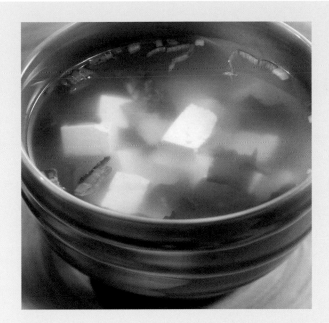

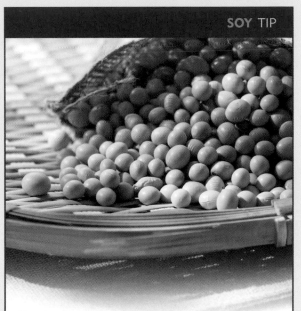

SOY TIP

Purchasing dry roasted soy beans is a simple way of choosing to add soy to diet. Soybeans are now available in the nut section of most grocery stores (if not, ask your store manager to order them). They may be eaten plain, salted, or barbecued. To lower the amount of salt, mix a bag of plain soybeans with a bag of salted ones. Easy to carry around as a daily treat, whether in the office or while shopping, on a hike, on the golf course, or on a trip, soybeans make for a delicious and healthful snack.

need to be much more prudent with their soy consumption. The use of isoflavone supplements should also be discouraged; studies indicate that these products may increase the risk of cancer instead of diminishing it!

CHAPTER 13 Tomatoes and Prostate Cancer: It's All in the Secret Sauce

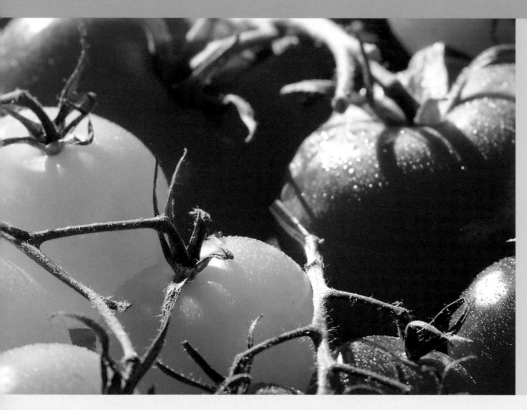

Lycopene

From its discovery in the sixteenth-century Americas by the first conquistadors, the humble tomato has progressively inserted itself into European culinary tradition, especially in Mediterranean countries, to become one of the world's most popular vegetables. Coming on top of what we now know about its real health benefits, we can only cheer the rise of the tomato!

Studies have shown that the incidence of prostate cancer is less widespread in regions where the population regularly consumes different kinds of dishes prepared with tomatoes. Men in Italy, Spain, and Mexico suffer less from prostate cancer than men in areas where fewer tomato-based dishes are eaten. These findings led researchers to suspect that tomatoes might contain substances that slow the development of this disease. It seems that this protection is linked to the presence of lycopene, a pigment found mostly in tomatoes, and the substance responsible for the tomato's characteristic rosy hue. According to some studies, persons having more elevated than average lycopene blood levels run a significantly lower risk of developing prostate cancer: about 25 to 30 per cent lower.

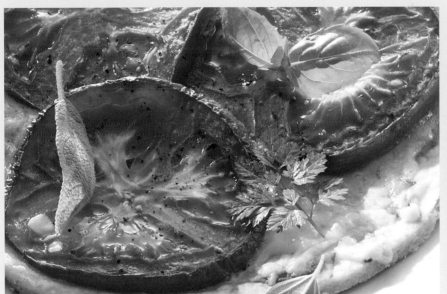 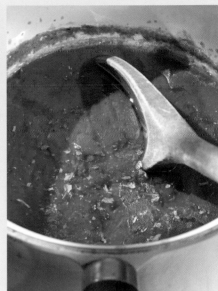

To attain blood lycopene levels high enough to interfere with the growth of precancerous cells in the prostate, it is important to eat cooked tomatoes! They should ideally be prepared in olive oil, as sauce, for example. Cooking tomatoes in oil increases lycopene content and allows the lycopene to be more easily assimilated into cells.

CHAPTER 14

Berries : The Power of the Little Guy

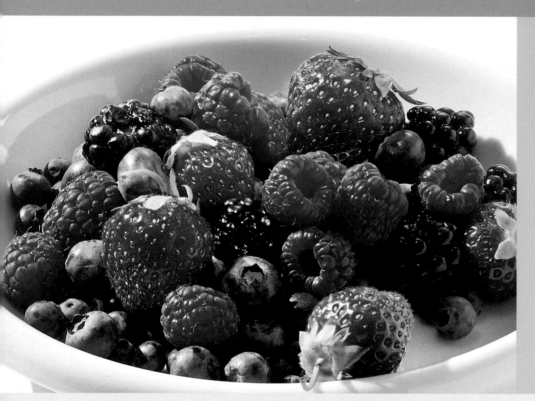

Ellagic acid

Although berries are best known for their exquisite flavour, they pack some unexpected punch : they are an exceptional source of very powerful anti-cancer molecules that may very well contribute to lowering the risk of developing certain types of cancers.

Ellagic acid, found in large amounts in raspberries and strawberries, and anthocyanidins, principally associated with blueberries, are able to selectively block the activity of at least two proteins essential to the development of cancer (PDGF and VEGF receptors). These molecules interfere with the formation of new blood vessels in the neighbourhood of the tumour, thus cutting off its supply routes, preventing the tumour from obtaining the oxygen and essential nutrients it needs to grow and spread. Proanthocyanidins, found in cranberries and blueberries, have extraordinary antioxidant strength; several studies have corroborated their potential to interfere with different phases of tumour development.

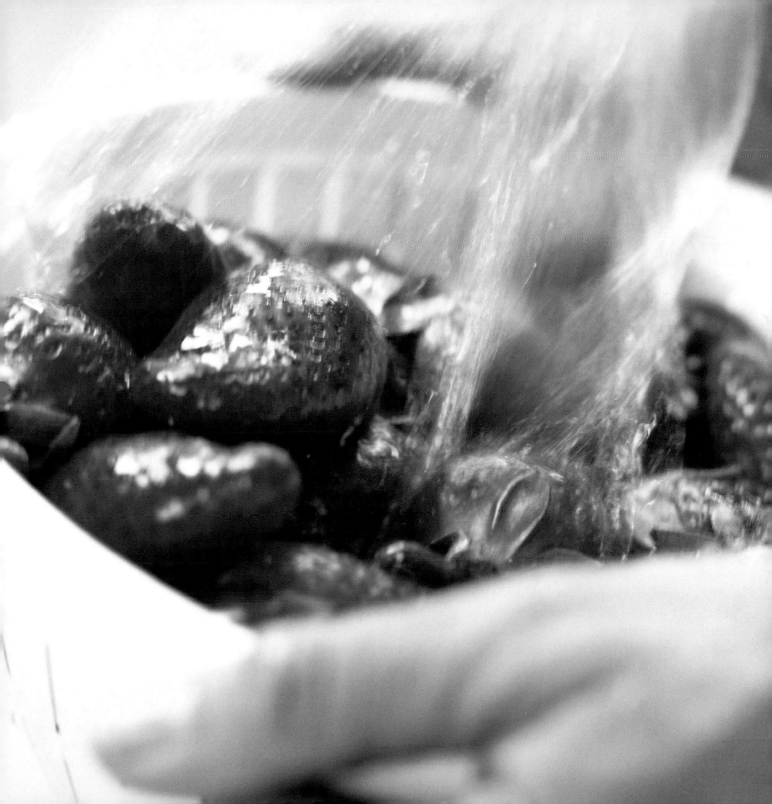

CHAPTER 15

Citrus Fruits : So Much More Than Vitamin C !

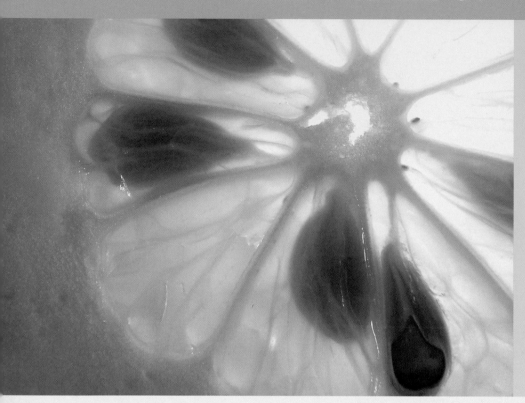

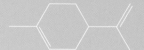

Limonene

Long considered luxury items, citrus fruits are now cultivated on a large scale all over the world, allowing us easy year-round access to these delicious bursts of sunshine at very reasonable cost. All the better for us : citrus fruits are not only an excellent source of vitamin C, they also contain significant quantities of monoterpenes and flavanones, two classes of anti-cancer compounds that play a key role in the beneficial effects associated with regular citrus fruit consumption.

Of all fruits studied, citrus fruits exhibit some of the strongest anti-cancer activity on record.

Numerous studies have shown that the consumption of citrus reduces by half the risk of developing certain kinds of cancers, in particular those of the digestive system (esophagus, mouth, and stomach). This effect is likely linked to the ability of the anti-cancer molecules present in citrus, monoterpenes and flavanones, to carry out two tasks : first, interfere with different processes, especially cancer cell growth, that are necessary for tumour development; and second, reduce inflammation, thus depriving tumours of an important stimulus for growth.

Another very important property of citrus is their

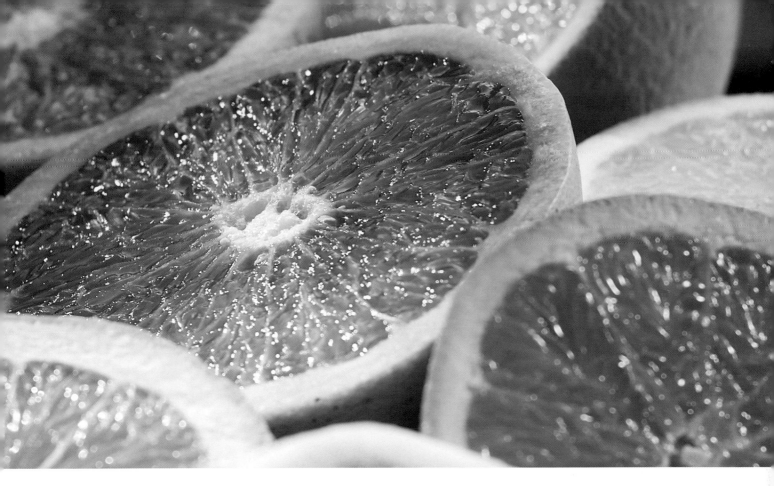

ability to increase the blood levels of other anti-cancer compounds also present in food. For example, citrus fruits, especially grapefruit, contain molecules that block the elimination systems (mediated by the enzyme cytochrome P450) of foreign molecules; this may considerably influence the levels of other molecules in the bloodstream. Although this characteristic of grapefruit can lead to unwanted side effects in the case of people who take certain types of medication, under normal conditions, the increase in absorption of anti-cancer compounds of food origin may have one very positive consequence : maximizing the anti-cancer potential of these molecules.

Drinking a glass of orange juice for breakfast is, of course, an excellent way to take in some needed vitamin C. More surprisingly, it also protects the body against the possible development of certain types of cancers!

CHAPTER 16

Green Tea : Drying Out Cancer

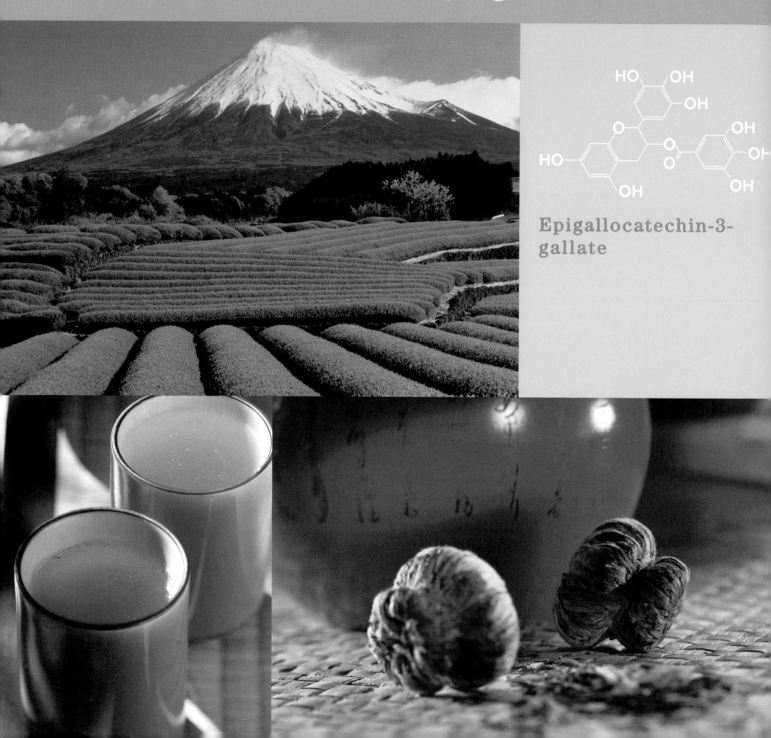

Epigallocatechin-3-gallate

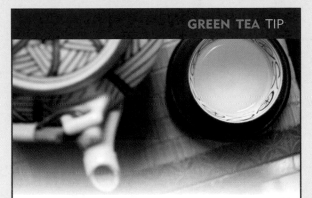

There are as many varieties of tea in the world as there are wines. The flavour of these teas varies considerably; it's in the trying that we realize which new flavours we prefer. Many differences exist between Chinese and Japanese teas, and between different types of Chinese teas or Japanese teas. Note, however, that satisfying oneself with tea from a tea bag is the equivalent of tasting cheap wine and concluding that all wines are undrinkable! Tea bags contain torn leaves, the residues of tea harvest. A true taste for tea can't be properly developed by trying only a low-quality product. Instead, try these three tips : drink tea brewed from real tea leaves in an attractive teapot; avoid stainless steel tea infusers that do not allow tea leaves to fully absorb water and thus express their full flavour; drink from an appealing cup. Drinking a cup of tea is a pleasure to be shared with family and friends, or enjoyed in a moment of solitary relaxation.

Green tea holds a place of prime importance in any diet planned with cancer prevention in mind. Of all foods, it contains one of the highest proportions of anti-cancer molecules. More than one-third of tea leaves by weight is made up of catechins, molecules that are able to target a large number of processes associated with the development of cancer cells! Green tea's high catechin content plays an extremely important role in the prevention of cancer; many studies have shown that its regular consumption decreases the risk of certain types of cancers, especially those of the bladder and the prostate. By reason of its unique properties and its relative abundance, EGCG, the most important catechin in green tea, may block certain mechanisms used by cancer cells to reproduce and invade surrounding tissue : it is able to prevent the formation of a new network of blood vessels by angiogenesis. Because angiogenesis is an essential prerequisite for the development of all cancers, the inhibition of this process, by the daily consumption of green tea, for example, constitutes one of the best strategies now available to us for preventing the progression of microtumours. Angiogenesis inhibition means that tumour formation is put on hold, or maintained in a latent state, without endangering the normal functioning of surrounding tissues.

The key to fully benefiting from the special properties of green tea is to choose the varieties that contain the highest amounts of catechins, and therefore of EGCG, and to consume these on a regular basis, so that EGCG blood levels stay high enough to attack precancerous cells over and over again. Choose Japanese green teas, richer in catechins, over Chinese teas; and brew the tea for eight to ten minutes, to extract the maximum quantity of these molecules. Prepared in this way, three daily cups of tea will allow you to take in an optimum catechin "allowance" for enabling effective protection against cancer.

CHAPTER 17

Red Wine : Methuselah's Daily Dose ?

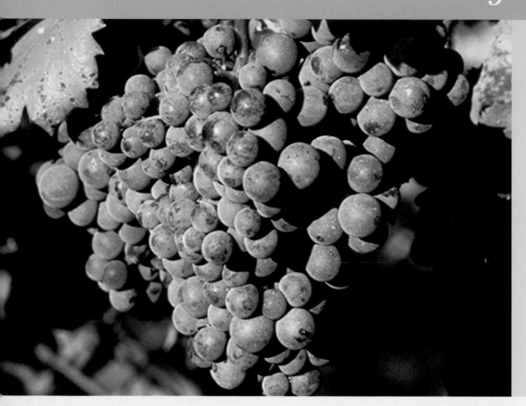

Resveratrol

Red wine is a very complex beverage containing thousands of different phytochemical compounds. One of these molecules, resveratrol, is found in appreciable quantities only in red wine, and seems to have multiple positive effects on the cardiovascular system and in cancer prevention.

Studies carried out to date suggest that resveratrol is one of the only molecules of dietary origin which can act simultaneously on more than one crucial phase of tumour development : it prevents both the appearance of new cancer cells and the growth to maturity of cancer cells already present. Although most of these exciting results were obtained in a laboratory environment, other studies suggest that this anti-cancer effect is also at work in the human body. Of course, the key to tasting the full benefits of red wine is moderation. Alcohol in high doses is very harmful to cells; heavy drinking considerably increases the risk of developing cancers such as mouth, liver, and breast cancer.

In addition to its protective effects against heart disease and cancer onset, resveratrol may slow down the aging process and help preserve brain function. Is red wine a fountain of youth ? Certainly not. It does

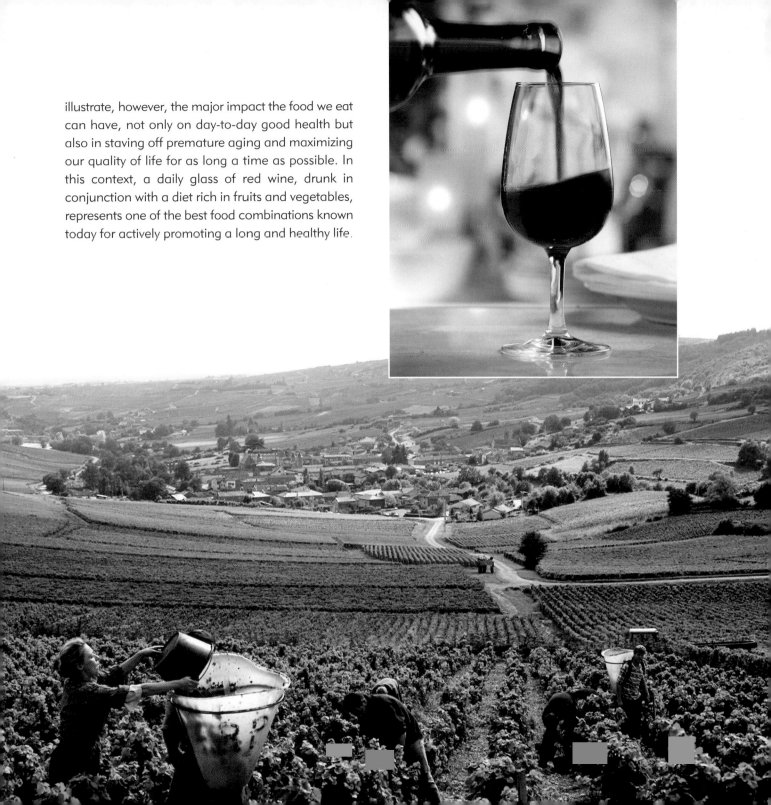

illustrate, however, the major impact the food we eat can have, not only on day-to-day good health but also in staving off premature aging and maximizing our quality of life for as long a time as possible. In this context, a daily glass of red wine, drunk in conjunction with a diet rich in fruits and vegetables, represents one of the best food combinations known today for actively promoting a long and healthy life.

CHAPTER 18

Chocolate : Passion and Prevention in One Dark Package

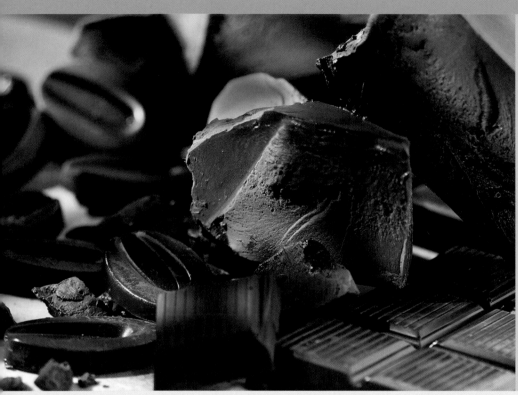

Proanthocyanidin

While pursuing other, less peaceful ends in sixteenth-century Mexico, the Spanish colonizers observed that the Aztecs consumed great quantities of what they called *xocoalt*, a very bitter beverage made from cacao (cocoa) beans. Without knowing it, they had stumbled upon what was fated to become a veritable object of gourmet desire!

Dark chocolate – made of 70 per cent cocoa mass – is an utterly delicious food with surprising and multiple benefits for health. Numerous trials have shown that cocoa mass contains large amounts of a certain class of polyphenols, the proanthocyanidins : molecules that possess potent health-promoting properties. These polyphenols are very similar to those found in other foods also known for their protective effect against cancer, especially green tea, berries, and onions. It follows that the molecules present in chocolate provide similar benefits. In fact, recent studies carried out on lab animals show that the addition to diet of cocoa mass extracts significantly slows down the growth of some cancers induced by carcinogenic substances. More research is needed to confirm the benefits of chocolate in cancer prevention, but the preliminary results are very

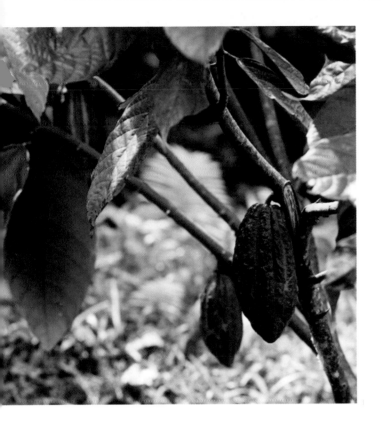

that should be eaten in moderation. The benefits associated with chocolate will be even greater if its regular consumption replaces that of other snack foods loaded with fats and sugars and without any health benefits whatsoever. In a cancer-fighting diet, there is no doubt that a daily twenty-gram serving of 70 per cent dark chocolate represents a simple, efficient, and delicious way of preventing the onset of cancer and cardiovascular disease. Dark chocolate is that rare but perfect example of a very good thing that's also very good for you!

CHOCOLATE TIP

A sweet treat that's also a healthy one : two squares of 70 per cent dark chocolate supply a quick sugar fix that's sure to boost energy levels ; they also provide an adequate amount of beneficial polyphenols, and an even greater hit of pure pleasure!

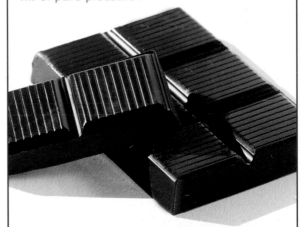

encouraging, and even more so when one considers that the regular consumption of chocolate should not be too problematic for people who are careful about what they eat! It should be noted, however, that previous studies have shown that the presence of milk will prevent the absorption of polyphenols from dark chocolate, thus neutralizing its positive effects. It may sound counterintuitive, but it seems better to enjoy dark chocolate without that accompanying glass of milk.

A common-sense caveat : all chocolate, including dark chocolate, is a calorie-rich food

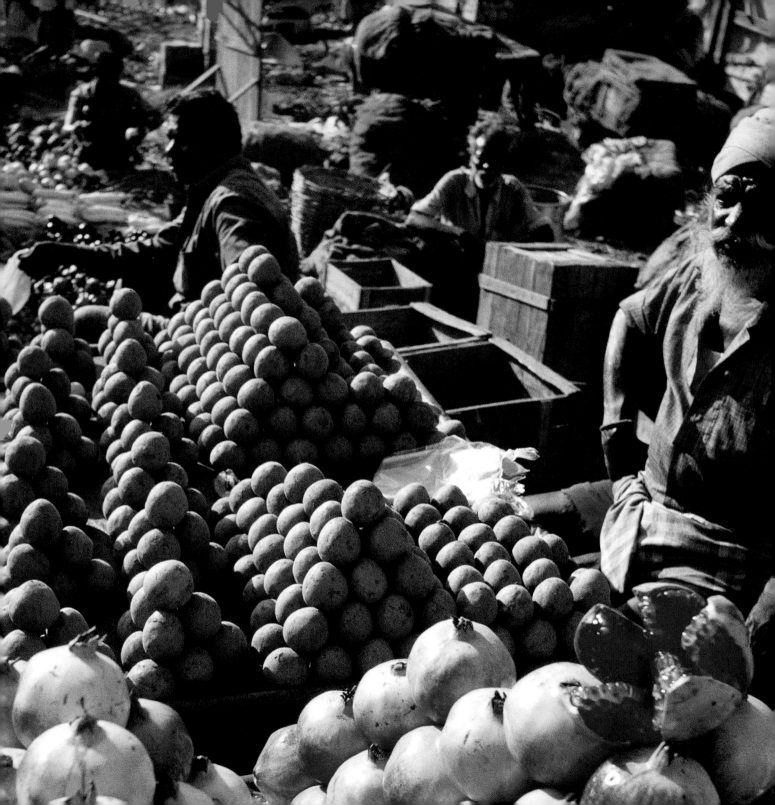

part THREE

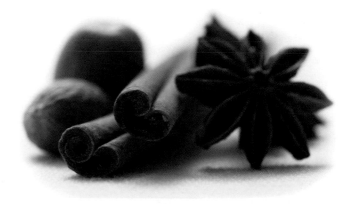

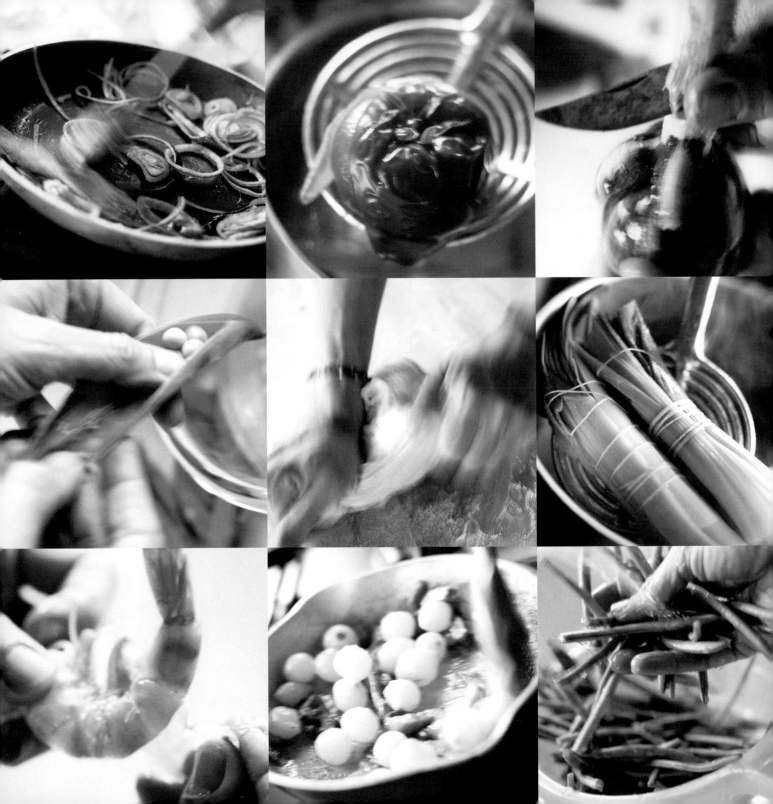

CHAPTER 19

Get Cooking!

Although the scientific theories that seek to explain the important role of diet in the prevention of cancer may be complex, and sometimes difficult to grasp, the practical application of these principles is often a very pleasant undertaking! As stated earlier, preventing cancer through diet is first and foremost a matter of the following : *learning* more about the world's great culinary traditions; and *benefiting* from this inestimable cultural heritage bequeathed to us by the millions of women who cared about the impact of diet on their families' health, and who multiplied their efforts to identify the food combinations that would optimize both pleasure and well-being. Accessing centuries-old cuisines is not just about understanding one cultural aspect of history's greatest civilizations; it also implies that we must seize the occasion to benefit from the positive impact that these traditions have on health.

To meet this twofold challenge, we asked a team of chefs to create recipes with the following in mind :

They were required to include fruits, vegetables, and spices whose credentials as important sources of anti-cancer molecules had already been well established by scientific research.

They were to respect the cultural authenticity of recipes by preferring ingredient combinations in line with culinary tradition.

They had to invent quick and easy-to-make dishes made from readily available ingredients.

Last but not least, our chefs were requested to produce a slew of recipes with one overriding common characteristic : they all had to be exceptionally delicious!

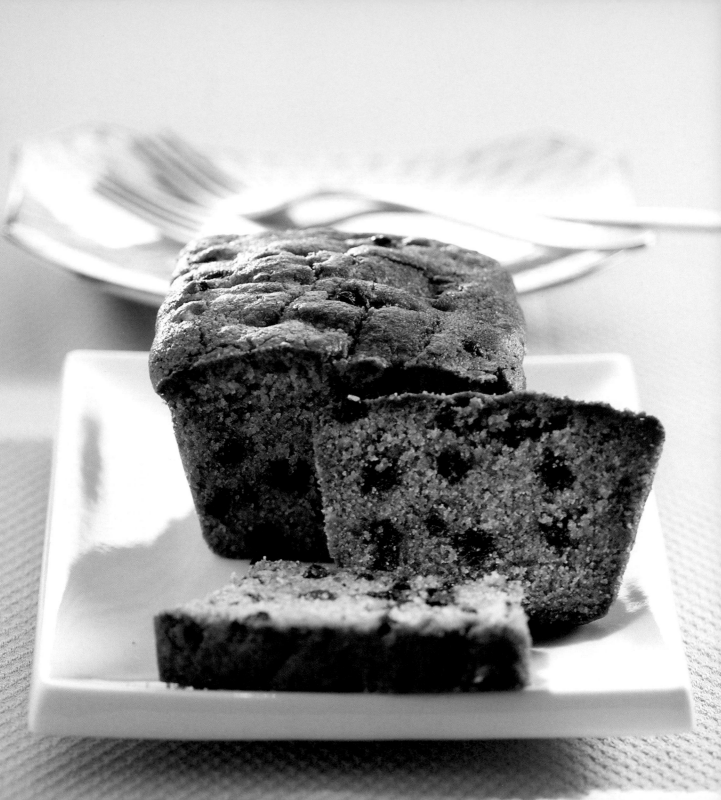

Wheat bran
and blueberry pound cake

Preparation time: 1 h 15   1 loaf
Difficulty: average

200 g (3/4 cup) sugar

175 ml (3/4 cup) vegetable oil

2 eggs

100 g (2/3 cup) flour

100 g (1 1/4 cups) wheat bran

150 g (1 cup) blueberries

Preheat the oven to 190°C (375°F).

Whisk together the sugar and oil in a bowl.

Whisk in eggs, one at a time.

Fold in the flour and wheat bran, and mix well.

Add the blueberries and mix carefully.

Transfer to a buttered and floured 23 x 13 cm (9 x 5 in) breadpan.

Bake in the oven for 35 to 40 minutes. Let cool in the pan 10 minutes before unmoulding.

 Philippe Castel, elected health-conscious chef by his peers in 2004

Translation: Gordon Cruise McBride

Maple
and orange-flavoured cranberry jelly

Preparation time: 20 minutes   4 servings
Difficulty: easy

Zests can be removed from citrus fruit using a zester or vegetable peeler. It is important to carefully remove the bitter white inner skin from the peel. Don't forget to wash the fruit thoroughly first

300 g (2 cups) cranberries

175 ml (3/4 cup) dark amber maple syrup

Zest of 1 orange

2 oranges, sectioned

Bring the cranberries and maple syrup to a boil.

Add the orange zest and reduce heat, simmering uncovered for 10 minutes.

Add the oranges and cook for five minutes over low heat.

 Éric Harvey, Chef-Instructor at the École hôtelière de la Capitale in Quebec

breakfasts and brunches

wheat bran pound cake

cranberry jelly

Muesli

Preparation time: 45 minutes
Difficulty: easy

Approximately 30 servings

This muesli will keep for one month at room temperature, and is a tasty and healthy alternative to junk food!

630 g (7 cups) whole grain oats

240 g (2 cups) sunflower seeds

125 ml (1/2 cup) olive oil

150 g (3/4 cup) buckwheat honey

60 g (1/2 cup) sesame seeds

240 g (2 cups) sliced almonds

1 tbsp (per portion) freshly ground flaxseed

50 g (1/4 cup) dried cranberries per serving

Milk to taste

Preheat the oven to 190°C (375°F).

Mix the oats, sunflower seeds, olive oil, and honey together in a large dripping pan. Sprinkle the sesame seeds on top.

Cook in the oven uncovered, stirring every 5 minutes if using a convection oven, or every 20 minutes in an ordinary oven.

When the cereal grains begin to brown evenly, add the almonds and continue cooking until the cereal grains are golden brown.

Remove from the oven and let cool completely before transferring to airtight glass or metal containers.

Serve in individual bowls, adding the flaxseed, cranberries, and milk to taste.

 Richard Béliveau

muesli energy boost crêpes

breakfasts and brunches

Energy
boost crêpes

Preparation time: 45 minutes
Difficulty: average

Approximately 8 crêpes

200 g (1 cup) crushed multigrain cereal (8 grains if possible)

100 g (1/2 cup) little millet

40 g (1/3 cup) flaxseed

100 g (2/3 cup) buckwheat flour

1/2 tsp baking powder

4 tbsp baking soda

1 pinch of salt

1 egg

125 ml (1/2 cup) milk

1 tsp vanilla

250 ml (1 cup) water

Grind the first three ingredients using a coffee grinder, and, with a spoon, mix together with all dry ingredients.

In a separate bowl, beat the egg together with the liquid ingredients using a fork.

Combine the two mixtures and mix well. Let sit 5 to 10 minutes while the batter thickens.

Grease a skillet and ladle in the desired quantity of batter. Cook over medium heat.

Cover the skillet to ensure that the inside of the crêpe cooks properly.

When the crêpe is cooked on one side, flip it using a spatula, and carefully monitor the heat. Calculate approximately 7 to 10 minutes total cooking time.

Cook the other crêpes in the same manner.

Serve these delicious energy boost crêpes with cottage cheese and small chunks of fresh or frozen fruit.

 Jean Vachon, Chef-Instructor at the École hôtelière de la Capitale in Quebec

Sweet chestnut,
cashew, and red wine loaf

Preparation time: 2 hours   1 loaf
Difficulty: average

The hazelnut or cobnut bush grows in abundance in the Italian regions of Sicily and Piedmont. Its nuts are known as "filberts" in some countries.

2 tbsp butter

1 onion, chopped

1 celery stalk, finely chopped

4 garlic cloves, crushed

350 g (2 1/3 cups) fresh or canned chestnuts, coarsely chopped

360 g (3 cups) ground cashews

100 g (3/4 cup) ground filberts

100 g (2/3 cup) sharp cheddar, grated

150 ml (2/3 cup) dry red wine

3 tbsp fresh parsley, chopped

1 tbsp cognac

1/2 tsp paprika

1 pinch of ground thyme

2 eggs

Salt and freshly ground pepper

GARNISH

Sprigs of fresh parsley

Tomato slices

Lemon slices

Butter a 23 x 13 cm (9 x 5 in) loaf pan.

Melt the butter in a skillet and cook the onions and celery for 7 minutes over medium-high heat.

Add the garlic and cook for another 2 to 3 minutes.

Preheat the oven to 180°C (350°F).

Remove the skillet from the heat and add all other ingredients, seasoning generously with salt and pepper.

Mix in a food processor until smooth, then transfer the mixture to the greased loaf pan.

Cover with aluminium foil and bake in the oven for 1 hour.

Remove the foil and bake for another 15 minutes.

Verify doneness; the middle of the loaf must be firm to the touch.

Remove the loaf from the oven and let stand for 4 to 5 minutes before unsticking the sides with a kitchen knife.

Turn out onto a hot plate.

Before serving, decorate with parsley sprigs, tomato, and lemon slices.

 Jean Vachon, Chef-Instructor at the École hôtelière de la Capitale in Quebec

breakfasts and brunches

sweet chestnut, cashew, and red wine loaf

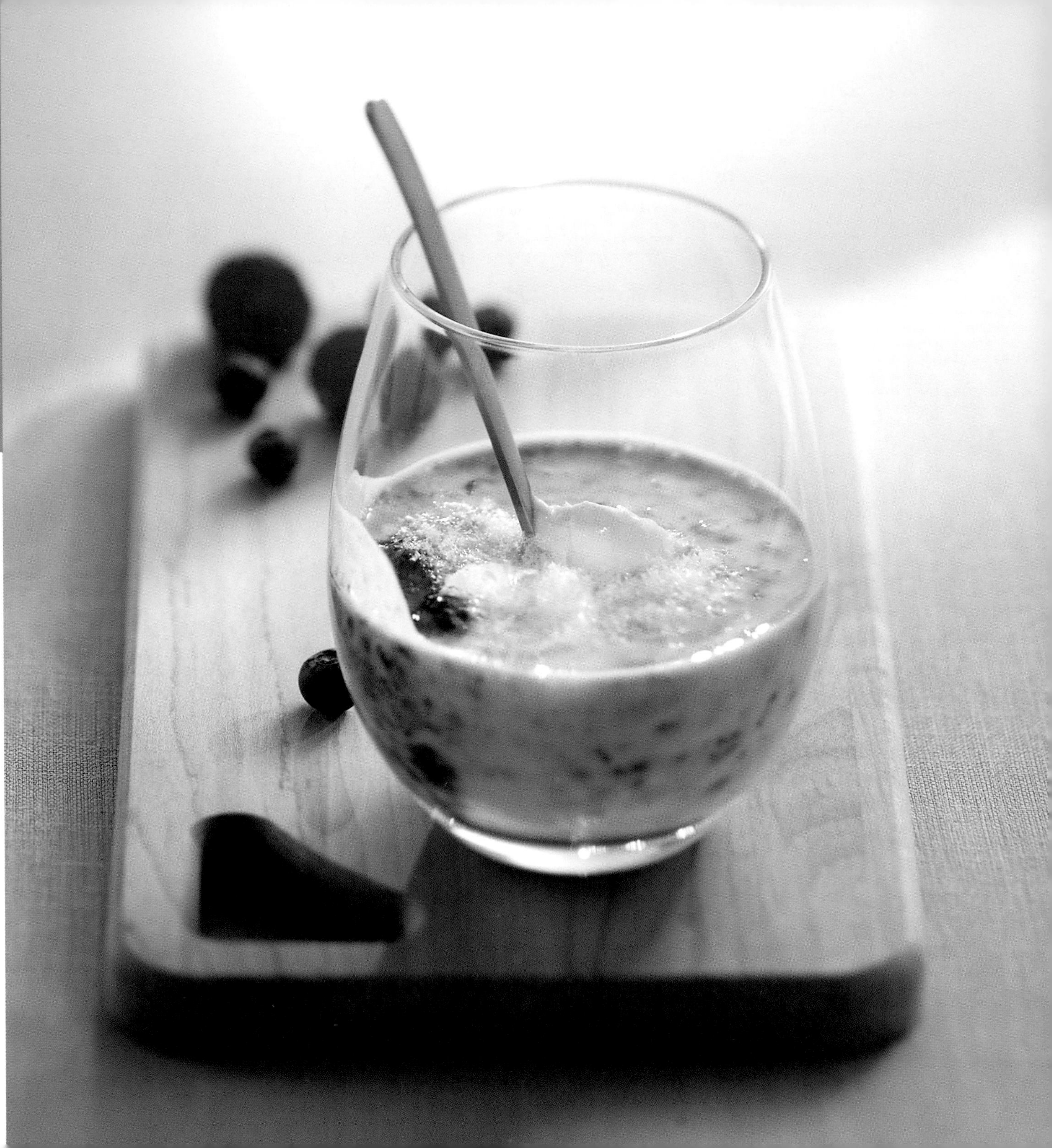

Fieldberry
smoothie

Preparation time: 5 minutes
Difficulty: easy

Approximately
1.5 litres

This refreshing smoothie is inspired by lhassi, a delicious drink that is highly popular in India. The traditional recipe highlights plain yogurt and mango, but this interesting variation includes yogurt and fieldberries. Use frozen berries when not in season, reducing the quantity of crushed ice.

1 kg (4 cups) plain yogurt

60 g (1/4 cup) sugar

175 ml (3/4 cup) water

250 ml (1 cup) purée of fieldberries, fresh or frozen

250 g (1 cup) crushed ice

Blend all ingredients together using a food processor or mixer until smooth. Serve chilled.

 Jean Vachon, Chef-Instructor at the École hôtelière de la Capitale in Quebec

Tasty
energy bars

Preparation time: 15 minutes
Difficulty: average

12 bars

250 g (2 3/4 cups) rolled oats

120 g (1 cup) sesame seeds

35 g (1/3 cup) poppy seeds

40 g (1/3 cup) flaxseed

70 g (1/3 cup) dried raisins

100 g (3/4 cup) pecans (pecan nuts)

1/4 tsp fresh ginger, chopped

1/4 tsp ground cinnamon

350 g (1 3/4 cups) honey

In a large bowl, mix together all ingredients except the honey.

Heat the honey in a small saucepan until a sugar thermometer reaches 117°C (243°F).

Pour the hot honey over the dry ingredients and mix well.

Transfer to a greased rectangular mould.

Let cool in the refrigerator before cutting into 12 equal bars.

 Éric Harvey, Chef-Instructor at the École hôtelière de la Capitale in Quebec

snacks

fieldberry smoothie

tasty energy bars

Minty
grapefruit surprise

Preparation time: 15 minutes
Difficulty: easy

4 servings

2 large grapefruits

1 bunch fresh mint

4 tbsp cane sugar

4 orange slices

Using a sharp knife, peel the grapefruit over a large bowl (to retain all the juice), taking care to remove the skin and the white rind from the fruit.

Cut the grapefruit into wedges and add them to the bowl with the juice.

Coarsely chop the fresh mint and add to the grapefruit. Cover and let steep for 1 hour in the refrigerator.

Wet the edges of 4 dessert cups or glasses with a bit of the grapefruit juice and rim with the cane sugar.

Serve the grapefruit wedges in frosted glasses and garnish each cup with an orange slice. Serve well chilled.

 Philippe Castel, elected health-conscious chef by his peers in 2004

Oat and ginger
shortbread cookies

Preparation time: 1 h 15
Difficulty: average

24 cookies

70 g (3/4 cup) rolled oats

240 g (1 cup) butter

240 g (1 cup) brown sugar

1 tsp ground ginger

225 g (1 3/4 cups) all-purpose unbleached flour

30 to 60 g (1/2 to 1 cup) crystallized ginger, finely chopped

Preheat the oven to 180°C (350°F).

Chop the rolled oats in a food processor and set aside.

Mix the butter and brown sugar together until creamy.

Add the ground ginger, rolled oats, flour, and crystallized ginger.

Pack the mixture into a large rectangular 30 x 25 cm (12 x 10 in) cake pan with your hands.

Using a knife, make incisions in the form of squares, diamonds, triangles, or rectangles on the surface of the mixture.

Bake in the oven for 30 to 35 minutes, until the top is golden.

Cut the bars along the incision marks while still hot, set aside and let cool completely before serving.

 Susan Sylvester, Chef-Instructor at the École hôtelière de la Capitale in Quebec

grapefruit surprise

shortbread cookies

snacks

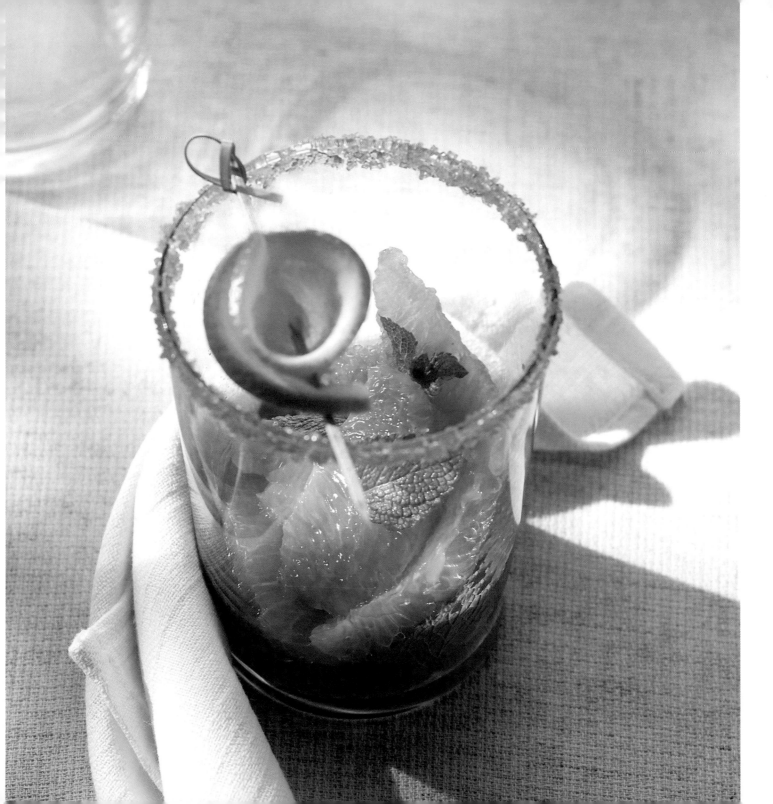

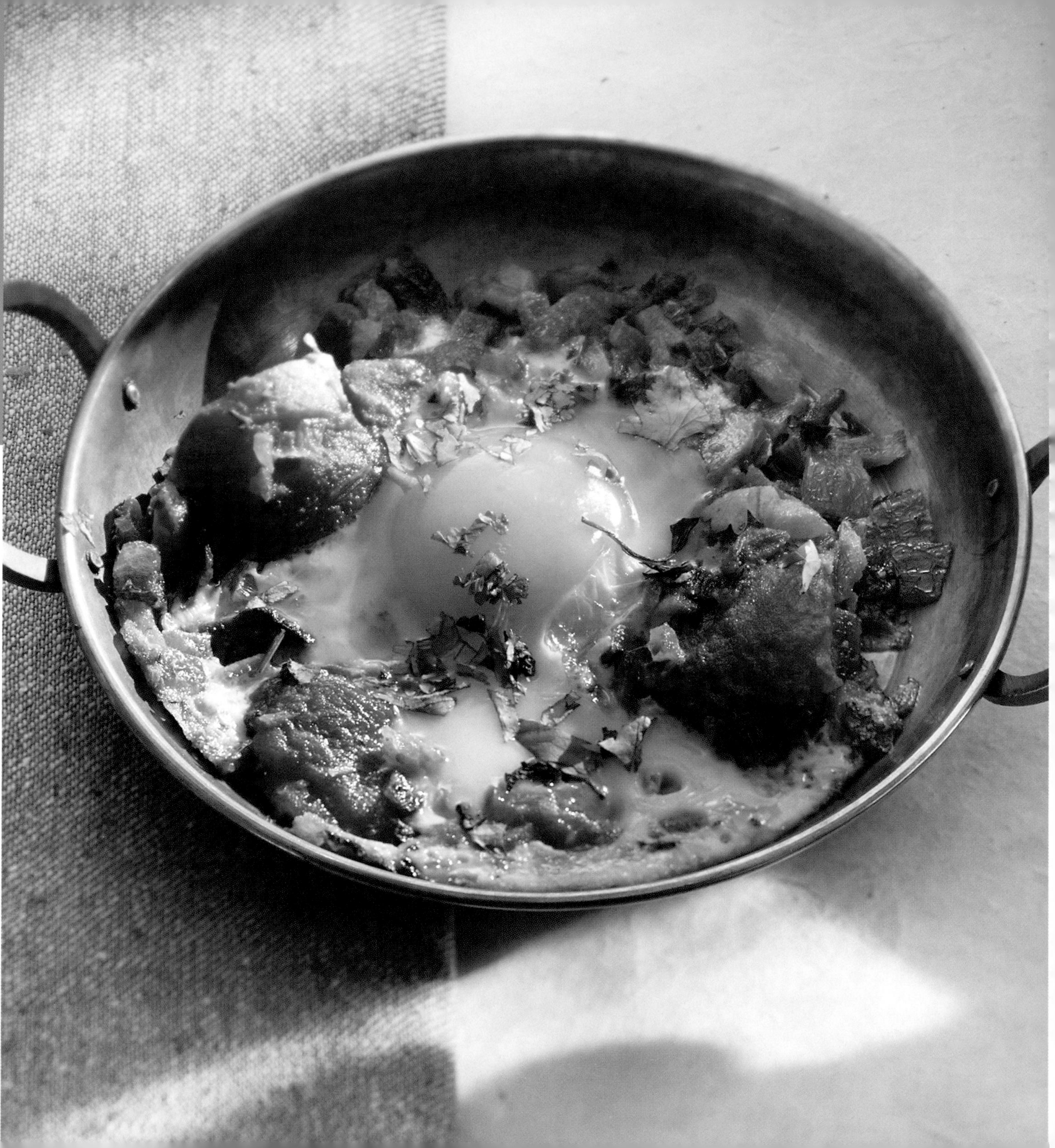

Indian-style
cumin and turmeric eggs

Preparation time: 30 minutes   2 to 4 servings
Difficulty: easy

Here's an original way to reintroduce eggs, so essential to our health, into our diet. This recipe provides a magnificent contrast of colours and flavours.

1 dash of olive oil

1 large onion, chopped

2 or 3 garlic cloves, minced

1 tsp ground turmeric

2 tsp ground cumin

340 g (2 1/4 cups) stewed canned tomatoes

Salt and freshly ground pepper

4 eggs

7 g (1/4 cup) fresh coriander, chopped

Heat the olive oil in a large skillet, and sweat the onions and garlic until they are translucent.

Add the turmeric and cumin, and stir for 1 to 2 minutes.

Add the tomatoes, and season to taste. Simmer for approximately 20 minutes, until the mixture thickens.

Make four "nests" in the mixture, and crack one egg into each nest, taking care not to break the yolk.

Continue cooking until the egg whites are cooked.

Garnish with the fresh coriander and serve immediately.

 Richard Béliveau

Blueberry
and ginger milk

Preparation time: 20 minutes   4 servings
Difficulty: easy

Silken tofu has the consistency of a flan. It is often used to make mayonnaises and low-fat creams. It is found in supermarkets and natural food stores, and in Asian grocery shops.

800 ml (3 1/3 cups) milk or natural soy milk

110 g (3/4 cup) silken tofu

300 g (2 cups) blueberries, fresh or frozen

1 tbsp fresh ginger, grated

60 ml (1/4 cup) maple syrup

1 pear, cut into large pieces (optional)

2 tbsp wheat germ (optional)

Blend the milk, tofu, blueberries, ginger, and maple syrup in a mixer until smooth, gradually increasing the speed of the mixer.

Pour into glasses that have been rimmed with lemon juice and cane sugar.

Optional: Spear the pear slices with 4 wooden fondue sticks, and coat the slices evenly with the wheat germ, covering all sides. Serve each glass with a pear "brochette."

 Steve McCandless, Chef-co-owner of the Bistro Le Clocher Penché in Quebec

snacks

cumin and turmeric eggs
blueberry and ginger milk

Nectar velouté
with fieldberries

Preparation time: 10 minutes **6 servings**
Difficulty: easy

This refreshing and nourishing drink provides you with all the anti-cancer properties of small fruits.

100 g (2/3 cup) strawberries

100 g (2/3 cup) raspberries

75 g (1/2 cup) cranberries

75 g (1/2 cup) blueberries

1 banana

70 g (1/3 cup) honey

300 g (1 1/4 cups) plain yogurt

GARNISH

6 ground cherries

6 fresh mint leaves

Mix all ingredients together using a food processor or mixer.

Pour into wine glasses and garnish each serving with a ground cherry and a mint leaf.

 Jean-Pierre Cloutier, Chef-proprietor of the Café-restaurant du Musée in Quebec

Vegetarian
tofu and lentil pâté

Preparation time: 1 h 30 **4 servings**
Difficulty: average

This pâté is excellent served with a tomato sauce. Accompany it with a spinach, lettuce, or endive salad.

110 g (1/2 cup) canned lentils, rinsed and drained

260 g (1 1/2 cups) firm tofu, grated

20 g (1/4 cup) wheat bran

10 g (1/3 cup) fresh parsley, chopped

40 g (1/4 cup) onions, finely chopped

50 g (1/2 cup) mushrooms, finely chopped

2 tbsp Dijon mustard

3 eggs

60 ml (1/4 cup) soy sauce

2 garlic cloves, minced

1/4 tsp black pepper

1 tsp ground turmeric

Preheat the oven to 200°C (400°F). Grease a bread pan with the olive oil.

Purée the lentils using an electric mixer or food processor.

In a large bowl, combine the lentils together with all the other ingredients.

Firmly press the mixture into the greased pan.

Bake in the oven for approximately 1 hour. Remove and let sit for 10 minutes before unmoulding.

 Marlène Gagnon, Chef-Instructor at the École hôtelière de la Capitale in Quebec

nectar velouté
with fieldberries

vegetarian
tofu pâté

snacks

Almond pâté

Preparation time: 45 minutes
Difficulty: average

6 to 8 servings

This pâté is delicious spread on small buns, biscuits, and rice cakes. It also makes an excellent accompaniment to sandwiches, with a few crispy lettuce leaves.

120 g (1 cup) almonds

60 g (1 cup) whole-wheat bread crumbs

75 g (1/2 cup) silken tofu

120 g (1 cup) red pepper, cubed

1 celery stalk, chopped

1 garlic clove (or to taste)

3 tbsp yeast

2 tbsp soy sauce

1/2 tsp dried sage

1/2 tsp dried thyme

1 tbsp fresh chives, chopped

GARNISH

Red pepper slivers

Celery sticks

Sprigs of fresh parsley

Finely grind the almonds with a mixer and blend well with the breadcrumbs.

Using a mixer, beat together the tofu, peppers, celery, and garlic.

Combine the almond mixture with the tofu in a large bowl. Add the yeast, soy sauce, and the fines herbes, and mix well.

Lightly grease a 23 x 12 cm (9 x 5 in) pan.

Line the insides of the pan with the pepper slices, celery sticks, and the parsley sprigs.

Transfer the almond mixture to the pan, pressing down well on the sides. Cover and let chill in the refrigerator for 1 hour before serving.

 Jean Vachon, Chef-Instructor at the École hôtelière de la Capitale in Quebec

snacks

almond pâté

Aromatic
Indian tea

Preparation time: 20 minutes
Difficulty: easy

2 litres

In India, this tea is called chai, and is part of a daily ritual for most inhabitants. To open the cardamon seeds, simply crush them with the flat side of a large knife.

1.5 litres (6 cups) water

8 slices fresh ginger

12 whole cloves

1 star anise (star aniseed)

1/4 tsp fennel seed

7 cardamom seeds, opened

1/2 cinnamon stick

3 bags green tea

500 ml (2 cups) milk

4 tbsp honey

Bring the water to a boil.

Reduce the heat and add the ginger and spices. Let simmer for 5 to 10 minutes.

Add the tea bags and steep for 5 minutes.

Add the milk and honey. Strain the tea and serve hot or cold.

 Jean Vachon, Chef-Instructor at the École hôtelière de la Capitale in Quebec

Portobello
and mozzarella sandwiches

Preparation time: 40 minutes
Difficulty: average

4 servings

If you can't find Portobello mushrooms in your area, you can make this recipe with other large-capped mushroom varieties.

4 portobello mushrooms

60 ml (1/4 cup) olive oil

Sea salt and freshly ground pepper

8 slices of sourdough bread

40 g (1/3 cup) mozzarella

150 g (1/2 cup) pesto, basil, or watercress

Alfalfa sprouts (optional)

Preheat the oven to 200°C (400°F). Remove the stems from the mushrooms, and sprinkle the mushroom caps with the olive oil. Season with salt and pepper to taste.

Arrange the mushroom caps on a baking sheet, top down, and grill (broil) for 12 to 15 minutes on high heat.

Toast the bread slices.

Cut the mushrooms into 1 cm (1/2 in) thick slices.

Cut the mozzarella into slices the same thickness as the mushrooms.

Combine the cheese and mushroom slices in alternate layers on the baking sheet, and bake in the oven for 5 to 6 minutes, until the cheese is runny.

Remove and serve on the 4 toasts, garnishing with the pesto/herb mixture, and cover with the other toast slices.

Garnish with alfalfa sprouts (optional).

 Steve McCandless, Chef-co-owner of the Bistro Le Clocher Penché in Quebec

aromatic
Indian tea

portobello
sandwiches

snacks

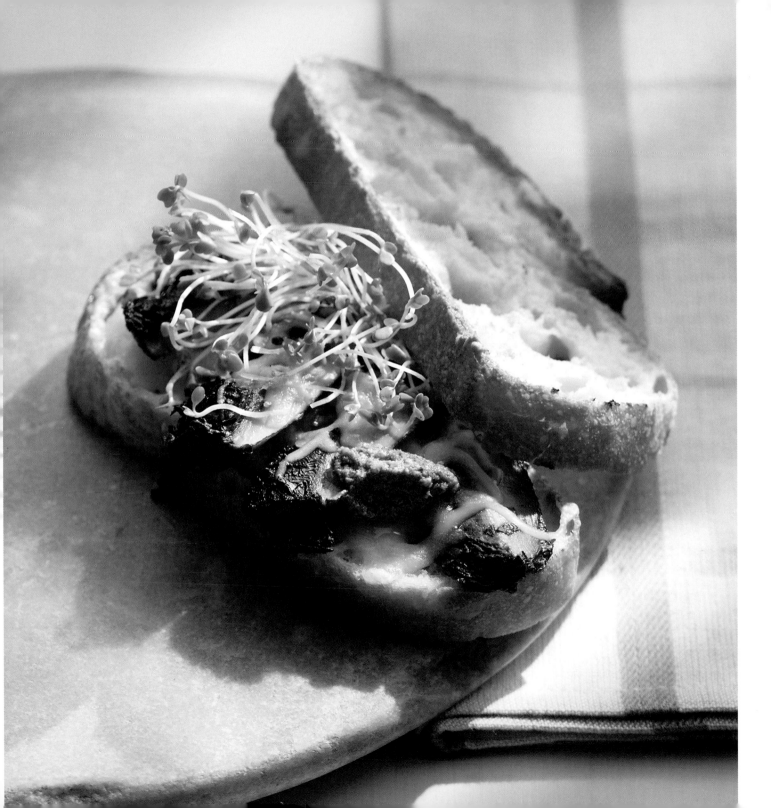

Garden
terrine

Preparation time: 2 hours   **8 to 12 servings**
Difficulty: average

200 g (1 cup) dried green lentils, washed and drained

500 ml (2 cups) cold water

1 leek

100 g (1/2 cup) carrots, sliced

1 onion, cut in large cubes

3 tbsp olive oil

75 g (1/3 cup) unsalted soybean, chopped

1 tbsp dried basil

2 tbsp brown sugar

Salt and freshly ground pepper

2 eggs

75 g (3/4 cup) wheat germ

75 g (1/2 cup) wheat flour

3 tbsp fresh parsley, chopped

1 tbsp garlic, chopped

Place the lentils in a pot with lightly salted water. Cover, bring to a boil, and cook over low heat for 30 minutes.

Slice the leek in two lengthwise and carefully wash it under cold running water, ensuring no sand remains in between the leaves. Chop coarsely.

Finely chop the carrots, onion, and leek in a food processor.

In a large bowl, blend together the lentils, olive oil, vegetables, soybeans, basil, and the brown sugar. Season with salt and pepper, mixing well.

In another bowl, blend together the eggs, wheat germ, flour, parsley, and garlic. Add this mixture to the first bowl and mix together well.

Transfer to a 23 x 13 cm (9 x 5 in) pan and cook in the oven at 180°C (350°F) for 40 minutes. Let stand to cool before serving.

 Christophe Alary, Chef-Instructor at the École hôtelière de la Capitale in Quebec, elected Chef of the Year 2004 by his peers

Edamame
with Guérande salt

Preparation time: 10 minutes   **Approximately 500 g**
Difficulty: easy

This is the easiest way to eat soybean. Edamame is a variety of soy that originates from East Asia. The term edamame means "bean on a branch." These green beans are eaten before they mature by pressing the inedible seedpod between the teeth. Edamame is one of the best available sources of isoflavones. You can also do as the Japanese do and eat them as snacks!

1 pack 500 g (1 lb) frozen edamames

Guérande salt or coarse sea salt

Bring a large pot of salted water to a boil and add the edamames. Calculate 5 minutes cooking time once the water returns to a boil.

Drain the beans, arrange on a serving dish, and season with salt to taste.

 Richard Béliveau

garden terrine

edamame with Guérande salt

snacks

Tofu
and flaxseed tartinade

Preparation time: 10 minutes   **4 servings**
Difficulty: easy

This spread is best served with crackers or raw vegetables, or in a sandwich with lettuce leaves.

150 g (1 cup) firm tofu

1 green onion, chopped

20 g (1/4 cup) celery leaves, chopped

80 g (1/3 cup) mayonnaise

4 tbsp flaxseed, ground

50 g (1/4 cup) carrots, grated

60 ml (1/4 cup) lime juice, freshly squeezed

1 tsp ground turmeric

1 tbsp hot mustard

1 tbsp soy sauce

Salt and freshly ground pepper

Chop the tofu in a food processor or with a grater.

Add the remaining ingredients and mix well.

.

 Marlène Gagnon, Chef-Instructor at the École hôtelière de la Capitale in Quebec

Marinated
cherry tomatoes

Preparation time: 1 h 10   **4 servings**
Difficulty: easy

Serve these tomatoes accompanied by mixed greens, spinach, endives, watercress, or alfalfa sprouts. You may substitute the cherry tomatoes with regular tomatoes, quartered.

20 cherry tomatoes, halved

VINAIGRETTE

2 garlic cloves, finely chopped

1 tsp maple syrup

7 g (1/4 cup) fresh parsley, finely chopped

2 tbsp red wine vinegar or your favourite vinegar

60 ml (1/4 cup) walnut oil

2 tbsp fresh lemon juice

2 tbsp fresh chives

Salt and freshly ground pepper

Whisk all the vinaigrette ingredients together.

Marinate the tomatoes in the vinaigrette at least 1 hour before serving.

 Marlène Gagnon, Chef-Instructor at the École hôtelière de la Capitale in Quebec

appetizers

tofu
tartinade

marinated
cherry
tomatoes

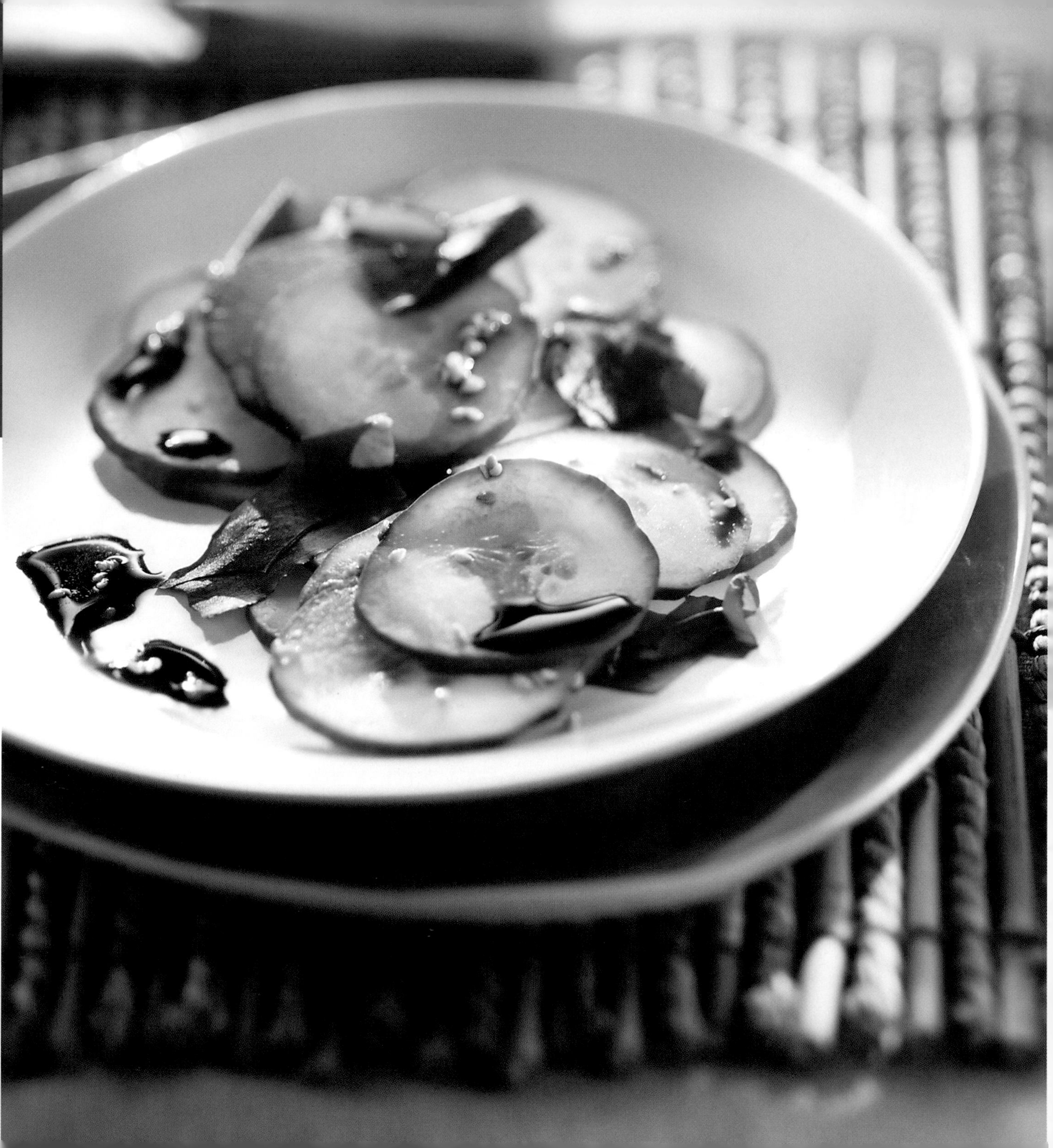

Cucumber
and wakame seaweed with sesame perfume

Preparation time: 45 minutes
Difficulty: easy

4 servings

The easiest way to toast sesame seeds is to spread them on a non-stick pastry sheet and toast them in the oven for 10 minutes at 180°C (350°F). Make sure they don't overcook, stirring after 5 minutes to ensure they don't burn. Store them in an airtight metal container.

1 English cucumber, washed and sliced fine lengthwise

Fine sea salt

100 g (3 1/2 oz) wakame seaweed, rehydrated in cold water for 5 minutes

Sesame seeds, grilled

VINAIGRETTE

60 ml (1/4 cup) soy sauce

60 ml (1/4 cup) rice wine vinegar

2 tsp sugar

2 tbsp dashi (see page 147)

Prepare the vinaigrette, mixing all the ingredients in a bowl. Arrange the cucumber slices in a sieve and sprinkle with salt. Let sweat for approximately 30 minutes to release the excess water.

Cut the seaweed into 2 cm (3/4 in) lengths.

Rinse and drain the cucumber slices and arrange on a serving plate.

Add the seaweed and sprinkle with the vinaigrette.

Sprinkle with the sesame seeds and serve.

 Jean Vachon, Chef-Instructor at the École hôtelière de la Capitale in Quebec

Thai
dumplings

Preparation time: 1 hour
Difficulty: average

20 dumplings

If you don't like cooking with oil, you can steam these dumplings. Serve with a Thai roll sauce, found on page 212.

200 g (7 oz) pork, chopped

2 tbsp green onions, finely chopped

2 garlic cloves, finely chopped

Freshly ground pepper

1 1/2 tsp fresh ginger, chopped or finely grated

4 tsp soy sauce

20 Chinese wonton pastry sheets

Cornstarch

Olive oil

60 ml (1/4 cup) water

In a large bowl, mix together the meat, green onions, garlic, pepper, ginger, and soy sauce.

Cut out 20 circles from the pastry.

In a small bowl, whisk the cornstarch in a bit of cold water.

Place a small quantity of the meat in the middle of a pastry round. Moisten the outer edges of the pastry with a bit of the cornstarch mixture. Fold over each dumpling, forming a half-moon shape, pressing edges firmly. Coat each dumpling with oil, using your fingers. Repeat this procedure to make 20 dumplings.

Place a bit of olive oil in a skillet, and fry the dumplings on high heat until they are cooked on both sides. Pour in the water and cover. Cook for 1 to 2 minutes and serve immediately.

 Jean Vachon, Chef-Instructor at the École hôtelière de la Capitale in Quebec

appetizers

cucumber and wakame seaweed

Thai dumplings

Multigrain
guacamole tasty-teasers

Preparation time: 15 minutes
Difficulty: easy

4 servings

To peel the tomatoes, remove the stem and make a small cross-shaped incision on the bottom of the tomato. Blanch them in boiling water for 10 seconds, remove and rinse under cold water to stop cooking. Peel the tomato skins using a small sharp knife. This tasty guacamole can be served with healthy crackers, or as a dip for fresh vegetables.

1 very ripe avocado, peeled and pitted

Juice of one lime

1 tbsp olive oil

3 tbsp ripe tomatoes, peeled, seeded, and cubed

2 tsp onions, finely chopped

Salt

2 dashes of Tabasco

12 multigrain oven-baked crackers

Purée the avocado, lime juice, and olive oil in a food processor.

Transfer to a bowl and add all other ingredients, except the crackers. Mix well and spread the mixture on the crackers.

 François Rousseau, Chef-Instructor at the École hôtelière de la Capitale in Quebec

Oriental
guacamole

Preparation time: 20 minutes
Difficulty: easy

4 servings

This guacamole is especially tasty served with raw vegetable crudités or on toasted pita bread. Sambal oelek is an Indonesian condiment made from hot peppers, salt, and vinegar. It is found in Asian groceries and gourmet supermarkets and boutiques.

2 avocados

80 g (1/2 cup) red onions, chopped

75 g (1/2 cup) ripe tomatoes, diced

3 tbsp sake (optional)

1/2 tsp garlic, chopped

2 tbsp fresh ginger, chopped

1/2 fresh lime juice

Zest of half a lime

1 tbsp fresh coriander, chopped

80 g (1/2 cup) green onions, finely sliced

2 tbsp olive oil

1/2 tsp sambal oelek or pepper paste

Cut the avocados in half, remove the pit, and separate the flesh using a spoon.

In a bowl, crush the flesh using a fork and add all other ingredients. Mix well together, and serve on your favourite crackers or tortilla chips.

 Florence Albernhe, Chef-proprietor of Le Grain de riz in Quebec

multigrain
tasty-teasers

oriental
guacamole

appetizers

Mexican
stuffed tomatoes

Preparation time: 1 hour　　　　　　　**8 servings**
Difficulty: average

Jalapeno pepper is grown mainly in Mexico. Its name is derived from the city of Jalapa, located in the State of Veracruz, Mexico. It is a rather girthy, green pepper, measuring approximately 5 cm. Its reputation in the kitchen has spread throughout the world, and it is now sold in most supermarkets.

1 avocado

Juice of 2 limes, freshly squeezed

60 g (1/2 cup) quinoa (Peruvian rice)

8 large, fresh, ripe tomatoes

100 g (1/2 cup) cucumber, seeded and chopped

60 g (1/2 cup) red peppers, seeded and chopped

8 small green onions, finely chopped

95 g (1/2 cup) cooked corn

110 g (1/2 cup) canned black beans, rinsed and drained

60 ml (1/4 cup) extra virgin olive oil

15 g (1/2 cup) fresh coriander, chopped

2 tbsp fresh jalapeno peppers, finely chopped

2 tbsp ground cumin

Salt and freshly ground pepper

Chop the avocado and sprinkle with 2 tbsp of the lime juice. Set aside the remaining juice.

Cook the quinoa as per package directions. Drain, let cool, and transfer to a large glass bowl.

Cut a slice off the top of each tomato to form a cap.

Press each tomato over the sink to remove the surplus water and some of the seeds.

Using a grapefruit spoon or a small knife, empty each tomato over a bowl, leaving a bit of the flesh on the sides without piercing the skin. Finely chop the flesh and add to the quinoa.

Add the avocado and its juices, the cucumbers, peppers, green onions, corn, and black beans. Sprinkle with the remaining lime juice and olive oil.

Add the coriander, peppers, and cumin. Season with salt and pepper, stirring carefully.

Let sit at room temperature for approximately 30 minutes, stirring occasionally to properly blend the flavours.

Season the tomatoes before stuffing them with the avocado mixture. Cap each tomato with the tomato slice and serve immediately.

 Anne L. Desjardins, food reporter and author

appetizers　　Mexican stuffed tomatoes

Kachumber
with lime juice

Preparation time: 10 minutes
Difficulty: easy
4 servings

Kachumber is the most popular salad in India. This appetizer is especially delicious served with Indian cucumber raita (see page 145).

2 red tomatoes

1 cucumber

1/2 Spanish onion

Juice of one lime, freshly squeezed

Salt and freshly ground pepper

1 tbsp hot red peppers, sliced in rounds (optional)

Fresh coriander or parsley, finely chopped (optional)

Cut the tomatoes into 1 cm (1/2 in) sections, yielding approximately 16 sections per tomato. Remove the seeds.

Cut the cucumber in four lengthwise, remove the seeds and cut again into 2.5 cm (1 in) sections.

Cut the onion into 1 cm (1/2 in) quarters.

Mix the tomatoes, cucumber, and onion together in a bowl. Add the lime juice, season with salt and pepper to taste.

Add the peppers and coriander just before serving, mixing delicately.

 Jean Vachon, Chef-Instructor at the École hôtelière de la Capitale in Quebec

kachumber
with lime juice
avocado
dip

appetizers

Avocado
and citrus dip

Preparation time: 30 minutes
Difficulty: easy
4 servings

4 tbsp sunflower seeds

2 avocados

4 tbsp flaxseed, ground

3 tbsp orange juice, freshly squeezed

3 tbsp grapefruit juice, freshly squeezed

3 tbsp lemon juice, freshly squeezed

2 tbsp olive oil

1 tsp salt

1 tsp ground cumin

1 tsp ground coriander

Grind the sunflower seeds in a food processor.

Cut the avocados in half, remove the stone, and separate the flesh with a spoon, setting aside.

Mix all ingredients together in a large bowl to obtain a smooth spread. Cover and refrigerate until ready to serve.

VARIATION: DIP AND PITA BREAD

60 ml (1/4 cup) olive oil

1 tbsp Cajun spices

4 pita breads

Mix the olive oil and spices together and brush the pita breads with the mixture. Cut into triangles and spread on a cookie sheet.

Cook in the oven at 180°C (350°F) for approximately 10 minutes, until the pita bread is golden and crispy. Serve the dip in a bowl, arranging the pita triangles in a decorative pattern.

 Marlène Gagnon, Chef-Instructor at the École hôtelière de la Capitale in Quebec

Indian
cucumber raita

Preparation time: 10 minutes
Difficulty: easy

4 servings

This sauce was created to quickly cool the taste-buds while eating very spicy dishes. Serve it as an appetizer, accompanied with nan or pita bread, or with spicy Indian dishes. To blanch the spinach, drop them into boiling water for 1 to 2 minutes, remove and squeeze out any extra liquid, then chop fine before mixing with the yogurt mixture.

250 g (1 cup) plain yogurt

1 tsp fresh mint, finely chopped

1/2 cucumber, peeled, seeded, and cut into julienne strips

Salt and ground white pepper

Ground cumin (to taste)

Dried fruit (to taste)

Spinach (to taste)

Ground nutmeg

Mix the yogurt, mint, and cucumber together in a bowl. Season to taste.

Add the other ingredients to taste.

Transfer to a serving dish and sprinkle with the nutmeg.

 Jean Vachon, Chef-Instructor at the École hôtelière de la Capitale in Quebec

Tofu
in soy sauce

Preparation time: 15 minutes
Difficulty: easy

4 servings

Bonito is a fatty fish related to the tuna. Bonito flakes can be found in Asian groceries, natural food stores, and many supermarkets. You can replace it with a small can of red sockeye salmon, drained and finely shredded. Spear the tofu cubes with toothpicks and serve them on a platter as an appetizer.

340 g (12 oz) firm silken tofu

Bonito flakes

Fresh chives, finely chopped, or dried chives

Japanese soy sauce (shoyu or soy sauce)

Remove the tofu from its package carefully so as not to break it.

Cut the block of tofu in half crosswise, taking care not to lose its shape. Then cut lengthwise, and again crosswise, to obtain small 1.5 cm (2/3 in) cubes.

Cover with the bonito flakes and sprinkle with the chives. Dribble the soy sauce on top and serve.

 Richard Béliveau

appetizers

cucumber raita

tofu in soy sauce

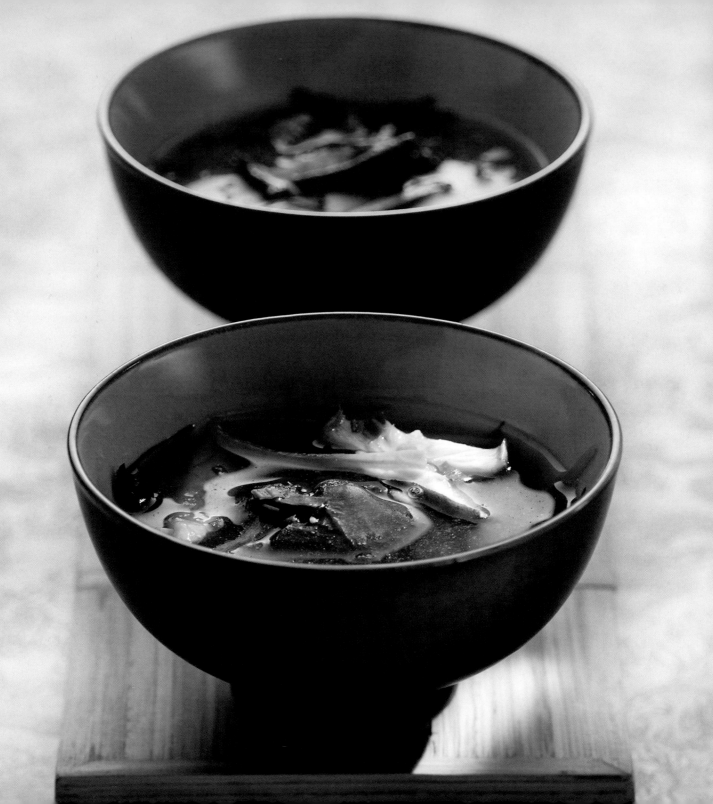

Miso
soup

Preparation time: 30 minutes
Difficulty: average

6 servings

Miso is a fermented soy paste rich in isoflavones. It comes in several grades, with colour ranging from white to red. In Japan this low calorie soup is eaten daily at breakfast, lunch, or evening meals. Miso can be kept for at least one year in a cool, dry place. Gai lon is also called Chinese broccoli, although it is not a true member of the broccoli family. Its long leaves are a dark green and its stems are very thin.

25 g (1 oz) wakame or arame seaweed

Stream of olive oil

120 g (3/4 cup) gai lon (Chinese broccoli) or curly kale, julienned

12 fresh shiitake mushrooms, finely sliced

2 litres (8 cups) chicken stock

3 tbsp red miso

3 green onions, finely sliced

Soak the seaweed for 5 to 10 minutes in a bowl of cold water.

Heat the olive oil in a large pot. Sauté the gai lon and mushrooms for 3 to 4 minutes over medium-high heat.

Pour in the stock, add the drained seaweed, and let simmer for 10 minutes without boiling.

Dilute the miso with a bit of the stock and add to the soup. Add the green onions and serve.

 Jean-Pierre Cloutier, Chef-proprietor of Café-restaurant du Musée in Quebec

Dashi

Preparation time: 15 minutes
Difficulty: easy

1 litre

Dashi is a stock originating in Japan, with a seaweed base. It can be used in the preparation of soups, vinaigrettes, sauces, and many other recipes. Kombu seaweed is highly prized by the Japanese, who use it abundantly in stocks and garnishes. It has a blade-like shape, with serrated edges.

1 litre (4 cups) water

2 tsp kombu seaweed

2 tbsp bonito flakes

Heat the seaweed in water slowly in a large saucepan.

Remove the seaweed just before the water boils, and add the bonito flakes.

Turn off the heat and let the flakes sink slowly to the bottom of the saucepan.

Strain the stock and serve.

 Susan Sylvester, Chef-Instructor at the École hôtelière de la Capitale in Quebec

soups and broths · miso soup · dashi

Turmeric-scented cauliflower soup

Preparation time: 1 hour
Difficulty: average

4 servings

1 tbsp vegetable oil

55 g (1/3 cup) onions, chopped

200 g (1 cup) celery, sliced

1 tbsp ground turmeric

2 tbsp flour

750 ml (3 cups) chicken stock, degreased

600 g (4 cups) cauliflower, separated into small florets

Salt and freshly ground pepper

In a saucepan, sweat the onions and celery slowly in the oil. Add the turmeric and cook for 1 minute.

Add the flour and stir well. Slowly pour in the stock, add the cauliflower, and bring to a boil.

Season with salt and pepper to taste. Let simmer 25 minutes.

Purée using a mixer and serve immediately.

 François Rousseau, Chef-Instructor at the École hôtelière de la Capitale in Quebec

Classic Andalusian gazpacho

Preparation time: 30 minutes
Difficulty: average

4 servings

2 slices of bread

4 tomatoes

1 cucumber, peeled

1 green pepper

1 red pepper

1 medium onion

2 garlic cloves

8 fresh basil leaves

80 ml (1/3 cup) olive oil

2 tbsp balsamic vinegar

Salt and freshly ground pepper

1 tsp Espelette pepper (optional)

12 black olives, chopped

GARNISH

Olive oil, balsamic vinegar

Soak the bread in a bit of water for 15 minutes.

Immerse the tomatoes in boiling water for approximately 30 seconds. Remove, peel, and cut in two, pressing the halves to remove the seeds and excess juice.

Chop the tomatoes, cucumber, peppers, and onion into small squares. Set aside approximately 4 tablespoons for the garnish. Using a food processor, purée the mixture, adding the garlic, basil, and drained bread.

Add the olive oil and vinegar, and season to taste. Add the Espelette pepper and mix well together.

Transfer to a large bowl, cover and let chill for 3 hours in the refrigerator.

Serve the gazpacho very chilled, with a stream of olive oil and a bit of balsamic vinegar. Garnish with the vegetable cubes and olives.

 Yves Moscato, Chef-co-owner of the restaurant 48 St-Paul, Cuisine_monde in Quebec

cauliflower soup

Andalusian gazpacho

soups and broths

Watercress
and leek soup

Preparation time: 1 h 15　　　　　　**4 servings**
Difficulty: average

1/2 tsp vegetable oil

1 medium onion, coarsely chopped

2 medium leeks, coarsely chopped

1.25 litres (5 cups) cold chicken stock

1 bunch watercress, coarsely chopped

1 large potato, cubed

Salt and freshly ground pepper

60 ml (1/4 cup) sour cream or plain skimmed yogurt

1 tbsp ground turmeric

Heat the oil in a large saucepan. Sweat the onions and leeks over medium heat, taking care not to brown.

Pour in the stock and bring to a boil. Add the potato cubes and season with salt and pepper to taste.

Cook for approximately 30 minutes over medium heat, add the watercress and continue cooking for another 4 minutes.

Blend the soup in a food processor and return to the saucepan. Bring to a boil, whisking constantly. Verify the seasoning as required.

Serve the soup in heated bowls. Garnish each bowl with 1 tablespoon of the sour cream or yogurt and approximately 1/2 teaspoon of turmeric.

 Philippe Castel, elected health-conscious chef by his peers in 2004

Thai
soup

Preparation time: 20 minutes　　　　　　**4 servings**
Difficulty: easy

Half a package of rice vermicelli 227 g (8 oz)

Olive oil

1 shallot, chopped

1/2 pack of red curry paste

125 ml (1/2 cup) water

280 ml (1 cup + 2 tbsp) chicken stock

1 medium onion, chopped into small cubes

8 tiger shrimp

250 ml (1 cup) coconut milk

125 ml (1/2 cup) milk

Lettuce leaves, julienned

Cook the vermicelli for 4 minutes in boiling water. Rinse and set aside.

Sauté the shallot in the oil for approximately 1 minute over high heat.

Stir the curry paste in a bit of cold water and mix with the shallot. Add the water and stock, and bring to a boil.

Add the onions and shrimp. When the shrimp are cooked, that is, firm and pink, add the coconut milk and the milk.

Place some of the vermicelli and lettuce in each bowl, and add the stock and 2 shrimp. Serve immediately.

 Olivier Neau, Chef-Instructor at the École hôtelière de la Capitale in Quebec

soups and broths

watercress soup

Thai soup

Broccoli
soup

Preparation time: 45 minutes   4 servings
Difficulty: average

Here is an excellent way to combine three of the functional foods that are highly effective against cancer: crucifers, onions, and turmeric. Eat this dish on a regular basis, replacing the broccoli with another crucifer (cabbage, cauliflower, curly kale, etc.). And you can freeze any leftover portions.

Olive oil

1 large onion, chopped

2 garlic cloves, minced

1 tsp ground turmeric

1 broccoli, separated into florets (peel the stems and cut into segments)

1 potato, quartered

1 litre (4 cups) chicken stock

1 tbsp dried parsley

1 tsp dried dill

Salt and freshly ground pepper

Heat the olive oil in a large saucepan. Sauté the onions and garlic over medium-high heat until they are tender.

Add the turmeric and stir for 2 minutes.

Add the potatoes and the stock. Incorporate the parsley and dill. Season with salt and pepper to taste. Let simmer for 30 minutes, then add the broccoli. Cook for another 10 minutes and remove from the heat.

Let cool, and purée until smooth and creamy.

      Richard Béliveau

broccoli
soup

cabbage
soup

soups and
broths

Cabbage soup
with soybeans

Preparation time: 1 h 30   6 to 8 servings
Difficulty: easy

Stream of olive oil

110 g (2/3 cup) onions, finely sliced

2 litres (8 cups) chicken stock

2 tbsp tomato paste

450 g (2 3/4 cups) Scotch kale, shredded

120 g (2/3 cup) soybeans, shelled and chopped

Salt and freshly ground pepper

Heat the onions in the olive oil in a saucepan.

Add the stock, tomato paste, and the kale. Bring to a boil and let simmer for approximately 30 minutes without boiling.

Add the soybeans and let simmer for 40 minutes. Season with salt and pepper to taste before serving.

      Jean-Pierre Cloutier, Chef-proprietor of the Café-restaurant du Musée in Quebec

Hearty
kale soup

Preparation time: 1 hour
Difficulty: average

8 to 12 servings

2 tbsp olive oil

1 large Spanish onion, finely chopped

4 garlic cloves, finely chopped

1 celery stalk, finely chopped

2 shallots, finely chopped

1 carrot, cut in rounds

2 litres (8 cups) degreased chicken or vegetable stock

1 tsp fresh thyme

1 tbsp ground turmeric

2 tbsp paprika

2 sweet potatoes, peeled and cut into small cubes

1.3 kg (8 cups) curly kale (kale) leaves, finely chopped

Salt and freshly ground pepper

Heat the olive oil in a large Dutch oven. Sauté the onions, garlic, celery, shallots, and the carrot over medium heat for 8 to 10 minutes, until the onions are translucent.

Add the stock, thyme, turmeric, and paprika. Bring to a boil.

Add the sweet potatoes and let simmer for 5 to 10 minutes, until they are almost cooked.

Add the curly kale and cook for several minutes until tender.

Pour the boiling soup into each serving bowl and season with salt and pepper to taste.

 Anne L. Desjardins, food reporter and author

Leek
soup

Preparation time: 1 hour
Difficulty: easy

4 servings

Olive oil

1 large onion, chopped

2 garlic cloves, minced

2 leeks, finely sliced (white and light green parts only)

4 potatoes, cut into large cubes

1.5 litres (6 cups) chicken stock

Salt and freshly ground pepper

Dried marjoram and parsley

Sauté the onion, garlic, and leeks in the olive oil until softened.

Add the potatoes and the stock. Season to taste and add the fines herbes.

Let simmer for 30 to 40 minutes and remove from the heat.

Allow to cool before processing in a mixer.

 Richard Béliveau

soups and broths

hearty kale soup

leek soup

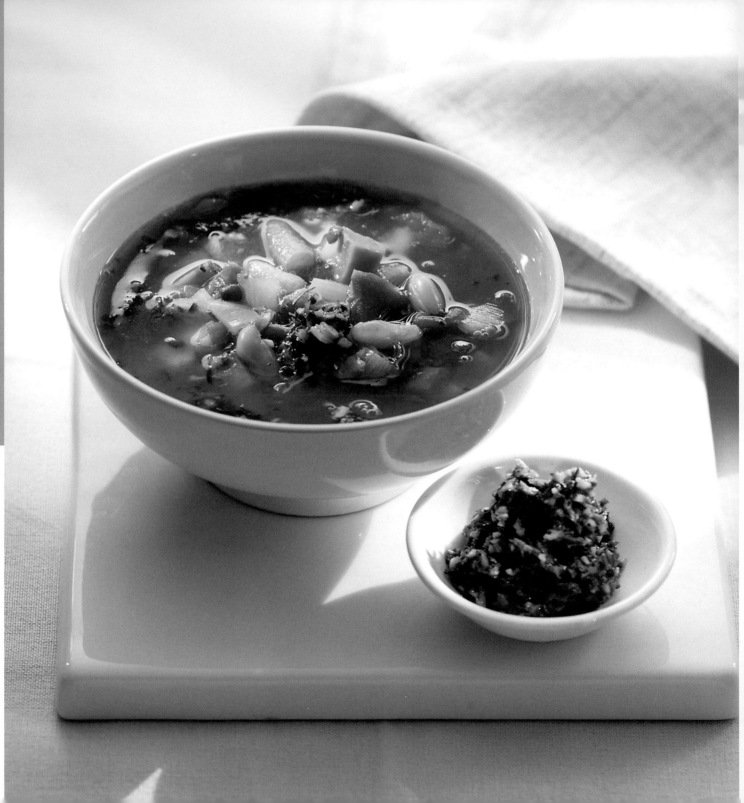

Mediterranean
bean soup

Preparation time: 1 h 15   4 servings
Difficulty: average

3 tbsp olive oil

100 g (2/3 cup) leeks, diced

80 g (1/2 cup) onions, diced

100 g (1/2 cup) carrots, diced

100 g (1/2 cup) zucchini, diced

50 g (1/4 cup) celery, diced

1.5 litres (6 cups) water

Salt

150 g (5 oz) potatoes

50 g (1/3 cup) green beans, cut into 2 cm (3/4 in) lengths

75 g (1/3 cup) canned white kidney beans, rinsed and drained

75 g (1/2 cup) ripe tomatoes, seeded and coarsely chopped

PISTOU

3 garlic cloves

160 g (1 cup) fresh basil

6 tbsp olive oil

Heat the olive oil in a large Dutch oven. Sauté the leeks, onions, carrots, zucchini, and celery for approximately 5 minutes over high heat.

Pour in the water and salt to taste. Add the potatoes and cook for 25 minutes on low boil.

Add the green beans, tomatoes, and white kidney beans, and cook for another 10 minutes.

To prepare the pistou, crush the garlic, and basil with a mortar and pestle, slowly incorporating the olive oil.

Add the pistou to the boiling soup and boil for an additional 2 minutes before serving.

 Jean Vachon, Chef-Instructor at the École hôtelière de la Capitale in Quebec

Onion and
garlic soup

Preparation time: 1 hour   6 servings
Difficulty: average

If you prefer a thicker soup, add 1 tbsp of flour to the onion and garlic mixture before adding the stock.

60 ml (1/4 cup) olive oil

8 medium onions, sliced in fine rounds

3 or 4 garlic cloves, finely chopped

1.5 litres (6 cups) beef stock

Salt and freshly ground pepper

2 tbsp dried parsley

2 tsp dried marjoram

6 slices of whole-wheat bread

200 g (1 1/3 cups) Gruyère cheese or cheddar, grated

Preheat the oven broiler.

Sauté the onions in the olive oil, stirring constantly until lightly golden.

Add the garlic and cook for 1 minute. Pour in the stock. Season with salt and pepper to taste, and add the parsley and marjoram. Bring to a boil and let simmer for 20 minutes uncovered.

Meanwhile, toast the bread in the oven or toaster. Remove the crusts and cut the bread slices to fit oven-proof soup bowls.

Pour the soup into the bowls, cover with a slice of bread, and top with the grated cheese.

Grill under the top broiler of the oven until the cheese bubbles and turns a golden colour.

 Richard Béliveau

soups and broths

Mediterranean bean soup

onion soup

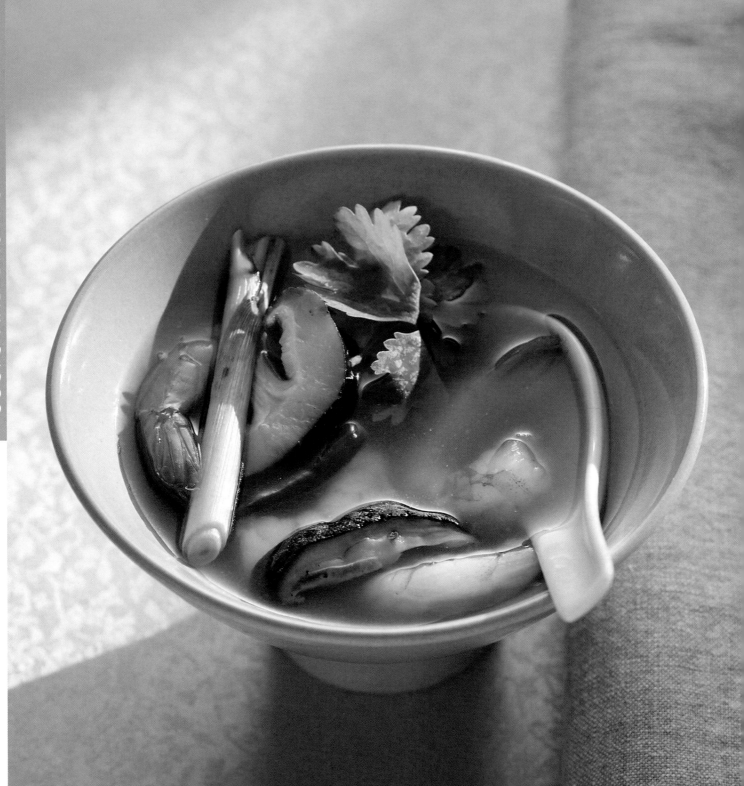

Spicy
shrimp soup

Preparation time: 30 minutes   4 servings
Difficulty: easy

Kafir, or combava, is a small lemon from India. The fruit is used in the kitchen, as are kafir leaves, which add a delicate flavour to many dishes. Galanga resembles ginger, and is used abundantly in South-East Asian cooking.

Nuoc-mâm is a Vietnamese sauce based on fish fermented in salt. It is used to flavour rice, vegetables and fish. There is a similar sauce in Thailand called Nam pla. These sauces can be found in Asian or specialty stores.

1 lemongrass shoot

1 tbsp olive oil

80 g (2 1/4 oz) fresh shiitake mushrooms, finely sliced

750 ml (3 cups) chicken stock, heated until hot

2 tsp fresh ginger or galanga, finely chopped

3 Kafir leaves (Kafir or combava) (optional)

Fish sauce (nuoc-mâm or nam pla)

8 large shrimp

1 or 2 hot peppers, finely sliced

3 tsp lime juice, freshly squeezed

Fresh coriander leaves

Cut the lemongrass shoot in 3 5-cm (2-in) lengths.

In a large saucepan, heat the mushrooms in a bit of the olive oil.

Add the hot stock, lemongrass, ginger, and the kaffir leaves. Add the fish sauce and cook for 10 minutes.

Add the shrimp and cook for 3 to 4 additional minutes.

Add the pepper slices and lime juice to a serving bowl. Pour in the soup, garnish with coriander and serve.

 Jean Vachon, Chef-Instructor at the École hôtelière de la Capitale in Quebec

Oriental-scented
broad bean soup

Preparation time: 2 h 30   6 servings
Difficulty: easy

A very hearty and nourishing soup that can be served as a main course.

Olive oil

2 onions, chopped

3 garlic cloves, minced

2 tsp ground turmeric

2 litres (8 cups) chicken stock

360 g (3 to 4 cups) broad beans, fresh or frozen

60 g (1/3 cup) barley

2 tbsp brined herbs, or fines herbes and salt to taste

Freshly ground pepper

Salt to taste (if you didn't use brined herbs)

In a large saucepan, sweat the onions and garlic in the olive oil until softened.

Add the turmeric and stir for 2 minutes. Then add the stock, and bring to a boil.

Add the broad beans, barley, brined herbs, and pepper, and let simmer approximately 2 1/2 hours, until the broad beans are cooked. Add any extra liquid (stock) at least 1 hour before the end of cooking.

 Richard Béliveau

soups and broths

spicy shrimp soup

broad bean soup

Cuban black bean soup

Preparation time: 40 minutes   **4 servings**
Difficulty: easy

You can replace the black beans with lentils. In place of chilli, cumin, and turmeric, use oregano, basil, thyme, and 2 bay leaves, and leave out the carrots. This soup follows in the tradition of the frequent use of legumes in all South American and West Indian cultures.

1 kg (5 cups – three 540 ml cans) black beans, rinsed and drained

340 g (2 1/4 cups – one 540 ml can) stewed canned tomatoes

Olive oil

2 onions, chopped

2 garlic cloves, minced

2 carrots, finely grated

4 tsp chilli seasoning

2 tsp ground cumin

1 tsp ground turmeric

Salt and freshly ground pepper

500 ml (2 cups) chicken stock

500 ml (2 cups) water

250 ml (1 cup) vegetable juice

Using a mixer, purée a third of the black beans with the tomatoes, and set aside.

Sauté the onions and garlic in the olive oil over medium-high heat until tender. Add the carrots and the chilli, cumin, and turmeric seasoning. Season with salt and pepper to taste, and stir constantly for 2 minutes.

Add the stock, water, vegetable juice, the remaining beans, and the tomato and bean mixture. Bring to a boil, partially cover the pot and cook for 40 minutes.

Cuban black bean soup

Balinese soup

soups and broths

Richard Béliveau

Balinese soup

Preparation time: 30 minutes   **6 servings**
Difficulty: easy

Pakchoi is a Chinese cabbage similar to Swiss chard. Its leaves and stems are eaten cooked.

10 green onions, finely chopped (set aside the green part)

425 ml (1 3/4 cups) coconut milk

3 to 4 tbsp soy sauce

2 tsp brown sugar

1 1/2 tsp curry powder

1 tsp fresh ginger

1 to 2 tsp garlic chilli paste

4 tomatoes (preferably Italian), cut into 6 pieces

1 yellow bell pepper, finely sliced

125 g (1 1/4 cups) mushrooms (preferably shiitake), sliced

7 g (1/4 cup) fresh basil, chopped

640 g (4 cups) pakchoi (green part only) or spinach

110 to 220 g (3/4 to 1 1/2 cups) silken tofu, cubed

Salt and freshly ground pepper

Cut the white part of the green onions into fine slices and set aside the green part for garnish.

In a heavy saucepan, mix together the coconut milk, soy sauce, brown sugar, curry, ginger, and chilli paste. Bring to a boil slowly.

Add the tomatoes, pepper, mushrooms, basil, and the green onions. Cover and cook for 5 minutes, stirring occasionally.

Add the pakchoi, cover and cook for approximately 5 minutes, stirring occasionally, until the vegetables are tender yet still crunchy.

Season with salt and pepper to taste.

Add the tofu 3 minutes before serving. Verify the seasoning and garnish with the reserved green onion.

Frances Boyte, dietitian and author of the book *Tofu tout flammé*, Éditions Trécarré, 2004.

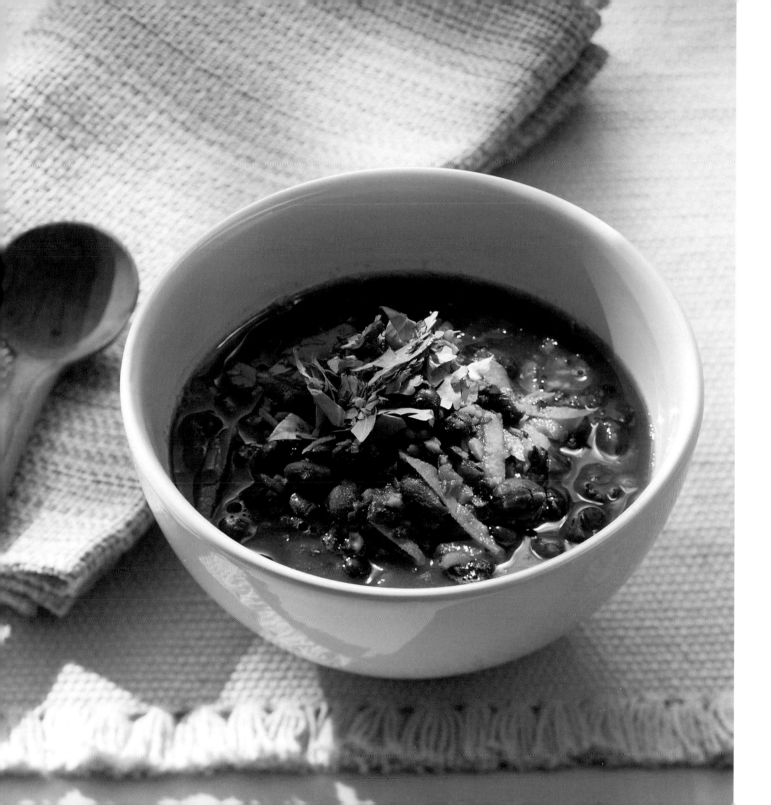

Tomato/apple soup

Preparation time: 45 minutes   4 servings
Difficulty: easy

You can replace the lovage with 150 g (3/4 cup) of diced celery and 30 g (1/4 cup) fresh chopped coriander. Serve this soup hot, garnished with fresh lovage, or cold with plain yogurt. Lovage is an aromatic plant that marries well with salads, soups, and meat-based dishes.

2 tbsp butter

1 onion, sliced

500 g (3 1/3 cups) ripe tomatoes, peeled, seeded, and cubed

4 Red Delicious apples, cubed

125 g (1 cup) fresh lovage leaves

1.25 litres (5 cups) chicken stock

Salt and freshly ground pepper

Heat the butter in a large saucepan and sauté the onion over medium heat.

Add the tomatoes, apples, and lovage, and stir, cooking for 2 to 3 minutes.

Pour in the stock and let simmer for 30 minutes.

Blend the soup with a hand mixer or electric mixer.

Season with salt and pepper to taste.

 Jean-Pierre Cloutier, Chef-proprietor of the Café-restaurant du Musée in Quebec

tomato/apple soup
red lentil soup
soups and broths

Red lentil soup

Preparation time: 50 minutes   8 servings
Difficulty: average

450 g (2 1/4 cups) dried red lentils, rinsed and drained

1.25 litres (5 cups) chicken stock or water

1 tsp ground turmeric

1 chunk of fresh ginger, measuring 2.5 cm (1 in), grated or finely chopped

300 g (2 cups) ripe tomatoes, diced

250 ml (1 cup) milk

Salt

60 g (1/4 cup) unsalted butter

160 g (1 cup) onions, finely sliced

2 tsp cumin seed

Freshly ground pepper

Fresh coriander, chopped

Put the lentils in a heavy saucepan. Add the stock, turmeric, ginger, and the tomatoes.

Bring to a boil, reduce the heat and let simmer for approximately 25 minutes, until the lentils are tender.

Purée using a food processor or mixer.

Return the soup to the saucepan and add the milk. Season with salt to taste, and cook over low heat.

Meanwhile, melt the butter in a skillet, and brown the onions with the cumin.

Pour the soup into 8 preheated bowls and add pepper to taste.

Place a bit of the butter and onion mixture in each bowl, and garnish with coriander.

 Jean Vachon, Chef-Instructor at the École hôtelière de la Capitale in Quebec

Lentil and carrot soup

Preparation time: 1 h 30
Difficulty: average

4 servings

100 g (1/2 cup) dried red lentils, washed and drained
250 g (1 1/4 cups) carrots, sliced
160 g (1 cup) Spanish onions, coarsely chopped
3 garlic cloves, whole
150 g (1 cup) ripe tomatoes, coarsely chopped
800 ml (3 1/4 cups) chicken stock
1 tbsp olive oil
1/2 tsp ground cumin
1/2 tsp ground coriander
1/2 tsp ground turmeric
Juice of one lemon, freshly squeezed
175 ml (3/4 cup) 3.25 % homogenized milk
Freshly ground pepper

In a large saucepan, mix together the lentils, carrots, onions, garlic, and the tomatoes. Add 3/4 of the stock and bring to a boil.

Reduce the heat, cover, and let simmer for approximately 30 minutes, until the lentils and vegetables are cooked.

Meanwhile, heat the olive oil in a skillet. Sauté the cumin, coriander, and turmeric for several minutes. Remove from the heat and add the lemon juice.

Process the soup in a food processor, and then strain.

Reheat and bring to a boil. Add the spices and the stock, and simmer for 10 minutes.

Stir in the milk, add pepper to taste, and serve.

 Jean Vachon, Chef-Instructor at the École hôtelière de la Capitale in Quebec

Spinach and pine nut velouté

Preparation time: 40 minutes
Difficulty: average

4 servings

3 tbsp olive oil
1 onion, finely chopped
2 tbsp flour
1 tsp ground turmeric
1 kg (2 lbs) fresh spinach, washed and patted dry
500 ml (2 cups) chicken or vegetable stock
2 egg yolks
125 ml (1/2 cup) 35 % whipping cream
125 ml (1/2 cup) milk
Juice of half a lemon, freshly squeezed
Salt and freshly ground pepper
2 tbsp pine nuts
50 g (1/3 cup) Parmesan cheese, shaved

Heat the olive oil in a large saucepan. Sauté the onion over medium-low heat until it becomes translucent.

Add the flour, turmeric, and spinach. Pour in the stock and cook for several minutes.

Process with a mixer until smooth.

In a small bowl, beat the egg yolks together with the cream and milk and add to the soup. Add the lemon juice, and salt and pepper to taste. Stir well.

Ladle the hot velouté into deep dishes and garnish with the pine nuts and Parmesan.

 Éric Villain, Chef-co-owner of the Bistro Le Clocher Penché in Quebec

soups and broths

lentil and carrot soup

spinach velouté

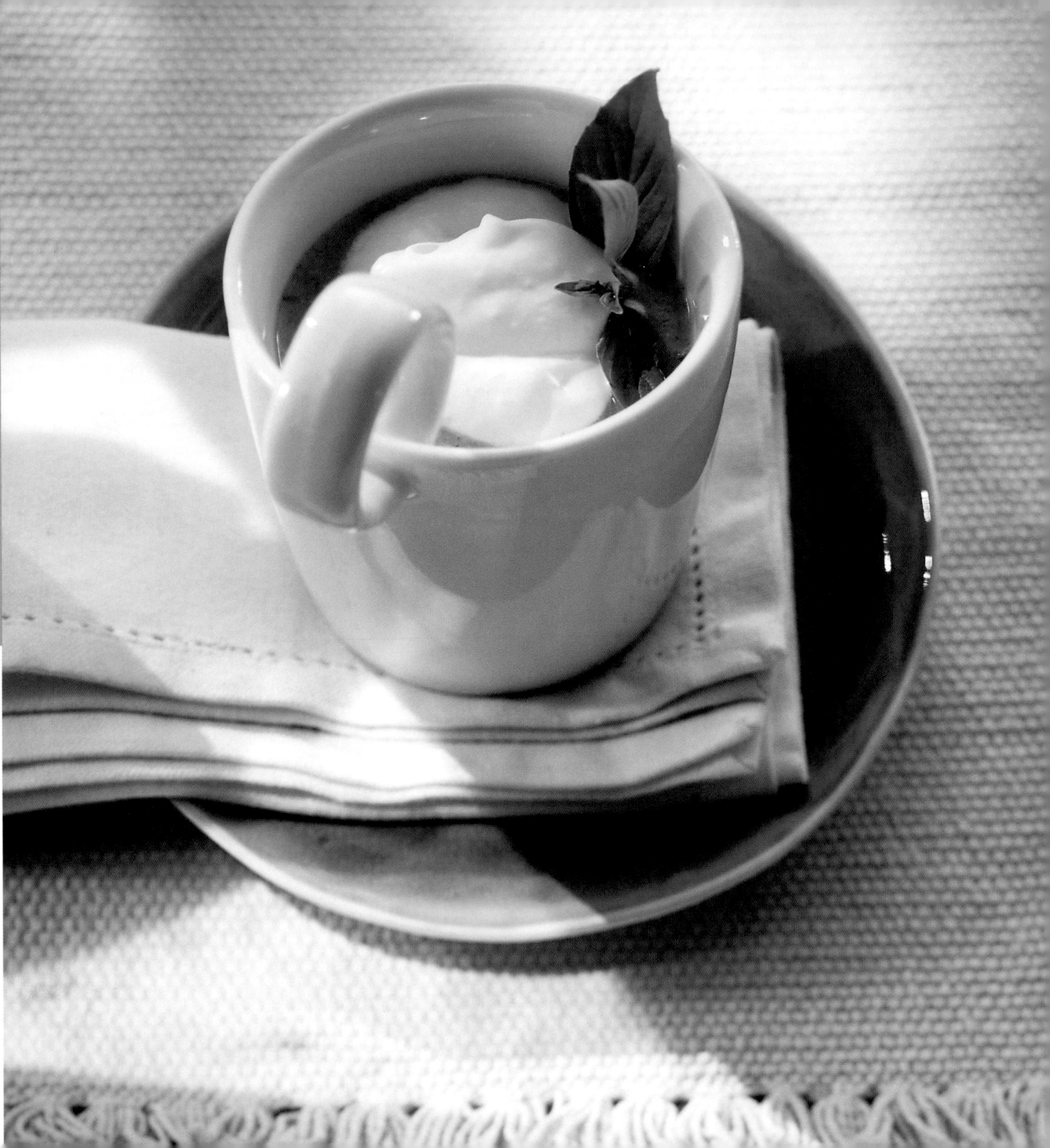

Mushroom
and cappuccino velouté

Preparation time: 45 minutes
Difficulty: average

6 servings

Thai basil has a slightly licorice flavour. If you can't locate any, select any fresh basil available in your region.

1/2 tsp olive oil

250 g (2 1/4 cups) fresh shiitake mushrooms or white mushrooms, thinly sliced

1 tsp garlic, finely chopped

2 shallots, sliced

1 litre (4 cups) chicken stock

1 tsp Thai basil (set aside 6 leaves for garnish)

Salt and freshly ground pepper

1/2 tsp sesame oil

250 ml (1 cup) milk, frothed

In a saucepan, sauté the mushrooms, garlic and shallots in the olive oil over medium-high heat.

Lower the heat, add the stock, and let simmer for 20 minutes.

Remove from the heat and add the basil. Blend the soup in a food processor, and season with salt and pepper to taste. Add the sesame oil to flavour.

Froth the milk and spoon on top of the velouté. Decorate each serving with a basil leaf.

 Florence Albernhe, Chef-proprietor of the restaurant Le Grain de riz in Quebec

Moroccan beef
and chickpea velouté

Preparation time: 1 h 30
Difficulty: average

8 servings

250 g (1/2 lb) 1 cm (1/2 in) beef cubes

2 onions, finely sliced

1 pinch of saffron

2 litres (8 cups) water or chicken stock

Salt and freshly ground pepper

2 celery stalks, diced

1 bunch fresh flat-leaf parsley, chopped

1 bunch fresh coriander, chopped

3 tbsp tomato paste

5 ripe tomatoes, peeled (see page 142), seeded, and diced

300 g (1 1/2 cups) canned chickpeas, rinsed and drained

50 g (1/3 cup) flour

Place the meat, onions, saffron, and water in a large saucepan. Season with salt and pepper to taste. Cover and let simmer for 20 to 30 minutes.

Add the celery, parsley, coriander, tomato paste, and the tomatoes. Let simmer for 20 minutes.

Add the chickpeas. Mix the flour with a bit of water and stir into the saucepan. Cook for several minutes to thicken, verify the seasoning and serve.

 Jean Vachon, Chef-Instructor at the École hôtelière de la Capitale in Quebec

soups and broths

mushroom velouté

beef and chickpea velouté

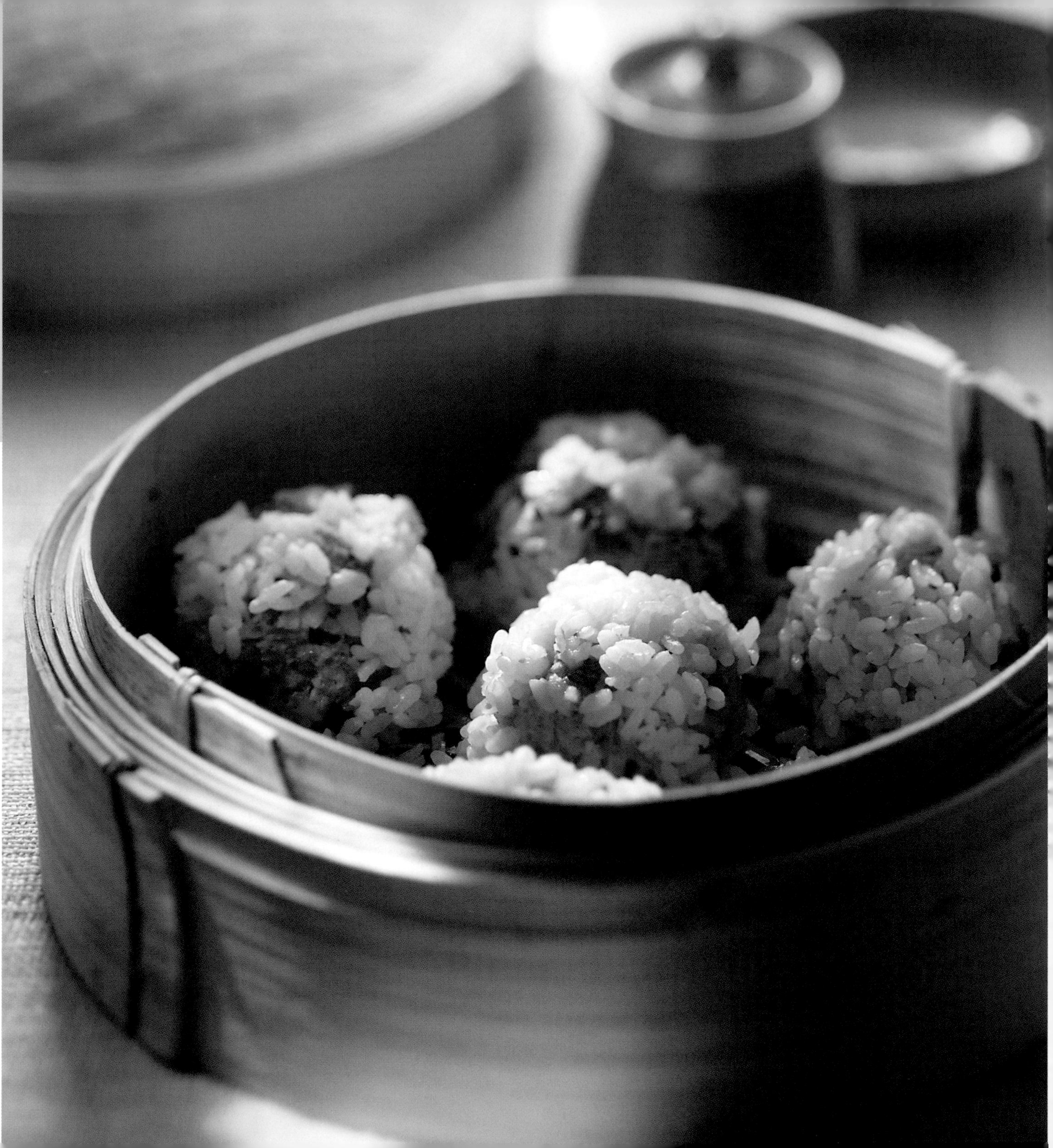

Pearled
meatballs

Preparation time: 2 h 30
Difficulty: average

Makes 18 to 20 meatballs,
or 6 servings

200 g (1 cup) sticky rice

350 g (12 oz) pork, chopped

1 egg, beaten

1 tsp light soy sauce

1 tsp salt

1/2 tsp powdered sugar

1/2 tsp fish sauce (nuoc-mâm or nam pla)

1 tsp fresh ginger, chopped

2 tsp cornstarch

6 large dehydrated Chinese mushrooms, rehydrated
and chopped

6 canned water chestnuts, chopped

15 g (1/2 cup) fresh coriander, chopped and several
sprigs for garnish

*Soak the rice for 2 hours in cold water. Drain and
spread over a clean dish towel to dry.*

*In a large bowl, combine the pork, egg, soy sauce,
salt, sugar, fish sauce, ginger, and cornstarch.*

*Add the mushrooms, water chestnuts, and coriander,
and mix well.*

*Shape the mixture into balls, moistening your hands
so the mixture won't stick to them.*

Roll the meatballs in the rice, pressing down firmly.

*Lightly oil a steamer basket or marguerite and
arrange the meatballs carefully.*

*Place the steamer over a pot of boiling water and
steam for 20 to 25 minutes.*

Garnish with sprigs of fresh coriander and serve.

 **Jean Vachon, Chef-Instructor at the
École hôtelière de la Capitale in Quebec**

Bocconcini
and strawberries
with ginger

Preparation time: 45 minutes
Difficulty: easy

4 servings

200 g (7 oz) bocconcini (fresh, ball-shaped
mozzarella cheese)

12 large strawberries

VINAIGRETTE

1 tbsp lemon juice, freshly squeezed

1 tsp black pepper, crushed

3 tbsp balsamic vinegar

1 tbsp maple syrup

60 ml (1/4 cup) walnut oil

1 tbsp fresh ginger, grated

1 tbsp water

Selection of lettuce leaves to taste (optional)

*Cut the cheese and strawberries into thick slices
and set aside.*

*In a small bowl, mix all of the vinaigrette ingredi-
ents together.*

*Marinate the cheese in half of the vinaigrette for
30 minutes.*

*Arrange the cheese slices and strawberries
alternately on a serving platter. They can also be
arranged around a bouquet of mixed lettuce.*

*Sprinkle with the vinaigrette and serve
immediately.*

 **Marlène Gagnon, Chef-Instructor at the
École hôtelière de la Capitale in Quebec**

first
courses

pearled
meatballs

bocconcini and
strawberries

Carpaccio of red tuna
with citrus and avocado quenelles

Preparation time: 40 minutes　　　　　**4 servings**
Difficulty: average

To make quenelles that are uniformly shaped, place a bit of the quenelle mixture in a moistened soup spoon, and shape it using a second spoon to form the top. This ensures that all quenelles are uniform in size.

1 orange

1 grapefruit

VINAIGRETTE

Salt and freshly ground pepper

Tabasco

2 tbsp fresh ginger, chopped

Juice of one lime, freshly squeezed

3 tbsp olive oil

250 g (1/2 lb) sushi grade red tuna

2 shallots, finely chopped

25 g (3/4 cup) fresh chives, finely chopped

1 large ripe avocado

4 tsp sesame oil

Sesame seeds

With a sharp knife, remove the peel and white skin from the oranges and grapefruit, and quarter them over a bowl, reserving the juice. Cut the fruit into small cubes and set aside.

Make the vinaigrette, mixing the reserved juice with a pinch of salt, pepper, tabasco, chopped ginger, 1 1/2 tbsp lime juice, and the olive oil.

Slice the tuna very fine and arrange on 4 individual serving plates. Season with salt and pepper and sprinkle with the vinaigrette. Decorate with the shallots, chives, and citrus cubes.

Cut the avocado in half, remove the stone, and separate the flesh using a spoon. Using a fork, purée the avocado in a bowl with the remaining lime juice and the sesame oil. Season with salt and pepper, and Tabasco to taste.

Form the avocado paste into a lovely quenelle and place in the centre of the tuna slices. Garnish with sesame seeds and serve.

 Jean-Luc Boulay, Chef-proprietor of the restaurant Le Saint-Amour in Quebec

carpaccio
of red tuna
with citrus
and avocado
quenelles

first
courses

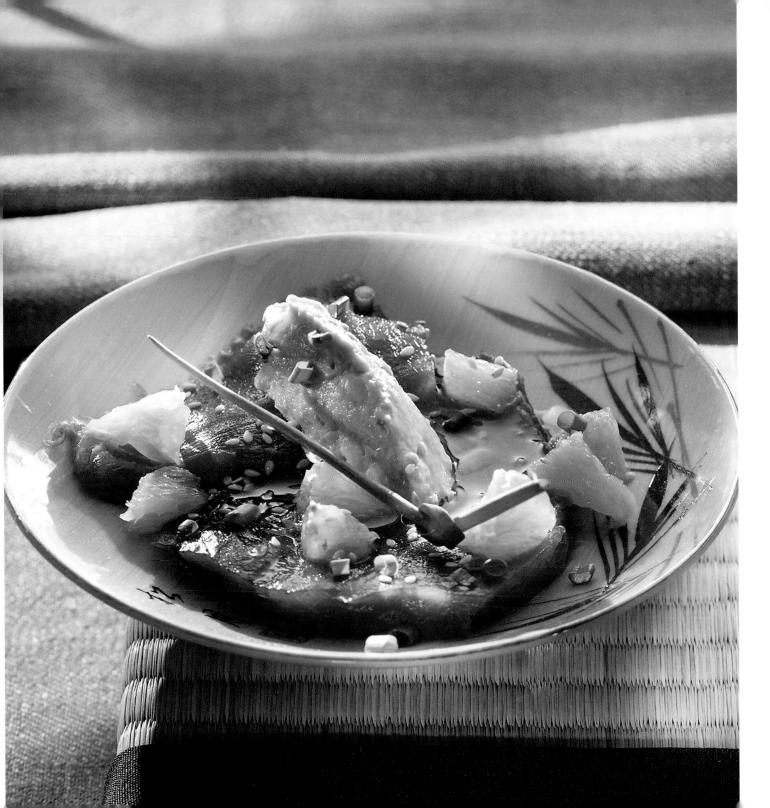

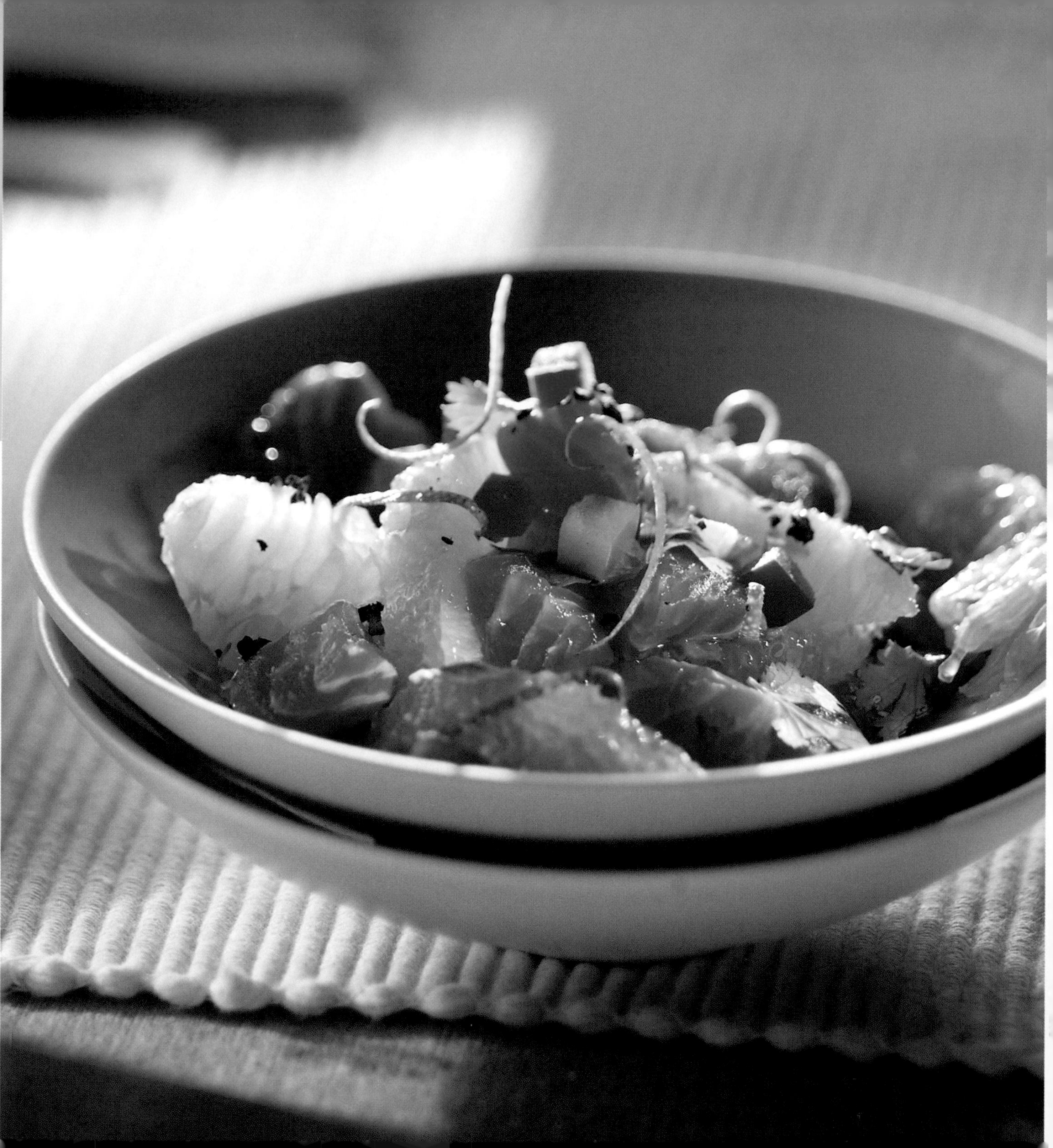

Citrus trout
ceviche

Preparation time: **20 minutes**
Marinade: **6 hours**
Difficulty: **average**

4 servings

*To make the orange and grapefruit suprêmes,
purchase thick-skinned citrus fruit if possible.
With a sharp knife, remove the peel and bitter
white skin from the underside, and quarter
them over a bowl, reserving the juice. Then cut
the wedges into thin slices.*

250 g (1/2 lb) raw trout, cubed

2 oranges, cut in suprêmes

1 pink grapefruit, cut in suprêmes

80 ml (1/3 cup) lemon juice, freshly squeezed

1/2 tsp lime zest, grated

10 g (1/3 cup) fresh parsley, chopped

30 g (1/4 cup) multicoloured peppers, diced

1 tbsp onions, sliced very fine

80 ml (1/3 cup) olive oil

Salt and freshly ground pepper

3 tbsp fresh coriander (garnish)

*Mix all ingredients together in a large glass bowl
and season to taste.*

Cover and marinate for 6 hours in the refrigerator.

*Serve in decorative cups and garnish with the
fresh coriander.*

**Benoît Dussault, Chef-Instructor at the École
hôtelière de la Capitale in Quebec**

Fish
cakes

Preparation time: **40 minutes**
Difficulty: **average**

4 to 6 servings

250 g (1/2 lb) lean white fish

1 tbsp red curry paste

1 tsp fish sauce (nuoc-mâm or nam pla)

40 g (1/4 cup) green beans, finely sliced

Oil for frying

Sprigs of fresh coriander

Finely chop the fish.

*In a large bowl, mix the fish together with the
curry paste, fish sauce, and green beans.*

*Shape the fish patties approximately 4 cm (1 1/2
in) in diameter and 1 cm (1/2 in) thick.*

*Heat the oil to 190°C (375°F) and fry the cakes
until they are golden brown.*

*Transfer to paper towels and remove any excess
oil.*

*Serve with the Thai cucumber sauce and garnish
with the fresh coriander sprigs.*

THAI CUCUMBER SAUCE

60 g (1/4 cup) sugar

1 pinch of sea salt

60 ml (1/4 cup) rice wine vinegar

50 g (1/4 cup) cucumber, diced

1 small hot pepper, finely sliced

*In a bowl, dissolve the sugar and salt in the rice
wine vinegar. Add the cucumbers and peppers,
and marinate for several minutes before serving.*

**Jean Vachon, Chef-
Instructor at the École
hôtelière de la Capitale
in Quebec**

first
courses

citrus trout
ceviche

fish
cakes

Grilled
3-spice sardines

Preparation time: 40 minutes
Difficulty: average

2 to 3 servings, depending on the size of the sardines

This recipe lends itself to cooking on the barbecue. A true festive summer treat that will please all guests.

6 whole sardines, fresh or thawed

2 tsp ground turmeric

2 tsp ground cumin

2 tsp ground coriander

Freshly ground pepper

80 ml (1/3 cup) olive oil

Mix the turmeric, cumin, coriander, and pepper together in a small bowl.

Preheat the oven broiler.

Scale the sardines under cold running water, simply rubbing them with your fingers. Gut the sardines, rinsing well, and cut off the fins.

Pat the sardines dry and rub them with the spices. Set aside for 10 minutes.

Sprinkle the sardines with the olive oil and place on a rack over a baking sheet covered with aluminium foil.

Cook in the oven under the top broiler for approximately 5 minutes for each side, until the skin turns a golden brown and blisters.

 Richard Béliveau

grilled sardines
feta-stuffed mushrooms

first courses

Feta-stuffed
mushrooms

Preparation time: 1 hour
Difficulty: average

6 servings

6 large mushrooms

1 tbsp olive oil

40 g (1/4 cup) onions, chopped

2 garlic cloves, minced

60 g (1/2 cup) sunflower seeds, coarsely chopped

60 ml (1/4 cup) red wine

25 g (1/3 cup) spinach, chopped

Salt and freshly ground pepper

90 g (2/3 cup) feta cheese, crumbled

3 tbsp walnuts, coarsely chopped

4 slices of stale whole-wheat bread, crust removed and cut into small squares

1 pinch of fresh thyme

Separate the mushroom stems from the caps. Finely chop the stems and set aside the caps.

Heat the olive oil in a skillet. Sauté the onions, garlic, and sunflower seeds over medium heat for 3 minutes.

Add the chopped mushroom stems and cook for 1 minute.

Pour in the wine and reduce until almost all the liquid is evaporated.

Add the spinach and cook for another minute. Season with salt and pepper to taste. Remove from the heat, add the feta and walnuts and set aside.

Using a food processor, grind the bread into breadcrumbs, mixing in the thyme.

Arrange the mushroom caps on an oiled or buttered cookie sheet, fill them with the spinach and feta stuffing, and top with the breadcrumbs.

Cook in the oven at 180°C (350°F) for 15 to 20 minutes, until the mushrooms are tender and the breadcrumbs brown. Serve immediately.

 Marlène Gagnon, Chef-Instructor at the l'École hôtelière de la Capitale in Quebec

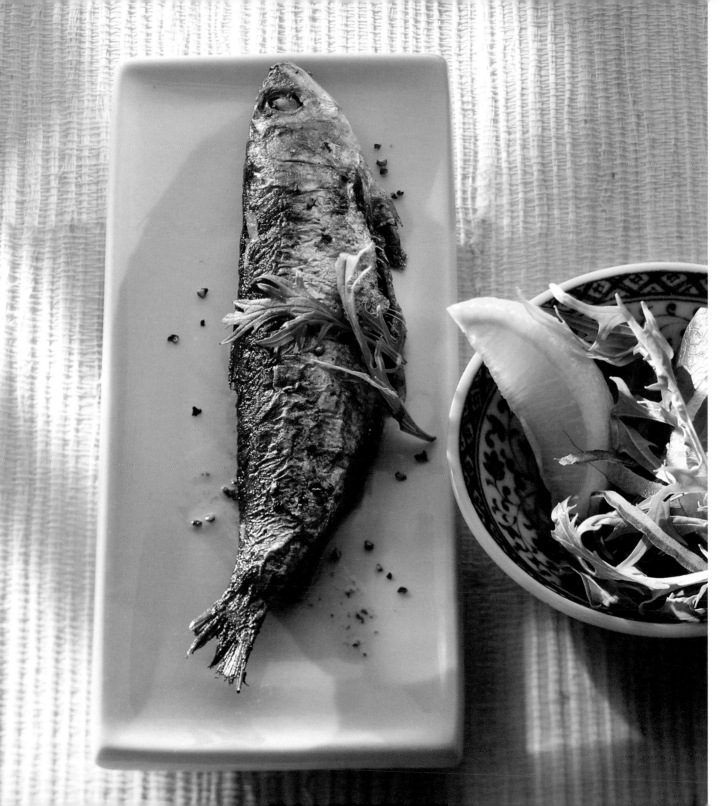

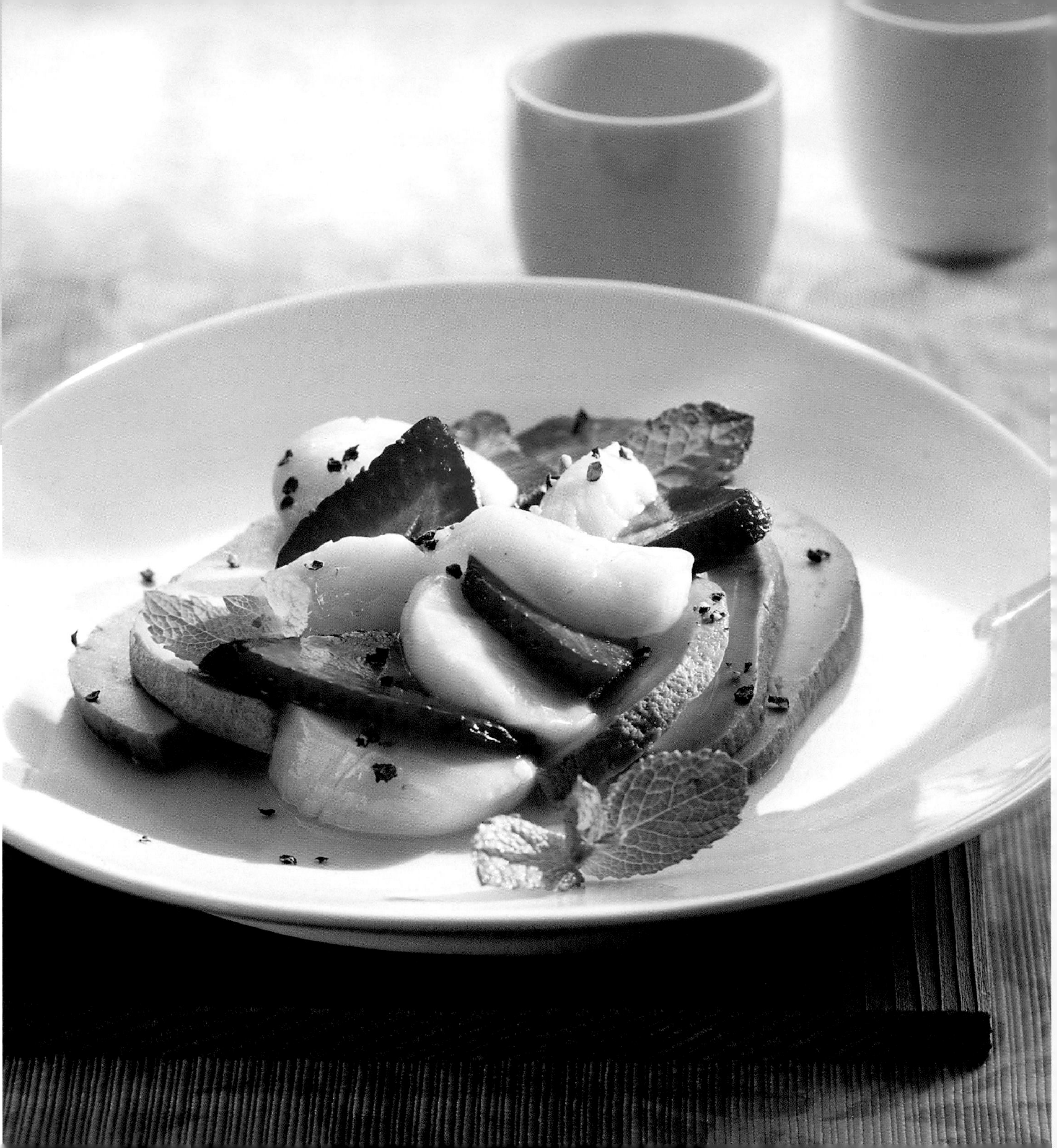

Scallop
and strawberry rosettes

Preparation time: 1 hour
Difficulty: average
4 servings

8 large scallops

8 very ripe strawberries, sliced

1 tsp sesame seeds, toasted (see page 141)

1 slightly firm avocado

4 fresh mint sprigs

4 whole strawberries, stems on

4 lime slices, twisted

MARINADE

2 tbsp lime juice, freshly squeezed

3 tbsp sesame oil

1 tsp fresh ginger, finely minced

Freshly ground pepper

Prepare the marinade, whisking together the lime juice, sesame oil, ginger, and pepper in a bowl.

Cut each scallop into three circles and place in the marinade. Cover and marinate 30 minutes in the refrigerator.

Decorate individual serving plates with the scallop rounds and the strawberry slices to form a rosette, pour over the marinade, and sprinkle with the sesame seeds.

Peel and slice the avocado into thin slices, and arrange in a fan shape around the scallops, and garnish each dish with mint sprigs, a whole strawberry, and a slice of lime.

 Yves Moscato, Chef-co-owner of the restaurant 48 St-Paul, Cuisine_monde in Quebec

Oriental herbed
tabbouleh

Preparation time: 30 minutes
Difficulty: easy
4 servings

250 ml (1 cup) boiling water

1 tsp salt

200 g (1 cup) precooked wheat semolina (couscous)

2 ripe tomatoes, seeded and diced

7 g (1/4 cup) fresh mint, finely sliced

7 g (1/4 cup) Thai basil, chopped

7 g (1/4 cup) fresh coriander, chopped

2 tbsp fresh ginger, minced

VINAIGRETTE

125 ml (1/2 cup) olive oil

1/2 tsp ground turmeric

Juice of one lemon, freshly squeezed

Salt and freshly ground pepper

Bring the water to a boil with the salt. Remove from the heat and pour over the couscous. Cover and let stand for 10 minutes.

In a small bowl, make the vinaigrette, whisking the olive oil, turmeric, and lemon juice together. Season with salt and pepper to taste.

Transfer the couscous to a large bowl, working with a fork to break up any lumps.

Add the tomatoes, mint, basil, coriander, and the ginger. Sprinkle with the vinaigrette, mix well and serve.

 Florence Albernhe, Jean-Pierre Cloutier, Chef-proprietors of Le Grain de riz in Quebec

first courses

scallop and strawberry rosettes

herbed tabbouleh

Glazed tomatoes in olive oil

Preparation time: 10 minutes
Marinade: 12 hours
Difficulty: easy

4 servings

You can serve these tomatoes on slices of black olive or dried tomato toast, and add a sliver of two-year-old cheddar. Bella tomatoes are sweet and juicy Italian vine tomatoes.

15 to 20 whole Bella tomatoes

3 tbsp extra virgin olive oil

1 tbsp basil pesto

Sea salt

Detach the tomatoes from the vine and rinse under cold water.

Heat the olive oil in a skillet. Add the pesto and cook for 30 seconds. Add the tomatoes and cook for approximately 2 minutes, stirring constantly, until the tomatoes begin to burst.

Transfer to a deep serving dish, season to taste and marinate at room temperature for 3 to 12 hours before serving.

 Christophe Alary, Chef-Instructor at the École hôtelière de la Capitale in Quebec, elected Chef of the Year 2004 by his peers

glazed tomatoes

spring rolls

first courses

Spring rolls

Preparation time: 45 minutes
Difficulty: average

4 servings

Stream of olive oil

150 g (1 1/2 cups) chanterelles or enoki mushrooms, sliced

80 g (2/3 cup) red peppers, finely sliced

80 g (1 cup) bean sprouts

2 green onions, finely sliced

15 g (1/2 cup) fresh mint, chopped

15 g (1/2 cup) fresh coriander, chopped

1 tsp sesame oil

Salt and freshly ground pepper

4 rice paper leaves

4 shoots fresh chives

Heat the olive oil in a skillet. Cook the mushrooms and the peppers over high heat, taking care not to overcook them. Use raw enokis.

Mix all other ingredients in a bowl, except the rice paper and chives, and let sit for 30 minutes at room temperature.

Soak the rice paper leaves in a large bowl of warm water for approximately 1 minute to soften.

Spread the leaves on a work surface and pat dry.

Divide the stuffing among the rice paper squares, turn up the edges and roll closed, pressing firmly.

Attach the rolls with the chive shoots.

 Jean-Pierre Cloutier, Chef-proprietor of Café-restaurant du Musée in Quebec

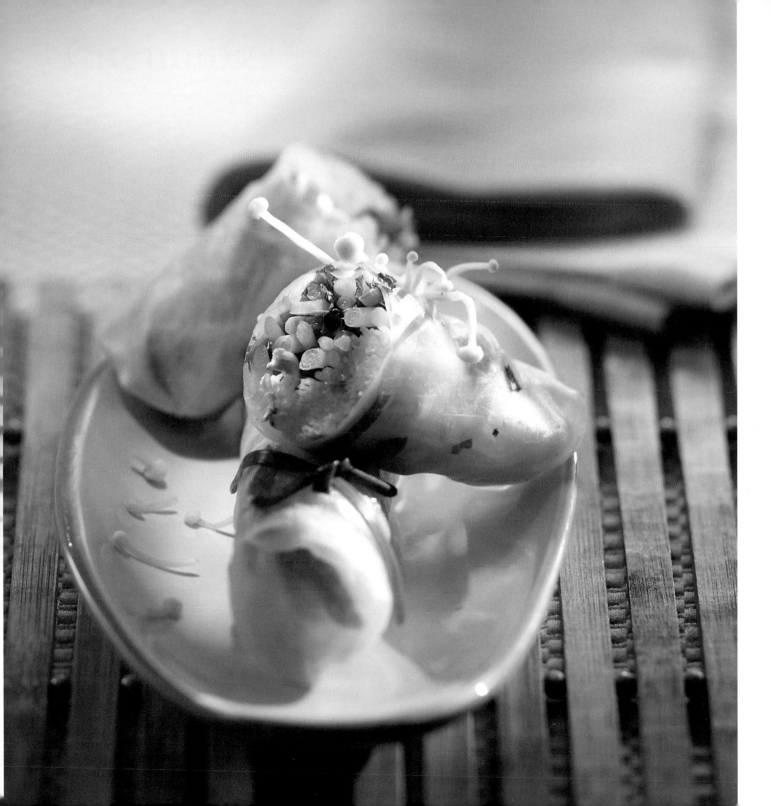

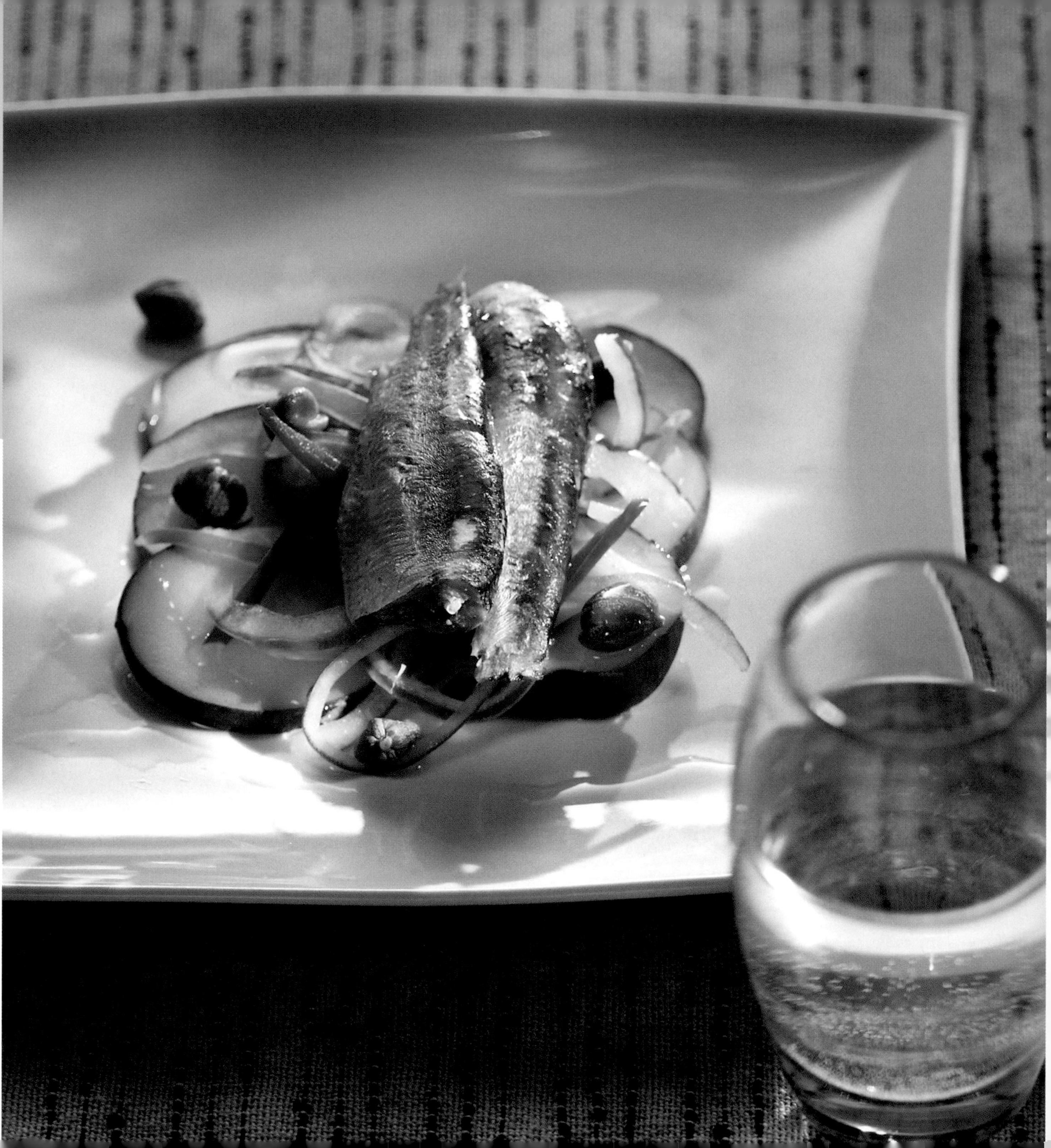

Warm sardines
on a bed of marinated onions

Preparation time: 30 minutes
Marinade : 3 hours
Difficulty: easy

4 servings

240 g (8 oz) sardines, canned

160 g (1 cup) red onions, finely sliced

40 g (1/3 cup) yellow, green, and red peppers, cut in strips

3 tsp capers

2 tbsp lemon juice, freshly squeezed

80 ml (1/3 cup) olive oil

250 g (1/2 lb) baby potatoes

Salt and freshly ground pepper

Mix the onions, peppers, capers, and lemon juice in a large bowl. Season with salt and pepper to taste.

Add the olive oil, cover, and marinate in the refrigerator for 3 hours.

Meanwhile, cook the potatoes in boiling salted water until tender. Cool, drain, and set aside.

When ready to serve, slice the potatoes into thin rounds, and arrange in the centre of an ovenproof dish. Cover with the drained onion mixture, without completely hiding the potatoes.

Place the sardines on top of the onions and sprinkle with the oil marinade.

Cook in the oven at 180°C (350°F) for 7 to 8 minutes.

Season generously with pepper and serve immediately.

 Benoît Dussault, Chef-Instructor at the École hôtelière de la Capitale in Quebec

Trio surprise
for crudités

Preparation time: 5 minutes
Difficulty: easy

1 serving

Arrange the dip bowls on a large serving platter with your favourite raw vegetables: mushrooms, cauliflower, broccoli florets, radishes, etc. To sweat leeks, cook them in a bit of olive oil over low heat until they release their natural liquid.

BASIC DIP

2 tbsp plain yogurt

80 g (1/3 cup) mayonnaise

2 tsp lemon juice, freshly squeezed

Salt and freshly ground pepper

TOMATO AND BASIL

4 tsp tomato paste

6 basil leaves, finely chopped

2 tsp sugar

HONEY AND CURRY

2 tsp curry powder

1 tbsp honey

GARLIC AND LEEK

2 tbsp leeks, finely sliced and sweated

1/2 garlic clove, minced

Using a food processor, combine the basic dip with the other flavoured dip ingredients.

 Jean-Pierre Cloutier, Chef-proprietor of Café-restaurant du Musée in Quebec

first courses

warm sardines on onions

trio surprise

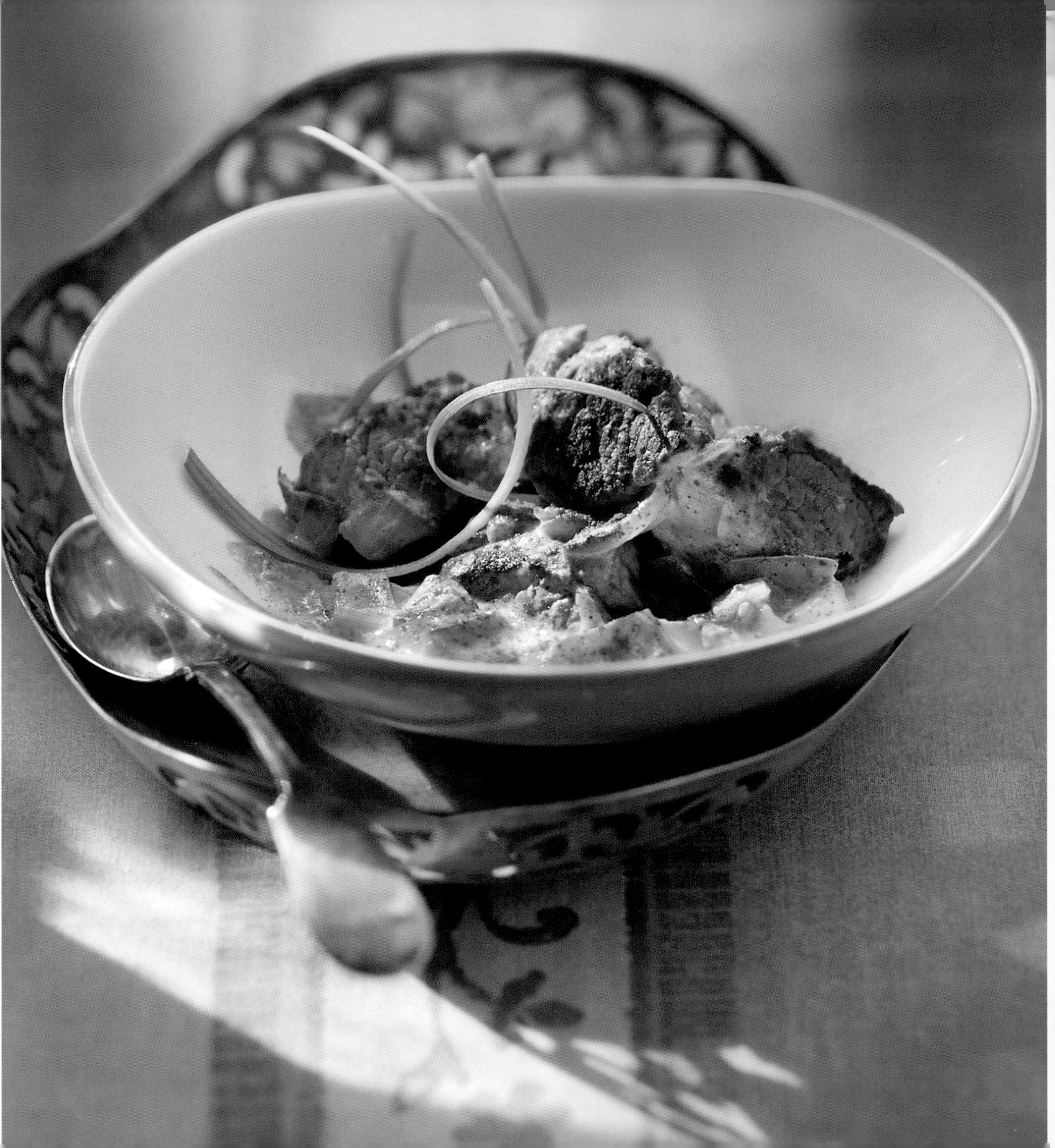

Spicy
Indian-style lamb

Preparation time: 2 hours
Difficulty: average

4 servings

You will receive many compliments when you serve this delicious dish with the rice pilaf recipe found on page 230.

700 g (1 1/2 lbs) lamb shoulder, cubed

1 1/2 tbsp olive oil

80 g (1/2 cup) Spanish onions, coarsely chopped

3 garlic cloves

2 tsp fresh ginger, finely chopped

1 tbsp hot red peppers

10 cardamom seeds

10 coriander seeds

4 whole cloves

1 1/2 tsp cumin seed

1 bay leaf

Salt and white pepper

125 g (1/2 cup) plain yogurt 8 % m.f. or more

1 tsp paprika (optional)

Heat the olive oil in a heavy saucepan and sear the meat on all sides. Add the onions and mix well. Sauté for 3 to 4 minutes.

Using a food processor or mortar, purée the garlic, ginger, peppers, cardamom, coriander, cloves, cumin, and bay leaf. Season with salt and pepper to taste. Mix in with the meat and cook for several minutes.

Slowly add the yogurt to the saucepan, mixing with the other heated ingredients, thus forming the braising liquid. Verify the seasoning and bring to a boil. Cover, reduce the heat, and simmer over low heat for approximately 1 h 15, stirring frequently.

Sprinkle with the paprika and serve.

**Jean Vachon, Chef-Instructor at the
École hôtelière de la Capitale in Quebec**

Korean-style
grilled beef

Preparation time: 50 minutes
Difficulty: easy

3 or 4 servings
(if served with other dishes)

The beef will be easier to cut into thin slices if you partially freeze it beforehand.

500 g (1 lb) beef steak (sirloin or other), finely sliced

4 green onions, chopped 2.5 cm (1 in)

MARINADE

60 ml (1/4 cup) soy sauce

2 tbsp sesame oil

2 tbsp sake or Sherry

1 tbsp sugar

2 tbsp de sesame seeds, toasted and ground (see page 141)

2 garlic cloves, finely sliced

2 tsp fresh ginger, grated

Salt and freshly ground pepper

Pepper flakes

Prepare the marinade by mixing together all its ingredients. Pour over the meat, cover, and marinate at least 30 minutes in the refrigerator.

Drain the meat well and cook with the onions over high heat in a ribbed skillet or wok.

**Susan Sylvester, Chef-Instructor at the
École hôtelière de la Capitale in Quebecc**

main
dishes

spicy Indian-
style lamb

Korean-style
grilled beef

Beef
with lemongrass

Preparation time: 20 minutes
Difficulty: easy

4 servings

Beef with lemongrass is delicious with perfumed steamed rice seasoned with fish sauce.

175 ml (3/4 cup) vegetable oil

160 g (1 cup) onions, finely sliced

2 tsp garlic, minced

2 tbsp lemongrass, chopped

2 tsp fresh ginger, minced

160 g (1 cup) green onions, finely sliced

500 g (1 lb) beef, Chinese fondue cut

60 ml (1/4 cup) fish sauce (nuoc-mâm or nam pla)

2 tsp sugar

2 tbsp sesame seeds, toasted

Salt and freshly ground pepper

Several leaves of fresh coriander

Heat the wok over high heat, add the oil and cook the onions, garlic, lemongrass, ginger, green onions, and beef over medium-high heat for 1 to 2 minutes.

Add the fish sauce, sugar, and sesame seeds. Season with salt and pepper to taste, and cook for 1 to 2 minutes over medium-high heat.

Serve immediately, garnishing with the coriander leaves.

 Yves Moscato, Chef-co-proprietor of the restaurant 48 St-Paul, Cuisine_monde in Quebec

beef
with lemongrass

Bengal
beef

main
dishes

Bengal beef

Preparation time: 45 minutes
Difficulty: average

6 servings

Kefir is a fermented milk that is sour tasting and bubbly. It is easy to digest, in addition to being an excellent source of protein. Kefir is drunk in large quantities in the Caucasus region.

This dish is especially succulent when married with Basmati rice. Experience nirvana with the rich combination of flavours!

60 ml (1/4 cup) olive oil
750 g (1 1/2 lbs) lean ground beef
4 onions, finely sliced
3 garlic cloves, minced
1 tbsp curry powder
1 tsp ground turmeric
1 tbsp flour
2 tsp salt
Freshly ground pepper
1/2 tsp ground cardamom
1 cube beef bouillon, crumbled
375 ml (1 1/2 cups) water
60 ml (1/4 cup) vinegar
100 g (1/2 cup) raisins
30 g (1/4 cup) pine nuts
60 g (1/2 cup) pistachio nuts, shelled
375 g (1 1/2 cups) yogurt or plain kefir

Heat the olive oil in a large, heavy saucepan. Cook the beef and set aside.

In the same saucepan, brown the onions and garlic for 20 minutes over medium-low heat. Add the curry and turmeric and cook slowly for 2 minutes.

Add the flour and salt, stirring well. Add a generous amount of pepper.

Add the cardamom, crumbled bouillon cube, water, vinegar, dried raisins, and the beef. Mix well, cover, and let simmer for 20 minutes. Add the pine nuts and pistachio nuts.

Serve in individual plates, topping each serving with approximately 4 tbsp of the yogurt.

 Richard Béliveau

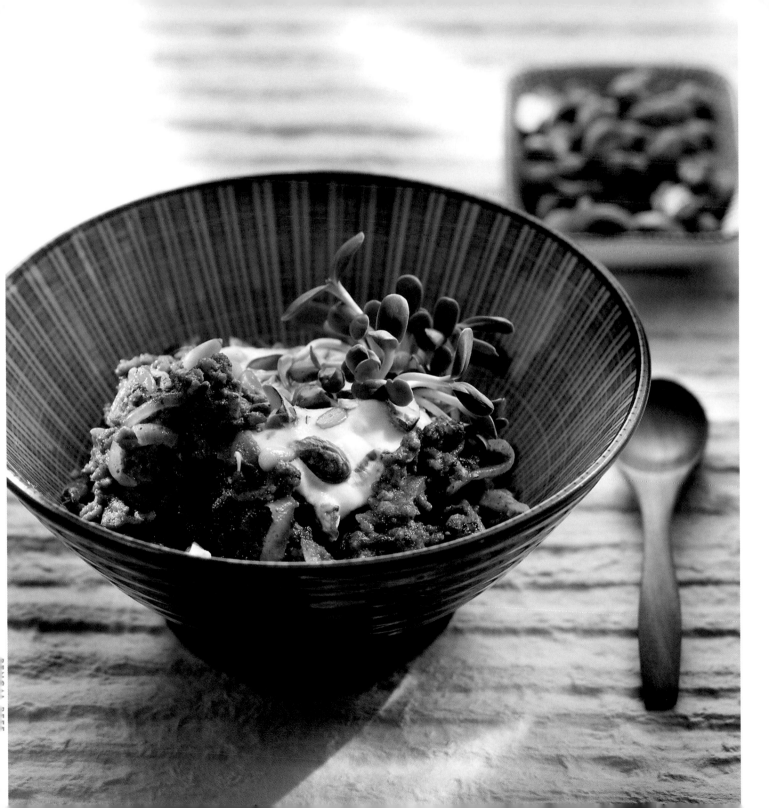

Yakitori chicken brochettes

Preparation time: 1 h 15
Difficulty: average

4 servings

This recipe lends itself perfectly to barbecue cooking. Mirin is a sweet rice wine from Japan. You can find mirin, sancho, and togarashi in Japanese grocery stores, most Asian markets, and at many sushi counters in supermarkets.

8 chicken legs, boned and cut into 2.5 cm (1 in) cubes

8 green onions

Sancho (Japanese pepper) or togarashi (dried red peppers)

8 lemon wedges

YAKITORI SAUCE

60 ml (1/4 cup) sake

80 ml (1/3 cup) soy sauce

1 tbsp sweet rice wine (mirin)

1 tbsp icing sugar

Mix all the sauce ingredients together in a saucepan. Bring to a boil, reduce the heat, and let simmer for 10 minutes uncovered.

Preheat the oven to 200°C (400°F).

Place a lightly oiled rack on a pastry sheet. Spread the chicken cubes on the rack and cook in the oven for approximately 10 minutes, until their juice runs and the chicken starts to brown.

Remove the chicken from the oven and mix well in the sauce. Return to the rack and cook the cubes for 1 minute each side, basting well with the sauce before turning. Remove and set aside.

Place the whole green onions on the rack the chicken was cooked on, and grill slowly for approximately 1 minute on each side, then cut into 2.5 cm (1 in) lengths.

Spear 4 chicken pieces onto each brochette, alternating with 3 green onion sections.

Place the brochettes on a rack and finish cooking in the oven at 140°C (280°F) for approximately 5 minutes, turning and basting the chicken with the sauce. You can also finish the cooking on the barbecue.

Arrange the brochettes on a serving plate, sprinkle with sancho or togarashi, and accompany with the lemon wedges.

 Susan Sylvester, Chef-Instructor at the École hôtelière de la Capitale in Quebecc

yakitori
chicken
brochettes

main
dishes

Tex-Mex chilli

Preparation time: 1 hour
Difficulty: easy

8 to 10 servings

Prepare this dish in advance and reheat just before serving. This recipe is a great idea when friends arrive and you'd rather spend more time with them than alone at the kitchen oven.

Olive oil

2 onions, chopped

3 garlic cloves, minced

1 red pepper, cubed small

1 green pepper, cubed small

250 g (1/2 lb) lean ground beef

1 1/2 tbsp chilli seasoning

1/2 tsp ground cumin

Salt and freshly ground pepper

500 g (2 1/4 cups – 1 540 ml can) red kidney beans, rinsed and drained

200 g (1 cup) rice

500 ml (2 cups) tomato sauce

250 ml (1 cup) water

340 g (2 1/4 cups – 1 540 ml can) stewed canned tomatoes

Heat the olive oil in a Dutch oven. Sauté the onions, garlic, and peppers over medium-high heat.

Add the meat and cook, stirring often.

In a small bowl, mix the seasoning and chilli, cumin and 3 tbsp of water to obtain a paste. Transfer this paste to the Dutch oven and stir well together. Season with salt and pepper to taste.

Add the beans, rice, tomato sauce, water, and the tomatoes. Cover and cook over low heat for 30 minutes without removing the cover.

Remove the cover, stir well, and continue cooking until desired thickness.

 Richard Béliveau

Fusilli al'arrabiata

Preparation time: 45 minutes
Difficulty: easy

4 servings

250 g (1/2 lb) small fusilli

1 tbsp olive oil

1 onion, chopped

2 garlic cloves, sliced

1/2 tsp hot chilli flakes

1 jalapeno pepper, finely chopped

175 g (1 3/4 cups) mushrooms, sliced

2 ripe tomatoes, peeled and diced

225 g (1 1/2 cups) canned crushed tomatoes

1 tbsp balsamic vinegar

1 pinch of sea salt

1 pinch of sugar

1 pinch of Cayenne pepper

8 to 10 fresh basil leaves, cut in thin strips

Heat the olive oil in a skillet and sauté the onion for 2 minutes over medium-high heat.

Add the garlic and the chilli flakes. Stir and cook for 1 minute.

Add the jalapeno pepper and the mushrooms. Stir and cook for 3 to 4 minutes.

Incorporate the tomatoes, vinegar, salt, and sugar.

Bring to a boil, reduce the heat and let simmer for approximately 10 minutes to reduce the sauce.

Add the Cayenne pepper and basil.

Cook the pasta in a large quantity of boiling water for 7 to 10 minutes until tender, but still firm (al dente).

Drain and mix well with the sauce.

 Jean Vachon, Chef-Instructor at the École hôtelière de la Capitale in Quebec

main dishes

Tex-Mex chilli
fusilli
al'arrabiata

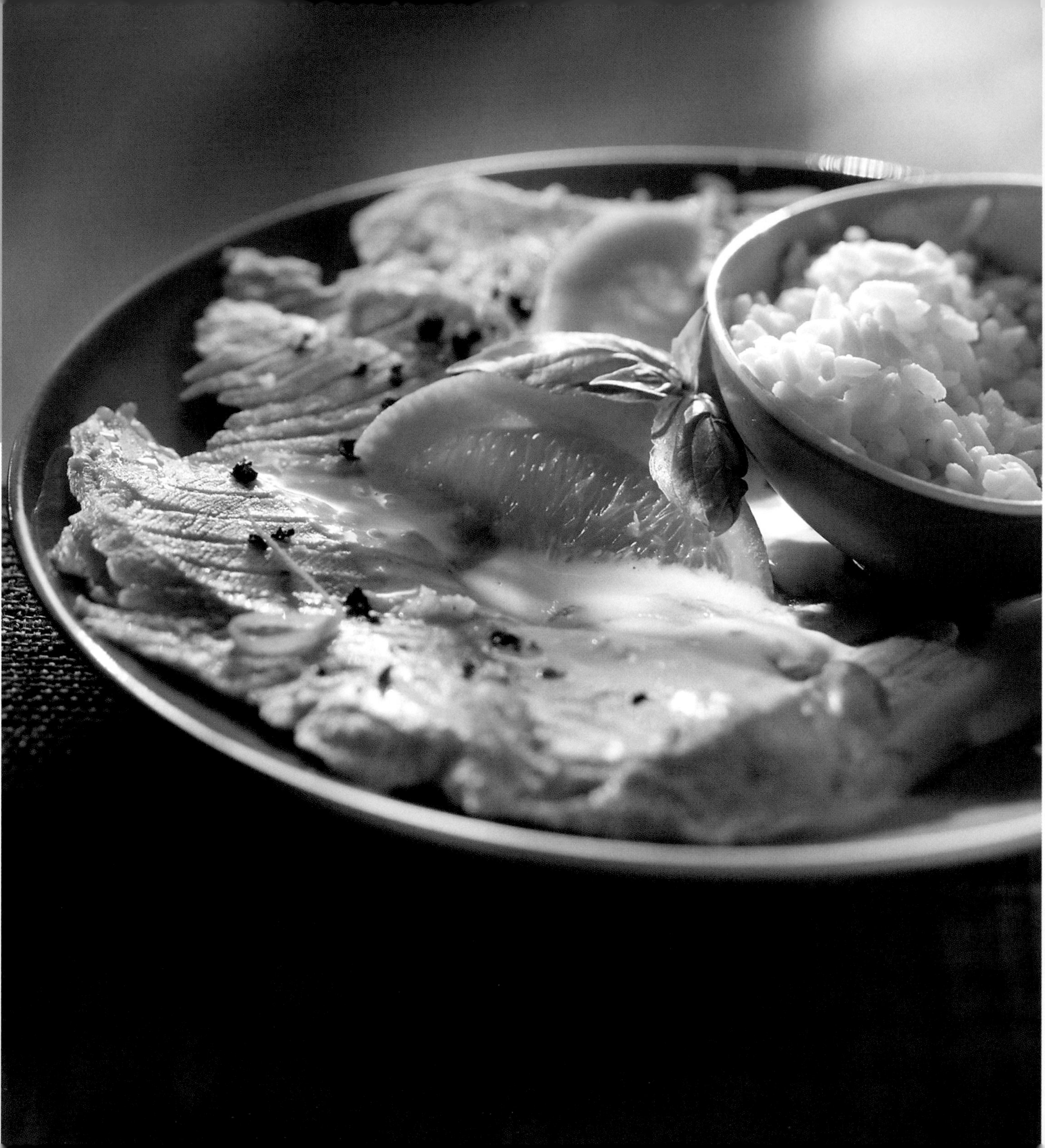

Poached
salmon escalopes in white wine

Preparation time: 30 minutes
Difficulty: average

4 servings

These escalopes are delicious when served with a good quality perfumed rice.

4 salmon escalopes

Zest of half an orange

80 ml (1/3 cup) white wine

CITRUS BUTTER

Juice of one orange, freshly squeezed

Juice of one lemon, freshly squeezed

2 tbsp shallots, shredded

2 tbsp honey

1 tbsp cornstarch

175 ml (3/4 cup) 15 % table cream

Salt and freshly ground pepper

Place the orange and lemon juice in a saucepan. Add the shallots and the honey, and reduce over medium-high heat until the liquid becomes syrupy.

Mix the cornstarch in with the cream. Pour into the saucepan and let simmer for 5 minutes on low heat. Season with salt and pepper to taste.

Preheat the oven to 180°C (350°F).

Grease a roasting pan or pie plate. Lay the escalopes on the bottom, and season with salt and pepper to taste. Add the orange zest and the wine, and cover with aluminium foil.

Bake in the oven for 10 to 15 minutes, until the salmon is cooked to taste. Coat with the citrus butter and serve immediately.

 Christophe Alary, Chef-Instructor at the École hôtelière de la Capitale in Quebec, elected Chef of the Year 2004 by his peers

Grilled
"Mount-Fuji" mackerel

Preparation time: 30 minutes
Difficulty: average

4 servings

4 small mackerel

Salt

1 lemon, sectioned

1 cucumber, julienned

4 lettuce leaves

1 tomato, cut in wedges

Daikon, finely grated

Soy sauce

Gut and clean the fish. Using a sharp knife, carefully make incisions in the skin and add a bit of salt.

Place the fish on the grill, skin side down, and grill until almost cooked. Turn with a spatula and grill until desired doneness.

Serve on individual plates, and garnish each plate with lemon wedges, the cucumber julienne, a lettuce leaf and tomato wedge.

Add the grated daikon in small Mount Fuji mounds and colour with a few drops of soy sauce before serving.

 Joe Nagata, Chef at the Japanese restaurant Ginko in Quebec

main dishes

poached salmon escalopes

grilled mackerel

Salmon fillets in a spinach crust

Preparation time: 45 minutes　　　　　**4 servings**
Difficulty: average

Prepare your fines herbes with your favourite herbs, or use whatever is available.

4 salmon fillets, weighing 150 g (5 oz) each

600 g (1 1/2 lbs) fresh spinach

Salt

Fresh fines herbes (basil, thyme, rosemary, tarragon, oregano, parsley), chopped

Parmesan, fresh grated

Juice of one lemon, freshly squeezed

Steam the spinach, press well to remove any excess liquid, and chop very fine. Heat to dry in a saucepan over medium-high heat. Season with salt to taste.

Spread the spinach on top of the salmon fillets, and add the fines herbes.

Place the fillets in an ovenproof dish and cook at 180°C (350°F) for approximately 20 minutes.

Sprinkle with a bit of Parmesan cheese and place under the broiler to brown. Remove and dribble with the lemon juice, and serve immediately.

 Philippe Castel, elected health-conscious chef by his peers in 2004

Teriyaki salmon

Preparation time: 20 minutes　　　　　**4 servings**
Marinade: 3 hours
Difficulty: easy

Japanese soy sauce is called shoyu when made with roasted cereals (rice, barley, or wheat) and fermented soybean..

4 Atlantic salmon steaks

125 ml (1/2 cup) sweet rice wine (mirin)

125 ml (1/2 cup) Japanese soy sauce (shoyu) or regular soy sauce

Whole green onions (white part only)

Mix the rice wine and soy sauce together in a small bowl.

Place the salmon steaks in a large Ziploc bag, pour in the rice wine mixture and seal well. Marinate in the refrigerator for 3 hours, turning the bag several times.

Cut the green onions lengthwise in 4 and soak for 30 minutes in a bowl of cold water.

Heat the oven broiler.

Remove the salmon steaks from the marinade and place them on a rack over a baking sheet. Broil for 5 minutes, turn the steaks and cook for another 5 minutes or until done.

Serve each portion decorated with the green onion, patted dry.

 Richard Béliveau

salmon fillets in a spinach crust

teriyaki salmon

main dishes

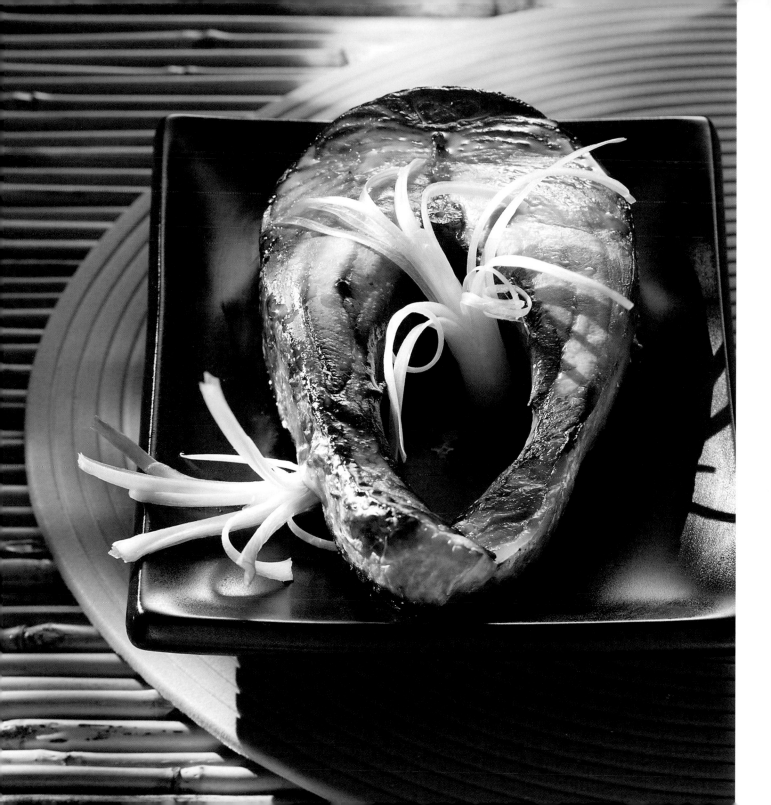

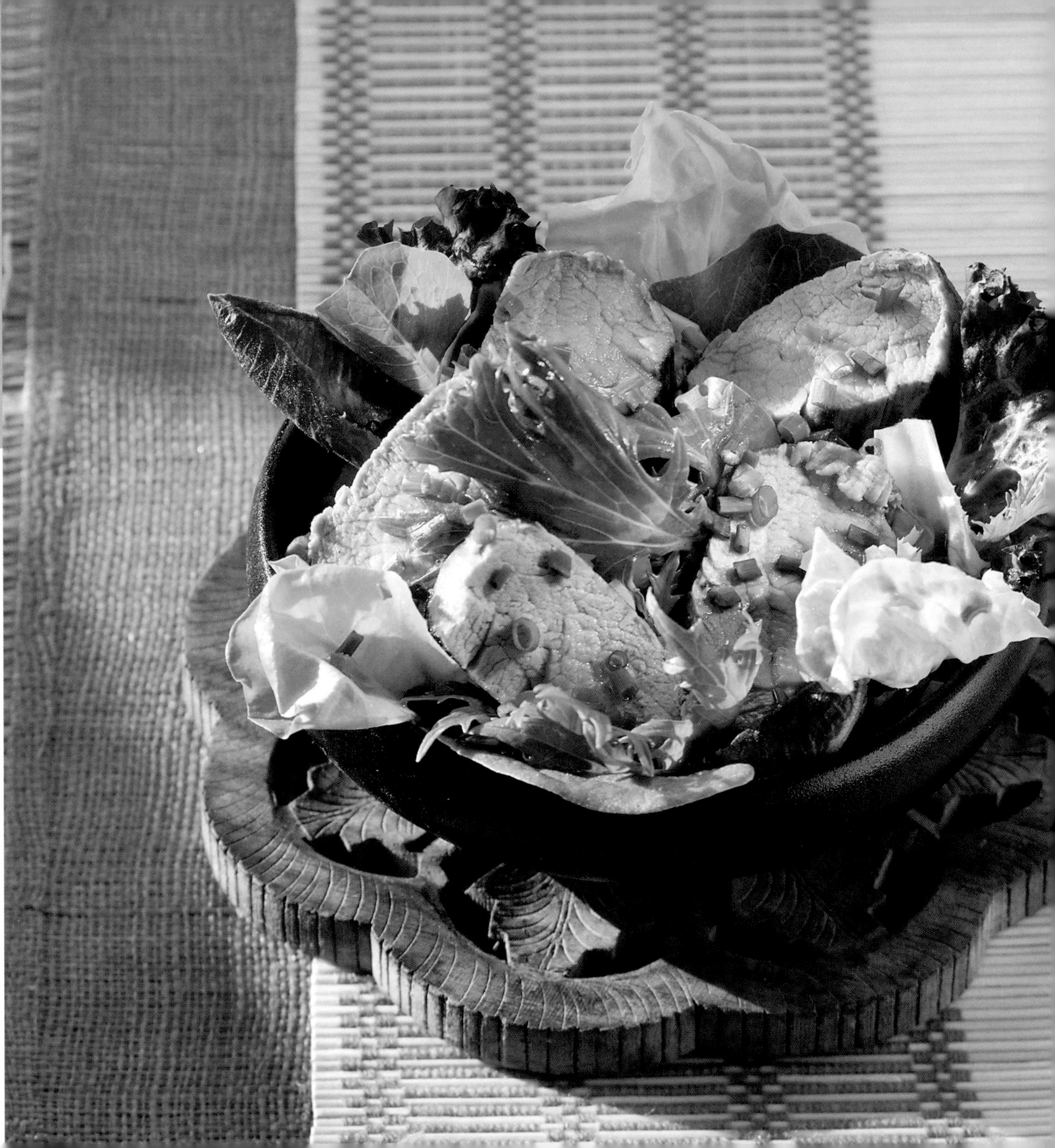

Indonesian pork
on a bed of mixed greens

Preparation time: 1 hour
Marinade: 1 to 2 hours
Difficulty: easy

4 servings

Pork is at its best when the cooked meat is pink, without being rare.

720 g (1 1/2 lbs) pork fillets

300 g (10 oz) very fresh greens (mixed greens)

MARINADE

Juice of one lime, freshly squeezed

2 tbsp Chinese soy sauce

2 tbsp dark brown sugar

2 or 3 garlic cloves, crushed

1 tbsp ground cumin

1 tbsp curry powder

1 tsp ground turmeric

1/2 tsp sambal oelek (see page 142) or hot chilli flakes

1 tbsp sesame oil

2 tbsp olive oil

VINAIGRETTE

125 ml (1/2 cup) olive oil

1 tsp Chinese soy sauce

1 tsp rice wine vinegar

1 tsp fresh chives, finely chopped

Freshly ground pepper

Mix all the marinade ingredients together in a bowl.

Place the pork fillets in a large Ziploc bag and pour in the marinade. Seal the bag and shake to completely coat the meat. Marinate in the refrigerator for 1 to 2 hours, turning frequently.

Remove the fillets from the marinade. In a non-stick skillet, sear the fillets on all sides over high heat. Remove and place on a rack over a shallow roasting pan.

Cook in the oven at 200°C (400°F) in the centre of the oven for approximately 35 minutes.

Mix all the vinaigrette ingredients together in a bowl, pour over the mixed greens, and toss delicately to cover.

Slice the pork fillets into thin slices and serve on the bed of mixed greens.

 Richard Béliveau

main dishes

Indonesian pork on a bed of mixed greens

Indian-flavoured
whitefish fillets

Preparation time: 45 minutes
Difficulty: easy

5 servings

5 whitefish fillets, approximately 125 g (4 oz) each

100 g (1/2 cup) carrots, grated

1 tomato, quartered

1 lime, sliced

MARINADE
1 garlic clove, minced

2 tsp garam masala (recipe page 213)

1/4 tsp chilli flakes

1/2 tsp ground turmeric

Salt

2 tbsp fresh coriander, finely chopped

2 tbsp vegetable oil

Juice of one lemon, freshly squeezed

Place the fish fillets on a lightly oiled baking sheet.

Prepare the marinade, mixing together the garlic, garam masala, chilli, turmeric, salt, and coriander. Incorporate the oil and the lemon juice, whisking well.

Using a pastry brush, coat the fish with the marinade. Cover and place in the refrigerator for approximately 30 minutes.

Preheat the oven to 200°C (400°F).

Cook the fish in the oven, basting often with the cooking juices.

When done, arrange on a serving platter and garnish with the carrots, tomato quarters, and lime slices. Serve immediately.

whitefish fillets

turbot fillets

main dishes

 Jean Vachon, Chef-Instructor at the École hôtelière de la Capitale in Quebec

Turbot fillets
on a bed of red lentils

Preparation time: 30 minutes
Difficulty: easy

4 servings

Serving suggestion: accompany with steamed broccoli florets and lentil shoots.

4 fresh turbot fillets, 125 g (4 oz) each

4 tbsp olive oil

200 g (1 cup) canned red lentils, rinsed and drained

1 shallot, finely chopped

1 tsp ground turmeric

3 garlic cloves, minced

500 ml (2 cups) chicken stock

25 g (3/4 cup) fresh chives, finely chopped

Salt and freshly ground pepper

Heat 2 tbsp of the olive oil in a skillet. Sauté the lentils, shallot, turmeric, and garlic for 2 to 3 minutes over medium-high heat.

Add the stock and cook slowly for 4 minutes. Season with salt and pepper to taste. Add the chives and set aside.

Using a sharp knife, carefully make several incisions in the skin of the turbot.

Heat the remaining 2 tbsp of olive oil in a skillet, and cook the fillets approximately 2 minutes on each side, until the flesh is opaque. Season with salt and pepper to taste.

Serve the fillets on a bed of red lentils.

 Jean-Luc Boulay, Chef-proprietor of the restaurant Le Saint-Amour in Quebec

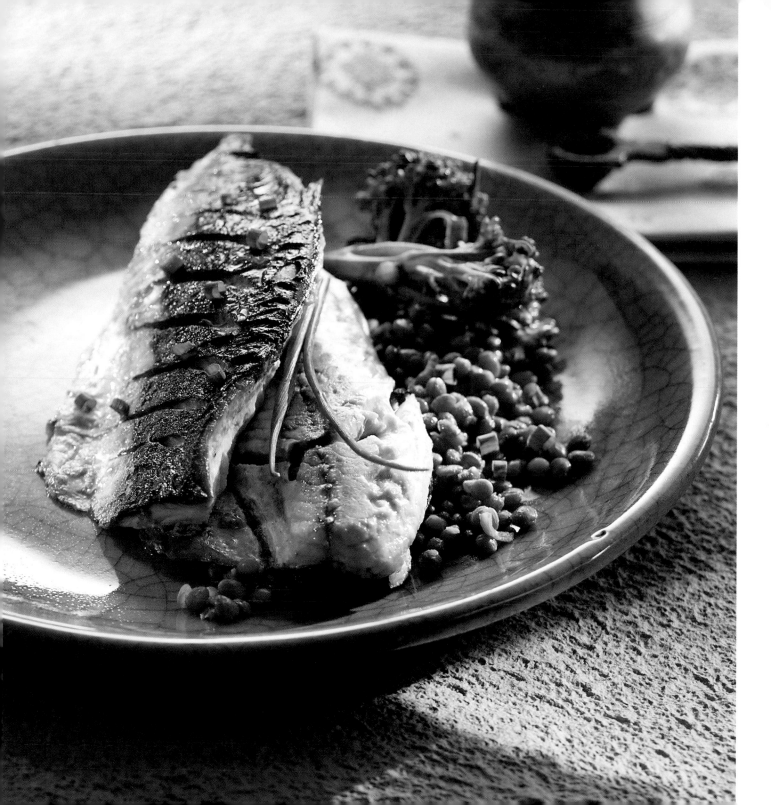

Chilled soba
noodles

Preparation time: 20 minutes
Difficulty: easy

4 servings

Soba noodles are made from buckwheat and common wheat. The Japanese have been making them since the fifteenth century.

250 g (1/2 lb) soba noodles

Green onions, chopped

Fresh coriander, chopped

Sesame seeds

VINAIGRETTE

6 tbsp soy sauce

2 tbsp rice wine vinegar

1 1/2 tsp sesame oil

1 tsp sugar

1 tbsp fresh ginger, chopped

Cook the noodles in boiling water as per package directions. Drain, cover, and set aside in the refrigerator.

Mix all the vinaigrette ingredients together in a small bowl. Verify the seasoning and pour over the cold noodles.

Garnish with green onions, coriander, and sesame seeds to taste.

Susan Sylvester, Chef-Instructor at the École hôtelière de la Capitale in Quebecc

Beijing
noodles

Preparation time: 30 minutes
Difficulty: average

6 servings

Vegetable oil

1 onion, sliced

375 g (3/4 lb) ground pork

4 garlic cloves, minced

1 tsp fresh ginger, chopped

1 tbsp sugar

1 tbsp hoisin sauce

2 tbsp soy sauce

2 tbsp white wine

2 tbsp water

400 g (14 oz) rice noodles

250 g (1/2 lb) bean sprouts, washed and drained

1/3 cucumber, in thin strips

8 radishes, finely sliced

3 pickles, finely sliced

4 green onions, chopped

Hoisin sauce is frequently used in Chinese cooking. It is made with fermented soybeans, spices, and dried peppers. It is thick in texture, with a reddish-brown colour.

Heat the oil in a wok and sauté the onion over high heat. Add the pork, garlic, and ginger. Cook for 3 minutes, and add the sugar, hoisin sauce, and soy sauce.

Add the wine and the water, and simmer for 5 minutes. Remove from heat and set aside.

Cook the noodles in boiling salted water as per package instructions, and drain well.

Shape the noodles into a nest in deep serving plates, and fill the centre with the meat mixture. Arrange the bean sprouts, cucumber, radishes, pickles, and green onions on the plates in a decorative fashion, and serve immediately.

Jean Vachon, Chef-Instructor at the École hôtelière de la Capitale in Quebec

chilled soba
noodles

Beijing
noodles

main
dishes

Sautéed
Indonesian noodles

Preparation time: 25 minutes   **4 servings**
Difficulty: average

Shrimp paste is a popular ingredient in Asian cuisine. Its use is optional in this recipe.

250 g (1/2 lb) Chinese wheat or egg noodles

Vegetable oil

3 garlic cloves, finely chopped

1 onion, sliced

2 tsp shrimp paste (optional)

1 pork chop, boned and cut into strips

250 g (1/2 lb) shrimp, peeled and deveined

2 celery stalks, sliced

2 cabbage leaves, sliced

Salt and freshly ground pepper

2 tbsp light soy sauce

Cook the noodles in boiling salted water as per package instructions. Drain well and set aside.

Heat the oil in a wok and sauté the garlic, onion, and shrimp paste over high heat. Add the pork and the shrimp, and cook for a few more minutes.

Add the celery and the cabbage, and season with salt and pepper to taste.

Mix with the noodles and sprinkle with the soy sauce.

 Jean Vachon, Chef-Instructor at the École hôtelière de la Capitale in Quebec

Soba noodles
with tuna and ginger

Preparation time: 25 minutes   **4 servings**
Difficulty: easy

250 g (1/2 lb) soba noodles

1 tbsp rice wine vinegar

1 tbsp marinated ginger, chopped

80 ml (1/3 cup) vegetable oil

2 tbsp soy sauce

1 tbsp sugar

1 tbsp sesame oil

340 g (12 oz) canned tuna, drained well

80 g (1/2 cup) green onions, finely sliced

40 g (1/2 cup) bean sprouts

2 tbsp sesame seeds, toasted (see page 141)

Cook the noodles in boiling water as per package instructions, and drain well.

In a small bowl, mix the vinegar, ginger, vegetable oil, soy sauce, sugar, and sesame oil together.

Place the noodles in a large serving bowl, and add the tuna, green onions, bean sprouts, and the sesame seeds. Toss with the vinaigrette, mixing well, and serve.

 Yves Moscato, Chef-co-owner of the restaurant 48 St-Paul, Cuisine_monde in Quebec

main dishes

sautéed noodles

soba noodles with tuna and ginger

Miso pasta
with vegetables

Preparation time: 30 minutes
Difficulty: average

4 servings

600 g (3 cups) favourite pasta, cooked

80 ml (1/3 cup) olive oil

150 g (2/3 cup) small broccoli florets

200 g (2 cups) mushrooms, finely sliced

70 g (1/3 cup) carrots, finely sliced

125 ml (1/2 cup) strong chicken stock

2 tbsp undiluted miso

1 tsp fresh ginger, grated

150 g (1 cup) ripe tomatoes, diced

120 g (2/3 cup) green zucchini, diced

2 green onions, finely sliced

3 tsp sesame seeds, toasted (see page 141)

4 tbsp fresh coriander, chopped

4 tsp flaxseed, ground

Heat the olive oil in a skillet. Cook the broccoli, mushrooms, and the carrots over medium-high heat.

Add the stock and the miso, and bring to a boil. Add the pasta, ginger, tomatoes, zucchini, green onions, and the sesame seeds, and simmer slowly until almost all the liquid has evaporated.

Add the coriander and the flaxseed. Verify the seasoning and serve.

 Benoît Dussault, Chef-Instructor at the École hôtelière de la Capitale in Quebec

miso pasta
with vegetables

lamb
kebabs

main
dishes

Lamb kebabs

Preparation time: 1 h 30
Difficulty: average

4 servings

This dish was introduced to India by the Muslims. It quickly became one of the most popular recipes in the country. You can make your own garam masala, or purchase it at the supermarket. Enjoy these kebabs with a mixed lettuce salad.

1 kg (2 lbs) lamb, chopped

1 large onion, coarsely chopped

1 chunk of fresh ginger, 5 cm (2 in), chopped

1 garlic clove, crushed

1 hot green pepper, finely chopped

1 tsp chilli seasoning

1 tbsp fresh coriander, finely chopped

1 tsp garam masala (recipe page 213)

2 tsp ground coriander

1 tsp ground cumin

1 tsp salt

1 egg, beaten

1 tbsp plain yogurt

1 tbsp vegetable oil

Mix all ingredients together in a large bowl, except the yogurt and the oil. Cover and refrigerate for 1 hour.

Preheat the grill.

Dust your hands with flour (to avoid sticking) and divide the mixture into 8 equal portions, rolling each portion into sausage shapes.

Spear the meat sausage onto skewers and place on a large plate. Cover and set aside in the refrigerator.

Lightly brush the brochettes with the yogurt and oil. Cook on the grill for 8 to 10 minutes, turning from time to time, until they are browned.

 Jean Vachon, Chef-Instructor at the École hôtelière de la Capitale in Quebec

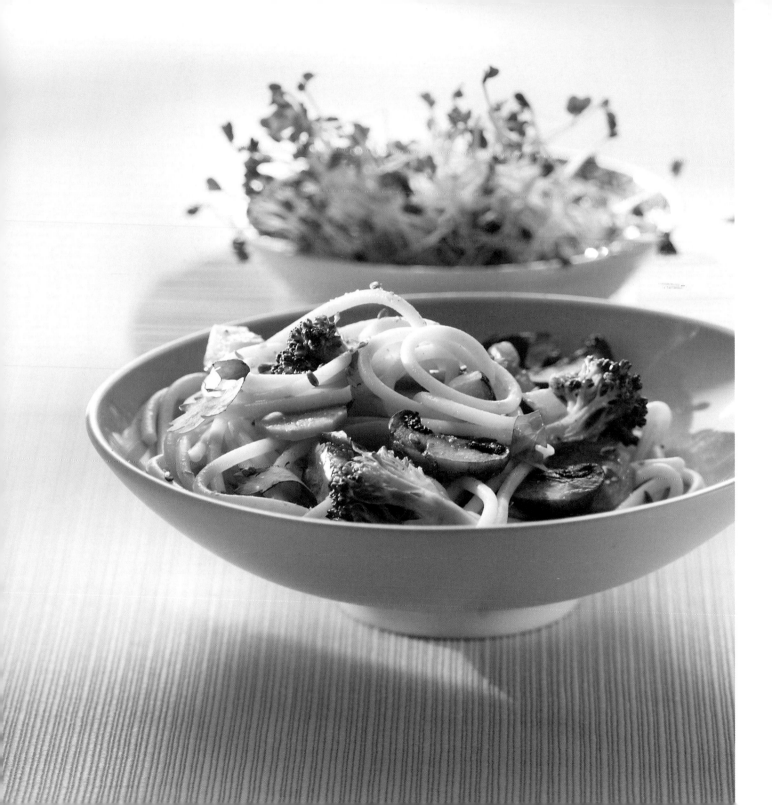

Pissaladière

Preparation time: 1 h 15
Difficulty: average

4 servings

Pissaladière is a speciality from Nice. This recipe replaces the traditional anchovies used in the dish with sardines.

1 bunch fresh parsley

2 sprigs of fresh thyme

1 bay leaf

8 whole black peppercorns

80 ml (1/3 cup) olive oil

1 kg (6 1/4 cups) onions, finely sliced

2 garlic cloves, minced

Salt and freshly ground pepper

400 g (14 oz) shortcrust pastry or 1 commercial pie crust

6 whole canned sardines

50 g (1/3 cup) black olives, finely sliced

Make a bouquet garni by combining the parsley, thyme, bay leaf, and peppercorns in a cheesecloth, and tie well together.

Heat the olive oil in a saucepan. Sweat the onions and garlic with the bouquet garni over low heat. Season with salt and pepper to taste.

Cover and cook for approximately 20 minutes, stirring frequently, without letting it brown. Remove the bouquet garni.

Roll out the pastry and line a greased pie tin.

Cover the pastry with the onions and place the sardines and olives on top. Cook in the oven at 180°C (350°F) for approximately 30 minutes.

Jean-Pierre Cloutier, Chef-proprietor of Café-restaurant du Musée in Quebec

Salmon
and leek papillotes

Preparation time: 30 minutes
Marinade : 1 hour
Difficulty: easy

4 servings

These papillotes are delicious when served with a ratatouille. A menu that will please all your guests!

150 g (5 oz) salmon or mackerel fillets, in strips

80 ml (1/3 cup) olive oil

115 g (3/4 cup) leeks, finely sliced

Juice of one lemon

MARINADE

2 garlic cloves, minced

Juice of one lemon, freshly squeezed

1 tbsp fresh parsley, chopped

2 tsp fresh oregano, chopped

1 pinch of red chilli flakes

Salt and freshly ground pepper

Heat the olive oil and cook the leeks over high heat. Deglaze the pan with the lemon juice.

In a large bowl, mix the leeks with all the marinade ingredients. Add the fish strips, cover, and refrigerate for 1 hour.

Cut 4 sheets of aluminium foil to 30 x 15 cm (12 x 6 in). Divide the fish strips and the leeks equally in the centre of each sheet, and form the papillotes by rolling up the outside corners like a candy wrapper.

Cook in the oven at 165°C (325°F) or on the barbecue for approximately 12 minutes.

Jean-Pierre Cloutier, Chef-proprietor of Café-restaurant du Musée in Quebec

pissaladière
salmon and
leek papillotes

main
dishes

Leek and goat cheese lasagna

Preparation time: 1 h 45
Difficulty: average

6 servings

6 to 8 lasagna pasta sheets

1 eggplant, sliced

2 red peppers, halved and seeded

3 tbsp olive oil

4 leeks, finely sliced

1 zucchini, sliced

200 g (7 oz) soft, unripened goat cheese, crumbled

50 g (1/3 cup) Parmesan, freshly grated

BÉCHAMEL SAUCE

60 g (1/4 cup) butter

100 g (2/3 cup) flour

900 ml (3 2/3 cups) milk

Salt and freshly ground pepper

Grated nutmeg

OLIVE OIL HINT Whenever possible, you should replace butter and other oils with olive oil (first cold pressing, if possible). It is the best fat for your good health, and can be used in cooked dishes as well as in uncooked dishes (vinaigrettes).

BASIC DIP RECIPE

First cold pressed **olive oil** (approximately 125 ml)
3 or 4 garlic cloves, crushed and peeled
Black pepper, salt, parsley, and **thyme** to taste
1/4 tsp **Espelette pepper**, crushed **chili** pepper, or **cayenne**.

Let sit for at least 30 minutes, and savour as a dip with chunks of good whole wheat bread. Can be kept for several weeks in the refrigerator, sealed in an airtight glass container.

Cook the pasta as per package directions.

Lightly salt the eggplant slices, arrange on a rack, and set aside to drain for approximately 20 minutes to remove their excess natural water.

Place the peppers on a roasting pan, skin side up, and broil in the oven until their skin blackens. Remove and let stand to cool before peeling and finely slicing.

Rinse the eggplant slices under cold water and pat dry with paper towel.

Heat the olive oil in a skillet and sauté the leeks, zucchini, peppers, and eggplant for approximately 5 minutes over medium-high heat.

In a saucepan, prepare the béchamel sauce by melting the butter over medium-low heat. Whisk in the flower and cook approximately 2 minutes, whisking constantly. Pour in the milk and cook over medium heat, whisking constantly until the sauce thickens. Season with salt and pepper, and ground nutmeg to taste.

Layer the lasagna sheets in a greased ovenproof dish, alternating with layers of the vegetables, goat cheese, Parmesan, and béchamel sauce. End with a final layer of sauce and sprinkle with the Parmesan.

 Jean Vachon, Chef-Instructor at the École hôtelière de la Capitale in Quebec

main dishes

leek and goat cheese lasagna

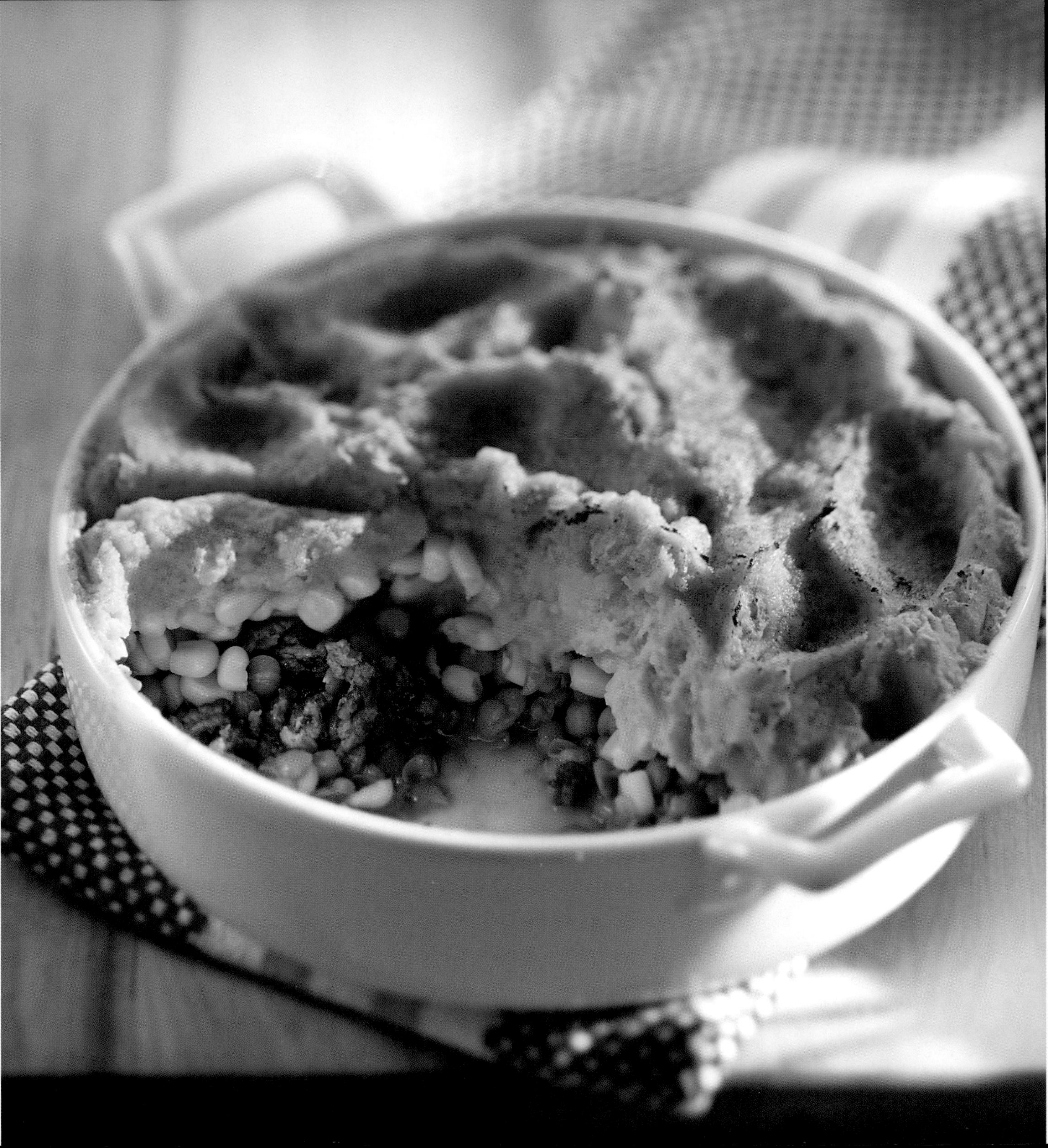

Shepherd's pie
with lentils

Preparation time: 1 h 15   4 to 6 servings
Difficulty: easy

Here's a new twist to a classic Quebec dish.

2 small potatoes, quartered
2 carrots, sliced
1 cauliflower, separated into small florets
Olive oil
3 or 4 garlic cloves
1 large onion, chopped
250 g (1/2 lb) lean ground beef
475 g (2 1/4 cups – 1 540 ml can) canned green lentils, rinsed and drained
1 tsp savory or dried thyme
1 tbsp dried parsley
Salt and freshly ground pepper
285 g (1 1/2 cups) cream or niblet corn
1 tsp butter, cut in squares

Preheat the oven to 180°C (350°F).

In a saucepan, cook the potatoes and the carrots for approximately 20 minutes. Cook the cauliflower in the microwave oven for 8 to 10 minutes (with 2 tbsp water), or steam them.

Meanwhile, heat the olive oil in a large skillet, and sauté the garlic and onion over medium-high heat for approximately 5 minutes, until they are tender. Add the beef and cook, stirring. When the meat is cooked, add the lentils, savory, and the parsley. Season with salt and pepper to taste. Stir for 2 to 3 minutes, remove from the heat and set aside.

Drain the potatoes, carrots, and cauliflower. Purée, and season with salt and pepper to taste.

Transfer the meat and lentil mixture to an ovenproof dish. Cover with the corn and then add a layer of the vegetable purée.

Dot with small pats of butter and bake uncovered in the oven for 30 minutes, or until the crust turns golden.

 Richard Béliveau

Sicilian-style
Spaghetti

Preparation time: 1 hour   4 servings
Difficulty: average

300 g (10 oz) spaghetti
3 tbsp olive oil
2 red peppers, diced
8 Italian tomatoes, diced
1 eggplant, diced
1 onion, chopped
2 garlic cloves, minced
80 ml (1/3 cup) water
80 ml (1/3 cup) red wine
30 g (1 cup) fresh basil, chopped (save a bit for the garnish)
30 g (1 cup) fresh flat-leaf parsley, chopped
50 g (1/4 cup) anchovies, diced small
12 black olives, finely sliced
2 tbsp capers
Salt and freshly ground pepper
Parmesan, freshly grated

Heat the olive oil and cook the peppers, tomatoes, eggplant, onion, and garlic for 10 to 15 minutes.

Add the water, wine, basil, and parsley. Bring to a boil, cover, and let simmer for 10 to 15 minutes.

Meanwhile, cook the pasta as per package directions.

Add the anchovies, olives, and the capers to the saucepan containing the peppers. Season with salt and pepper to taste, and cook for several minutes.

Serve over the pasta and garnish with freshly grated Parmesan and the remaining basil.

 Jean Vachon, Chef-Instructor at the École hôtelière de la Capitale in Quebec

main dishes

shepherd's pie
with lentils

Sicilian-style
spaghetti

Turmeric-curry
chicken

Preparation time: 40 minutes   **4 servings**
Difficulty: easy

Serve this dish with Basmati rice or another whole cooked cereal.

4 whole chicken breasts, 150 g (5 oz) each, fat and skin removed

2 tbsp olive oil

3 garlic cloves

4 shallots, sliced

2 tsp curry powder

1 tsp ground turmeric

2 tbsp fish sauce (nuoc-mâm or nam pla)

2 tbsp brown sugar

500 ml (2 cups) coconut milk

Freshly ground pepper

Heat the olive oil in a large skillet. Sauté the garlic and shallots 2 to 3 minutes over medium heat. Add all other ingredients and mix well. Let simmer slowly for approximately 20 minutes.

Slice the cooked chicken into thin strips and serve immediately.

 Florence Albernhe, Chef-proprietor of Le Grain de riz in Quebec

Cashew
chicken

Preparation time: 30 minutes   **4 servings**
Difficulty: easy

300 g (10 oz) chicken breast, cut in strips

Flour

175 ml (3/4 cup) corn or peanut oil

10 green onions

4 red peppers, dried, cut 1 cm (1/2 in)

2 tbsp garlic, crushed

60 g (1/2 cup) cashew nuts, unsalted, toasted

80 g (1/2 cup) onion, sliced

3 tbsp oyster sauce

3 tbsp soy sauce

2 tbsp sugar

Dust the chicken strips with flour. Heat the oil in a wok and cook the chicken over medium-high heat. Remove from the oil and drain on paper towels.

Fry the onions in the same oil. Add all other ingredients except the chicken, and simmer for 2 to 3 minutes. Add the chicken to the sauce, stir to mix well, and serve immediately.

 Jean Vachon, Chef-Instructor at the École hôtelière de la Capitale in Quebec

tumeric-curry
chicken

cashew
chicken

**main
dishes**

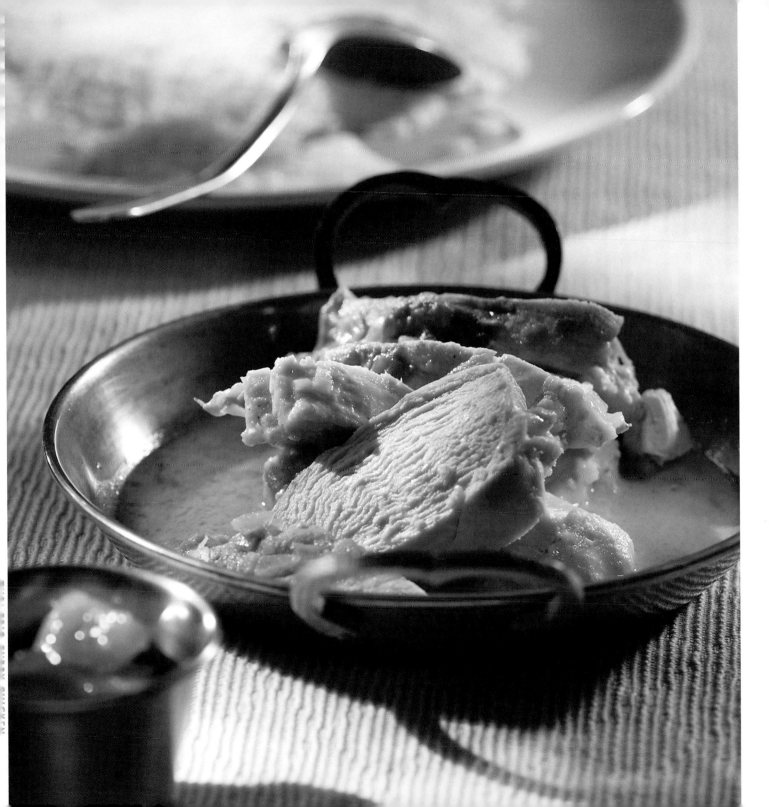

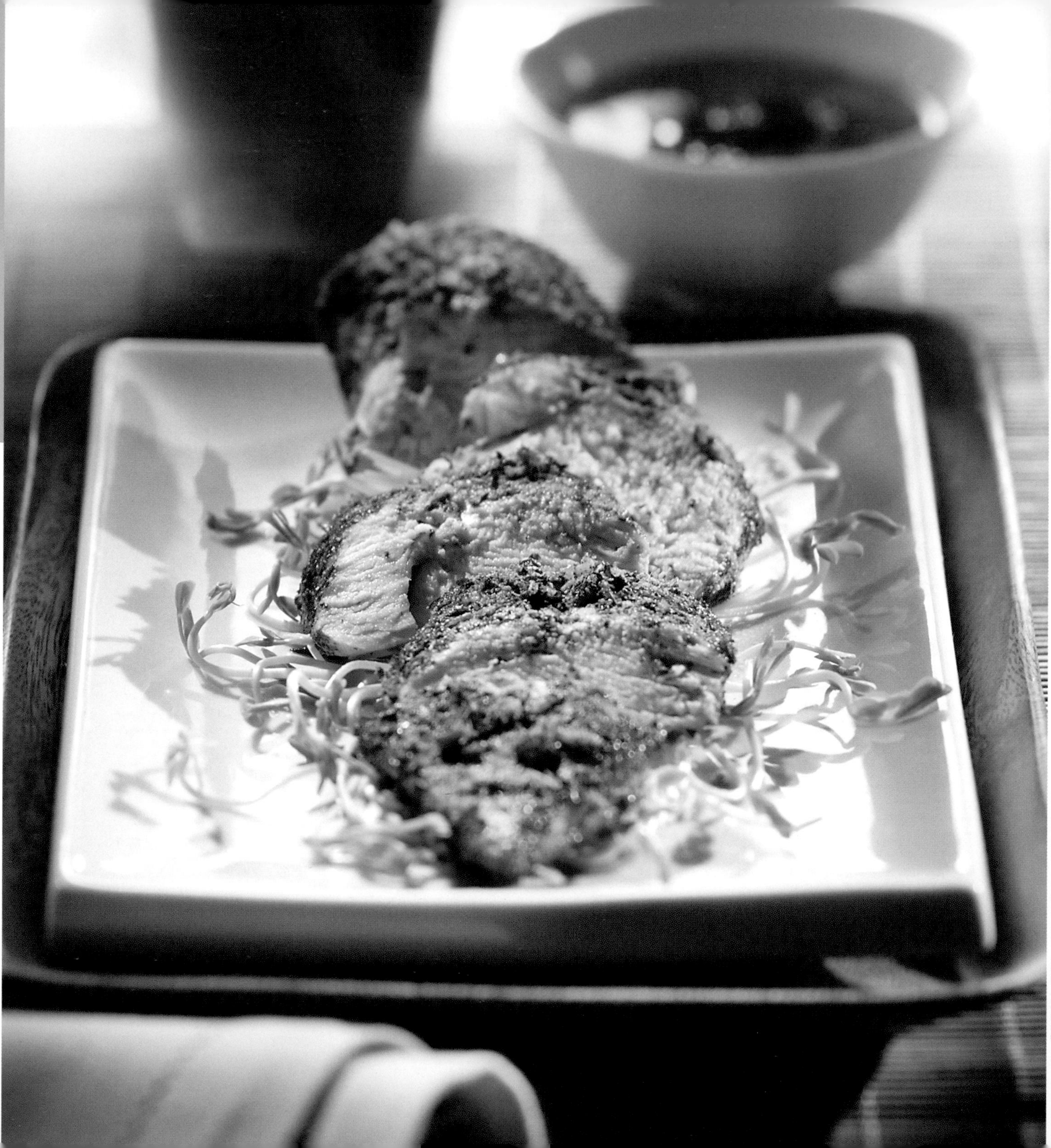

Green tea–crusted chicken

Preparation time: 40 minutes
Difficulty: easy

4 servings

This crust can be kept up to three weeks in an airtight container in the refrigerator. Sencha tea is a green tea from Japan that is gaining in popularity around the world. After harvesting, the leaves are steamed and rolled.

4 whole chicken breasts, 150 g (5 oz) each, fat and skin removed

2 tbsp olive oil

COATING

2 tbsp Japanese green tea (preferably Sencha) not infused

2 tbsp fresh mint

60 g (1/4 cup) lemongrass, ground

3/4 tsp salt

3/4 tsp brown sugar

2 tbsp orange zest

2 tbsp lemon zest

2 tbsp fresh ginger, grated

1/2 tsp ground cumin

Mix all the coating ingredients in a bowl.

Coat the chicken breasts well with the mixture.

Heat the oil in a large skillet, and sear the chicken for 2 minutes on each side.

Transfer to an ovenproof dish and cook in the oven at 180°C (350°F) for approximately 15 minutes, according to thickness.

 Florence Albernhe, Chef-proprietor of Le Grain de riz in Quebec

---

Sautéed chicken with peanuts

Preparation time: 30 minutes
Difficulty: easy

4 to 6 servings

Serve this chicken on a bed of steamed perfumed rice.

500 g (1 lb) chicken (breasts), finely sliced

2 tbsp cassava starch (tapioca)

160 g (1 cup) snow peas, stemmed

60 ml (1/4 cup) vegetable oil

80 g (1/2 cup) onions, cut in strips

60 g (1/2 cup) red peppers, cut in strips

2 tbsp green curry paste

4 tbsp fish sauce (nuoc-mâm or nam pla)

1 tbsp brown sugar

15 g (1/2 cup) fresh basil, shredded

60 g (1/2 cup) toasted peanuts, chopped

Dust the chicken strips with the starch and plunge in boiling water for 45 seconds.

Blanch the snow peas in boiling water in another saucepan for 1 minute, drain and rinse under cold water to stop cooking.

Heat the wok over high heat, pour in the oil, and sauté the snow peas, onions, peppers, and chicken strips for approximately 10 minutes.

Incorporate the curry paste, fish sauce, brown sugar, basil, and half the peanuts. Mix well.

Garnish with the remaining peanuts and serve immediately.

 Jean Vachon, Chef-Instructor at the École hôtelière de la Capitale in Quebec

main dishes

green tea–crusted chicken

sautéed chicken with peanuts

Salmon pavé
on crispy cabbage

Preparation time: 40 minutes   4 servings
Difficulty: easy

1 piece of salmon, 600 g (1 1/4 lbs)

1 kg (6 cups) Scotch kale (green cabbage), sliced

3 tbsp olive oil

1 tbsp cumin seed

Salt and freshly ground pepper

175 ml (3/4 cup) tomato sauce

1 garlic clove, finely chopped

Blanch the kale for 1 minute in boiling water. Cool under running water and drain well.

Heat the olive oil in a skillet. Sauté the cabbage over high heat with the cumin for 1 to 2 minutes. Season with salt and pepper to taste.

Cut the salmon into 4 equal fillets. Season with salt and pepper to taste, and steam until done.

Heat the tomato sauce and add the garlic.

Form a nest with the cooked cabbage in the centre of individual warmed serving plates, top with portions of salmon, and coat with a stream of the tomato sauce.

 Jean-Luc Boulay, Chef-proprietor of the restaurant Le Saint-Amour in Quebec

Arctic char
tartare

Preparation time: 25 minutes   4 servings
Difficulty: easy

You can replace the Arctic char with trout or salmon. Why not garnish this dish with 4 slices of black radish or cocoyam fried in 3 tbsp of vegetable oil and 2 tsp of lumpfish caviar?

1 320 g (11 oz) Arctic char fillet (very fresh), cubed small

1 egg yolk

1 tbsp Dijon mustard

2 tbsp old-fashioned strawberry vinegar or other vinegar

2 tbsp olive oil

Salt and freshly ground pepper

1 green onion, finely chopped

5 strawberries, cut into small cubes

8 dill sprigs, chopped

Whisk the egg yolk, mustard, and vinegar together in a bowl. Incorporate the olive oil very slowly, whisking vigorously to make a mayonnaise. Season with salt and pepper to taste. Cover and set aside in the refrigerator.

Combine the fish, green onion, strawberries, and dill together in a large bowl.

Incorporate the mayonnaise and stir until the mixture is smooth. Verify the seasoning and serve.

 Jean-Pierre Cloutier, Chef-proprietor of Café-restaurant du Musée in Quebec

salmon pavé
arctic char
tartare

**main
dishes**

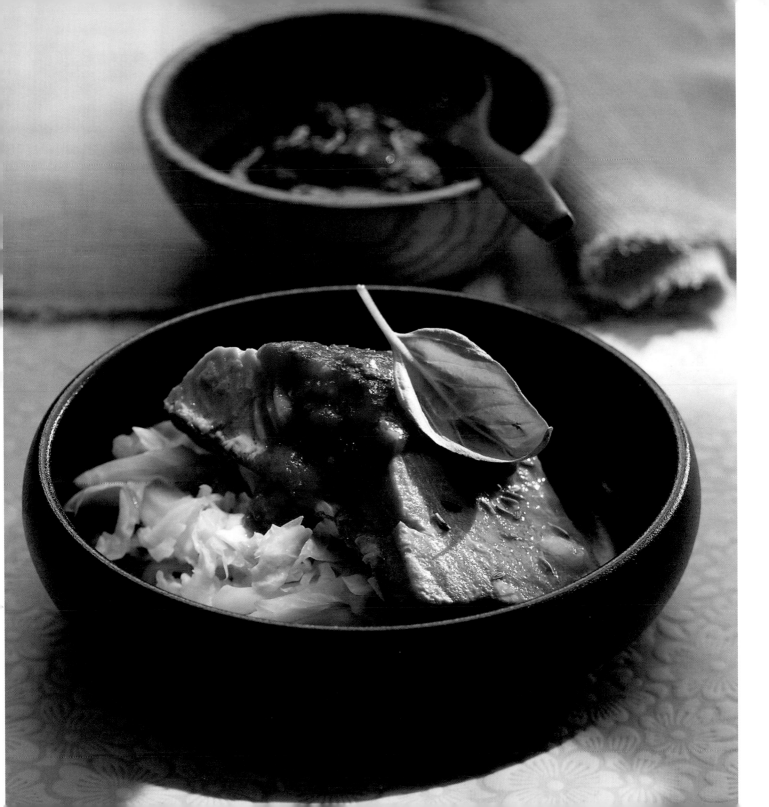

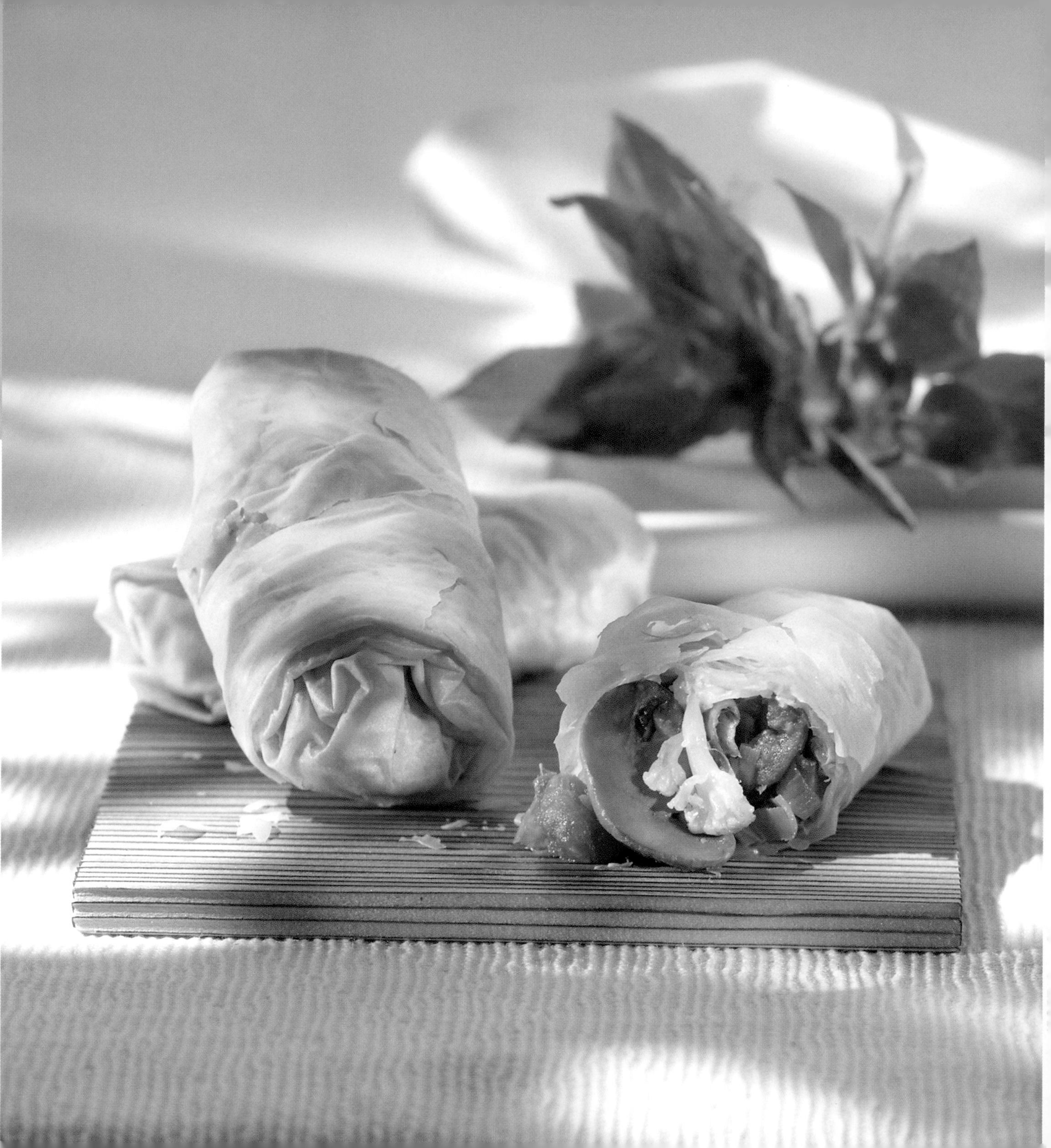

Beet greens pie

Preparation time: 1 hour
Difficulty: average

4 servings

3 tbsp olive oil

1 small onion, sliced

1 garlic clove, finely chopped

Approximately 250 g (1/2 lb) beet greens or Swiss chard, cut in sections

7 g (1/4 cup) fresh flat-leaf parsley, chopped

Juice of half a lemon, freshly squeezed

1 homemade or commercial pie crust

80 ml (1/3 cup) milk

2 eggs

1 pinch of ground nutmeg

60 g (1/2 cup) pine nuts, toasted (see page 206)

2 tbsp dried tomatoes, chopped

Salt and freshly ground pepper

Preheat the oven to 180°C (350°F). Heat the olive oil in a skillet over medium heat. Sauté the onion and garlic until they turn translucent.

Add the beet leaves, parsley, and lemon juice. Season with salt and pepper to taste. Cook over medium-high heat for several minutes to soften the leaves. Remove from the heat and set aside to cool.

Line a 25 cm (10 in) pie tin with the pastry, cover with aluminium foil, and weigh down with dried peas. Cook in the oven for 10 minutes. Remove the peas and the paper, and cook an additional 10 minutes (the crust must be dry without browning).

Mix the milk, eggs, and nutmeg together in a bowl. Add the beet leaves, pine nuts, and the dried tomatoes. Season with salt and pepper to taste.

Pour the mixture into the pie crust and bake in the over for approximately 20 minutes.

Serve hot, warm, or cold.

 Susan Sylvester, Chef-Instructor at the École hôtelière de la Capitale in Quebecc

Vegetable strudels

Preparation time: 1 hour
Difficulty: average

4 servings
or 12 strudels

2 tbsp olive oil

1 leek (green and white parts), sliced

2 garlic cloves, minced

1/2 medium cauliflower, separated into very small florets

100 g (1 cup) white mushrooms, finely sliced

1 medium tomato, diced

1 tbsp garam masala (recipe page 213)

1 tsp chilli seasoning

1 tbsp ground turmeric

Salt and freshly ground pepper

60 g (1/4 cup) butter, melted

12 phyllo pastry sheets

Heat the olive oil in a skillet. Sauté the leek, garlic, and cauliflower over medium heat for approximately 3 minutes, stirring constantly.

Add all other ingredients, except the butter and phyllo pastry. Cook over medium heat for 5 to 7 minutes.

Spread out the phyllo pastry and brush each sheet with the melted butter. Fold each sheet in four.

Spoon a bit of the vegetable garnish onto the centre of each sheet, and roll to form a cigar shape, taking care to seal in the garnish. Brush the exterior with the melted butter.

Arrange the strudels on a baking sheet and cook in the centre of the oven at 180°C (350°F) for 15 to 20 minutes. Serve hot.

 Marlène Gagnon, Chef-Instructor at the École hôtelière de la Capitale in Quebec

main dishes

beet greens pie

vegetable strudels

Tomato pie

Preparation time: 45 minutes
Difficulty: easy

4 servings

This dish is especially good accompanied by a spinach salad.

1 homemade or commercial 23 cm (9 in) savoury pie crust, uncooked

4 tbsp Dijon mustard

150 g (1 cup) cheese (mozzarella, cheddar, or Swiss), grated

4 ripe tomatoes, sliced

Salt and freshly ground pepper

2 garlic cloves, minced

7 g (1/4 cup) fresh chives, chopped

7 g (1/4 cup) fresh basil, chopped

A stream of olive oil

Preheat the oven to 180°C (350°F).

Brush the bottom of the pastry shell with the mustard. Add the cheese and top with the tomato slices. Season with salt and pepper to taste, and add the garlic.

Cook in the oven for 20 to 30 minutes, until the pastry turns golden.

Remove from the oven, add the chives and basil, and sprinkle with the olive oil.

 Marlène Gagnon, Chef-Instructor at the École hôtelière de la Capitale in Quebec

Pakchoi pie

Preparation time: 1 h 30
Difficulty: average

6 servings

Toast the pine nuts in a dry, non-stick skillet, shaking constantly until well toasted. You can also roast them on a baking sheet in the oven 180°C (350°F), stirring every 3 minutes until they reach the desired colour. Take care not to burn them.

300 g (1 3/4 cups) pakchoi

2 tbsp olive oil

200 g (1 1/4 cups) leek white, sliced

100 g (2/3 cup) onions, finely sliced

200 g (1 cup) yellow apples, sliced

30 g (1/4 cup) pine nuts, toasted

3 tbsp raisins

3 eggs, beaten

400 g (14 oz) homemade shortcrust pastry or 2 commercial pie crusts

Sesame seeds

Cook the pakchoi 1 minute in boiling water. Drain and press firmly to extract the water, and chop coarsely.

Heat the olive oil in a saucepan. Sauté the leek, onions, and apples for 10 minutes over medium-high heat.

Add the pakchoi and cook until all the liquid is evaporated. Incorporate the pine nuts, raisins, and eggs, and mix well.

Line a pie plate with half the pastry. Spread the vegetable mixture in the pie plate and cover with the second layer of pastry. Seal well, pinching outside edges firmly.

Brush the top with an egg wash and sprinkle with sesame seeds. Bake in the oven for 45 minutes at 180°C (350°F).

 Philippe Coudroy, Chef-Instructor at the École hôtelière de la Capitale in Quebec

tomato
pie
pakchoi
pie

main
dishes

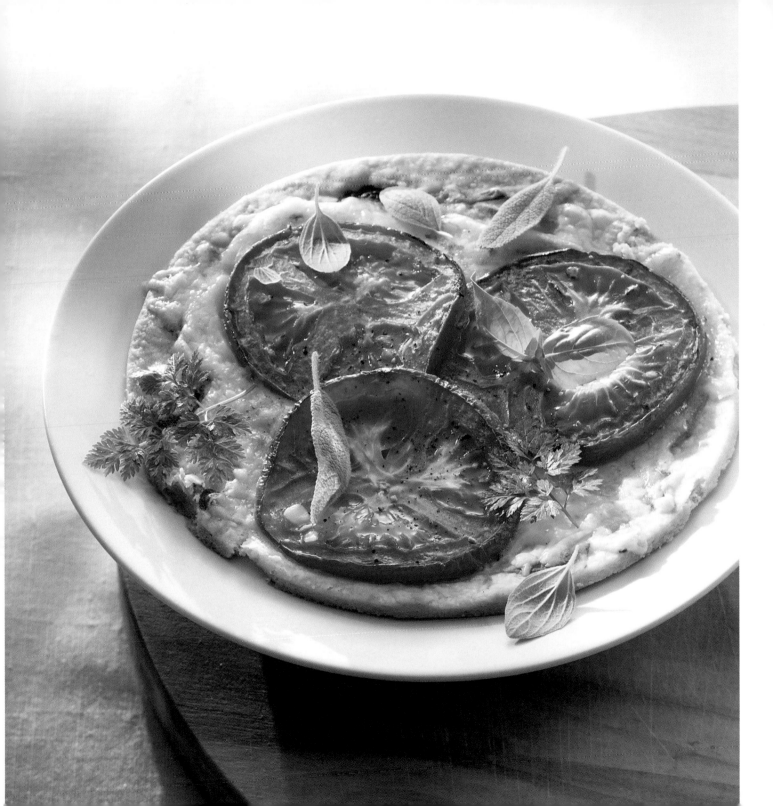

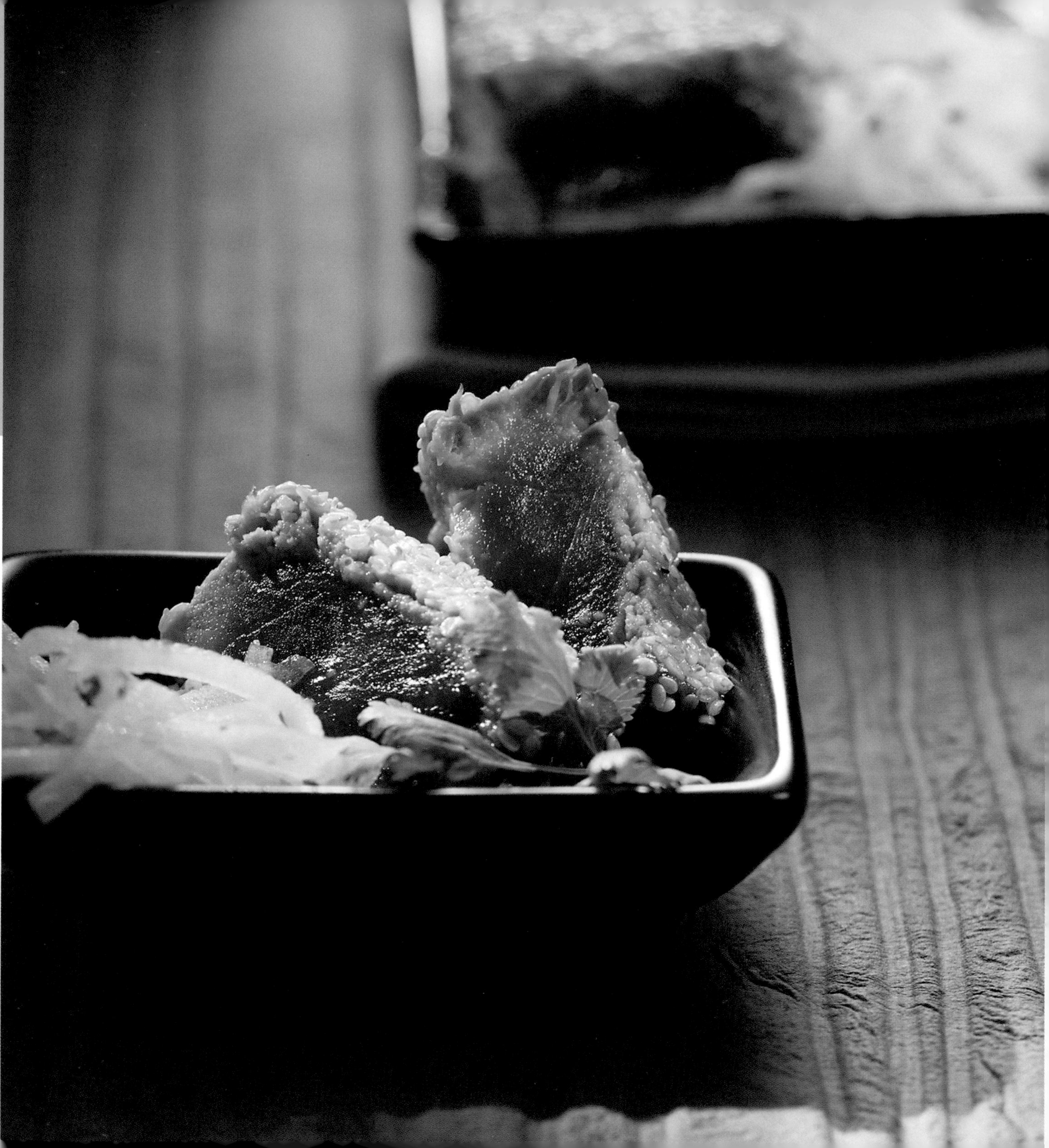

Tian
of Savoy cabbage

Preparation time: 1 h 15   **8 servings**
Difficulty: average

1 Savoy cabbage (core removed)
1 tbsp vegetable oil
600 g (1 1/4 lbs) minced veal
Salt and freshly ground pepper
3 garlic cloves, minced
4 carrots, grated
2 tbsp fresh parsley, chopped
4 potatoes, finely sliced
100 g (2/3 cup) Gruyère cheese, grated

Separate the cabbage leaves individually.

Fill a large stock pot with water and bring to a boil. Immerse the first 8 cabbage leaves in the water and boil for 1 to 2 minutes. Remove and set aside in a large bowl.

Chop the remaining leaves, taking care to remove the centres (hardest part of the leaf).

Sear the meat in the oil. Season with salt and pepper to taste.

Add the garlic and mix well. Then add the chopped cabbage and carrots. Season with salt and pepper to taste. Cook, stirring frequently, for approximately 5 minutes, until all the cooking liquid has evaporated. Add the parsley at the end of cooking.

Line a deep mould with 4 of the blanched cabbage leaves and half the potatoes. Cover with half of the cheese, and add half of the cooked cabbage mixture. Sprinkle with the grated cheese.

Cover again with another layer of potatoes, and add the remaining cooked cabbage. Cover all with the 4 remaining blanched cabbage leaves.

Press the mould firmly and cover with aluminium paper.

Place the mould on a pastry rack and bake in the oven for 35 to 40 minutes at 180°C (350°F).

 Christophe Alary, Chef-Instructor at the École hôtelière de la Capitale in Quebec, elected Chef of the Year 2004 by his peers

Tuna tataki
on a bed of daikon

Preparation time: 45 minutes   **4 servings**
Difficulty: average

Daikon is a delicately flavoured variety of Japanese radish, highly prized in Japan.

250 g (1/2 lb) sushi grade red tuna
225 g (1 1/2 cups) daikon, grated or finely julienned
2 tbsp orange juice, freshly squeezed
6 tbsp olive oil
2 tbsp fresh coriander, finely chopped
Salt and freshly ground pepper
60 ml (1/4 cup) soy sauce
50 g (1/4 cup) honey
2 tsp ground ginger
30 g (1/4 cup) sesame seeds
1 tsp sesame oil

In a large bowl, mix the daikon together with the orange juice, 2 tbsp olive oil, and the coriander. Season with salt and pepper to taste. Cover and set aside in the refrigerator.

Simmer the soy sauce, honey, and ginger in a small saucepan until it reaches a syrupy consistency.

Coat the tuna with the sesame seeds.

Heat 4 tbsp of olive oil over high heat in a non-stick skillet, and sear the tuna for 1 minute on all sides.

Remove from heat and cut the tuna into thin slices, and arrange on a serving dish. Coat with the caramelized soy mixture, and serve with the cooled daikon and 3 or 4 drops of sesame oil.

 Christophe Alary, Chef-Instructor at the École hôtelière de la Capitale in Quebec, elected Chef of the Year 2004 by his peers

main dishes

tian of Savoy cabbage

tuna tataki on a bed of daikon

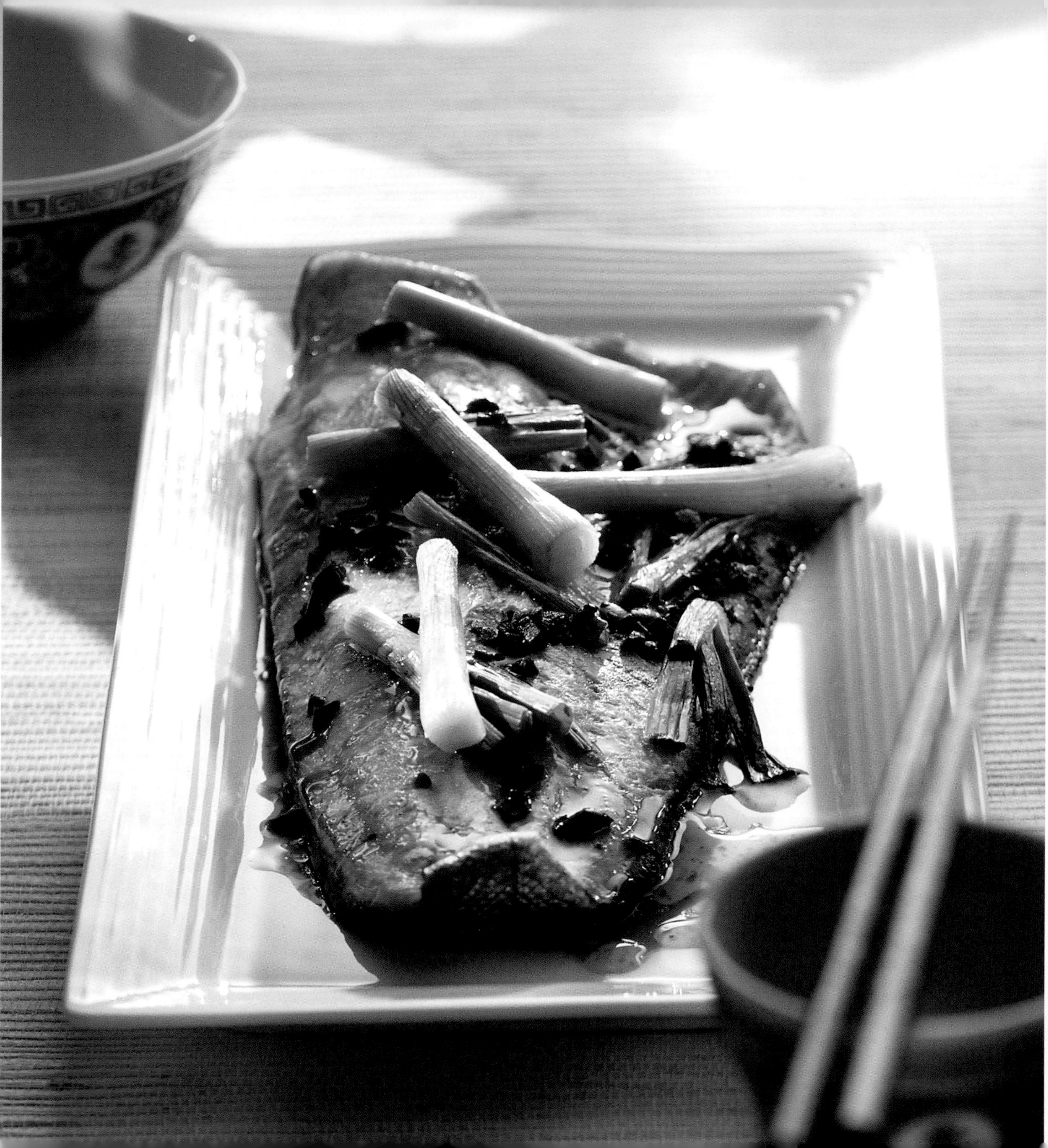

STEAMED CHINESE-STYLE TROUT

Seaweed-
stuffed tofu

6 servings

Preparation time: 45 minutes (+ 2 hours wait time)
Difficulty: average

Dried seaweed (ogonori, ao tosaka nori, aka tosaka nori, wakamc)

1 onion, finely sliced

2 blocks of firm tofu

1 green onion, cut small

1/2 tomato, cubed or finely sliced

VINAIGRETTE

Salt and freshly ground pepper

1 tsp rice wine vinegar

1 tsp lemon juice, freshly squeezed

1 tbsp balsamic vinegar

1 tsp soy sauce

1 tbsp olive oil

2 tbsp sesame oil

Hichimi pepper

Soak the seaweed for 5 to 10 minutes in cold water. Drain, pat dry, and cut into bite-size pieces.

Prepare the vinaigrette, mixing all ingredients together.

Separate the onion rings from each other in a bowl of cold water. Drain and pat dry.

Wrap the tofu chunks in paper towel, and weigh them down without crushing them, to extract as much water as possible. Set aside to drain for 2 hours. Then spoon out a hole in each of the tofu chunks with a small spoon, and chop the separated tofu together with the green onions.

Mix the tomato and the onion together with the seaweed, and stuff the tofu blocks with this mixture. Arrange on a serving platter and sprinkle with the vinaigrette (or serve in individual bowls), and top with the tofu and green onion mixture.

 Joe Nagata, Chef at the Japanese restaurant Ginko in Quebec City

Steamed
Chinese-style trout

4 servings

Preparation time: 45 minutes
Difficulty: average

Fermented black beans are used as a condiment in Asian cooking. You can find them in Asian groceries or natural food stores. They can be kept for at least one year in a cool, dry location.

4 trout fillets, 240 to 360 g (1/2 to 3/4 lb) each, cleaned well

1 tbsp fermented black beans

2 tbsp soy sauce

3 tbsp Sherry

1 tsp sesame oil

1 tbsp fresh ginger, finely chopped

1/2 tsp sugar

2 green onions, cut in 5 cm (2 in) lengths

Place the fish fillets in a deep dish.

Rinse the black beans under cold water and chop coarsely. Mix with the soy sauce, Sherry, sesame oil, ginger, and sugar, and pour over the trout. Sprinkle with the green onions.

Bring water to a boil in a double boiler. Place the dish with the fish in a steamer, ensuring that the plate does not touch the sides of the steamer. Cover and cook approximately 8 minutes per centimetre or half inch thickness. Verify doneness by inserting a knife in the back of the fish.

Turn off the heat, remove the cover, and let the steam dissipate before removing the plate. Serve the fish with the cooking juice.

 Susan Sylvester, Chef-Instructor at the École hôtelière de la Capitale in Quebec

main
dishes

seaweed-
stuffed tofu

steamed
trout

Thai spring roll sauce

Preparation time: 30 minutes
Difficulty: average

Approximately 750 ml

Use this sauce with dumplings (see recipe on page 141).

625 ml (2 1/2 cups) water

240 g (1 cup) sugar

1 tbsp sake

3 tbsp rice wine vinegar

2 tsp fresh ginger, finely grated

100 g (1/2 cup) carrots, fine julienne

1 tsp hot pepper seeds, or to taste

2 tsp garlic, finely chopped

1/2 tsp soy sauce

Mix 500 ml (2 cups) of the water with the sugar, and boil until caramelized. Deglaze with the sake and rice wine vinegar.

Add the ginger, carrots, pepper seeds, and garlic, and let the mixture reduce over low heat for approximately 2 minutes.

Add 125 ml (1/2 cup) of water, verify the seasoning and add the soy sauce.

 Jean Vachon, Chef-Instructor at the École hôtelière de la Capitale in Quebec

Satay sauce

Preparation time: 15 minutes
Difficulty: easy

500 ml

This sauce is the perfect accompaniment to chicken, pork, or shrimp brochettes. Tamarind purée is prepared with the tamarind pulp that is both sweet and sour. This paste is now sold in most grocery stores.

2 tbsp vegetable oil

2 tbsp red curry paste

1 tbsp frozen lemongrass

2 tbsp tamarind purée

375 ml (1 1/2 cups) coconut milk

120 g (1/2 cup) crunchy peanut butter

60 g (1/4 cup) sugar

2 tbsp unsalted peanuts, finely chopped

Heat the oil in a non-stick saucepan. Add the curry paste, lemongrass, and the tamarind purée, and cook over high heat for 1 minute.

Add the coconut milk, peanut butter, and sugar, and bring to a boil. Lower the heat and simmer uncovered for 2 minutes.

Sprinkle with the chopped peanuts and serve immediately.

 Jean Vachon, Chef-Instructor at the École hôtelière de la Capitale in Quebec

Thai spring roll sauce
satay sauce

sauces and seasonings

Garam masala

Preparation time: 15 minutes
Difficulty: easy

Approximately 125 ml

It is very important to clean the coffee grinder thoroughly before grinding the spices.

2 tbsp cumin seed

2 tbsp coriander seeds

2 tbsp black peppercorns

1 tbsp cardamom seeds

1 tsp whole cloves

1 cinnamon stick, crumbled

1 tsp ground nutmeg

1/2 tsp saffron

In a non-stick skillet, grill all the spices except the nutmeg and saffron for 5 minutes, stirring constantly to avoid burning.

Transfer to a bowl. Add the saffron and nutmeg, and set aside to cool.

Grind the mixture in a coffee grinder, or crush in a mortar.

Conserve the garam masala in an airtight container in a cool, dry location.

 Jean Vachon, Chef-Instructor at the École hôtelière de la Capitale in Quebec

Curry-coco
sauce

Preparation time: 15 minutes
Difficulty: easy

4 servings

This exotic sauce adds a burst of flavour to grilled lamb chops or chicken.

1 tsp cornstarch

175 ml (3/4 cup) coconut milk

1 tbsp vegetable oil

1 tbsp fresh ginger, chopped

1 shallot

80 ml (1/3 cup) 15 % table cream

1/2 tsp curry powder

Salt

Mix the cornstarch in the coconut milk.

Heat the oil in a small saucepan, and add the ginger and shallot. Sauté for 30 seconds, and add the coconut milk and the cream.

Add the curry, bring to a boil, reduce the heat and simmer for 5 minutes. Season with salt to taste.

 Christophe Alary, Chef-Instructor at the École hôtelière de la Capitale in Quebec, elected Chef of the Year 2004 by his peers

sauces and seasonings

garam masala
curry-coco sauce

Peanut
sauce

Preparation time: 25 minutes   Approximately 500 ml
Difficulty: average

This sauce is a marvel with chicken. Kecap manis is a dark, rich Indonesian soy sauce that is sweeter than Chinese or Japanese soy sauce. It can be replaced with Chinese soy sauce, to which is added a touch of brown sugar. Palm sugar is made with the sap of certain palm tree species.

250 ml (1 cup) vegetable oil

60 g (1/2 cup) peanuts

125 ml (1/2 cup) coconut milk

2 tbsp shallots, finely chopped

1 tbsp garlic, finely chopped

1/2 tsp sambal oelek (see page 142)

1 tbsp lime juice, freshly squeezed

1 tbsp kecap manis

Palm or brown sugar

Heat the oil in a large wok or skillet and brown the peanuts over medium-high heat.

Remove and purée the nuts in 60 ml (1/4 cup) of coconut milk, using a food processor.

Sauté the shallots and garlic in the wok over medium-high heat for approximately 1 minute without browning. Add the peanut paste, the remaining coconut milk, the sambal oelek, lime juice, and kecap manis.

Cook until thickened and add the palm sugar to taste. Add a bit of coconut milk if the sauce is too thick.

Christophe Alary, Chef-Instructor at the École hôtelière de la Capitale in Quebec, elected Chef of the Year 2004 by his peers

peanut sauce

maghreb couscous

sauces and sea-sonings

Maghreb
couscous

Preparation time: 30 minutes   4 to 6 servings
Difficulty: easy

Indicated measurements for the fines herbes, oranges, nuts, and dried fruit are approximate. Adapt them to your preferred taste.

250 ml (1 cup) chicken stock

1 pinch of ground turmeric

400 g (2 cups) precooked wheat semolina (couscous)

3 tbsp olive oil

Juice of 2 or 3 lemons or limes, freshly squeezed

1 tomato

1 celery stalk, chopped

2 green peppers, cut in thin strips

1 or 2 carrots, grated

Approximately 20 g (2/3 cup) mixture of flat-leaf parsley, mint, coriander, and fresh basil, chopped

Approximately 90 g (3/4 cup) mixture of nuts, dates, and dried raisins, chopped

1 or 2 oranges, chopped

Salt and freshly ground pepper

6 tbsp extra virgin olive oil

Bring the stock to a boil. Add the turmeric, stir well, and remove from the heat.

Add the couscous and the olive oil, mix well and allow to puff up for 10 minutes.

With a fork, break up the couscous and transfer to a large bowl.

Sprinkle with the lemon juice and mix well with all the other ingredients

Jean Vachon, Chef-Instructor at the École hôtelière de la Capitale in Quebec

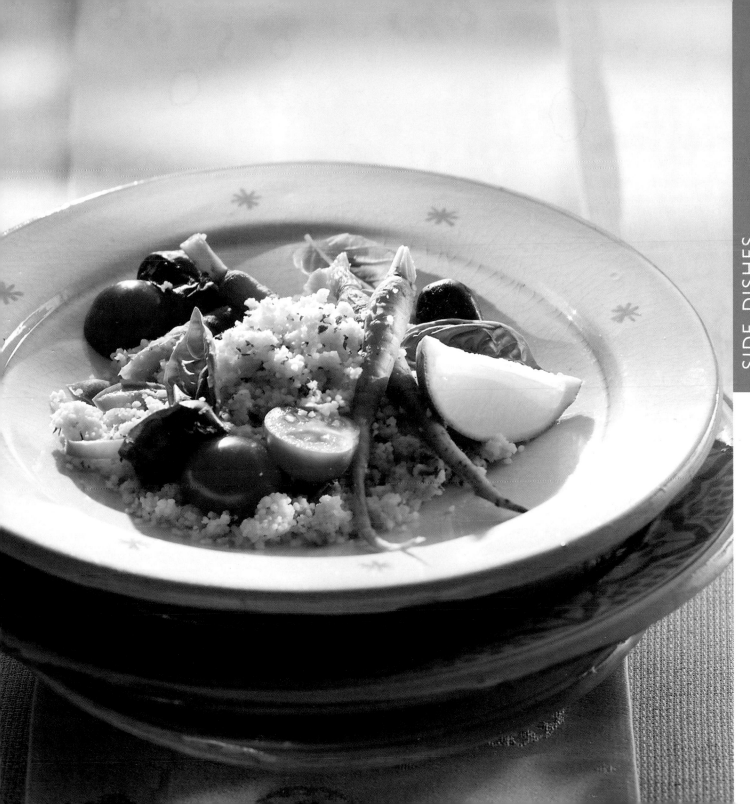

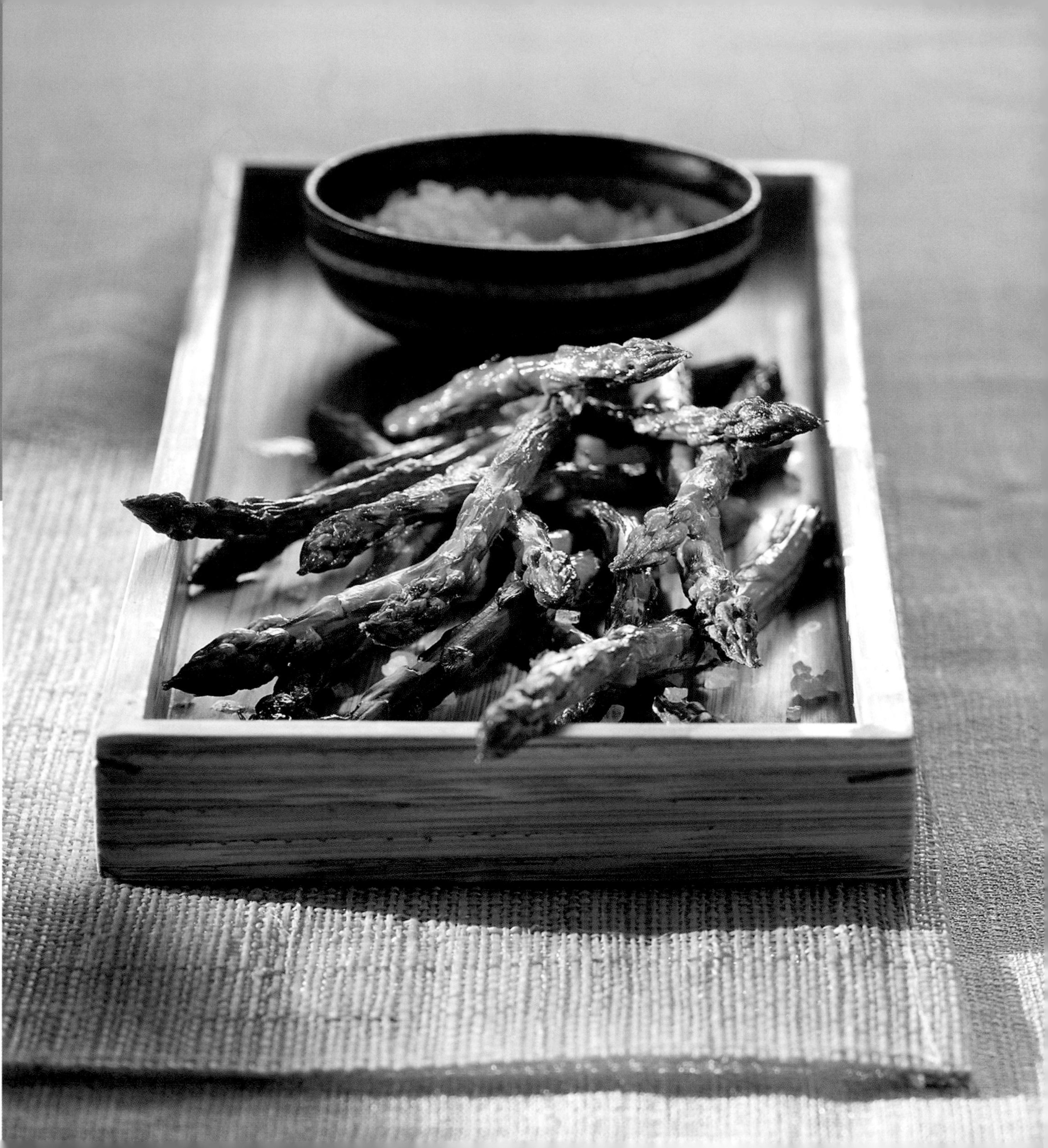

Baked asparagus

Preparation time: 15 minutes
Difficulty: easy

4 servings

If you don't have any Guérande sea salt handy, ordinary salt will do fine. Reserve the hard sections of the asparagus to add to a vegetable soup.

1 bunch very fresh asparagus
1 tbsp olive oil
Guérande sea salt and freshly ground pepper

Preheat the oven broiler.

Clean the asparagus under cold running water. Break off the soft part of the stems from the hard lower section and pat dry.

Place the asparagus spears in a Ziploc bag, add the olive oil, close tightly, and shake well to coat thoroughly.

Remove from the bag and arrange in one layer on a baking sheet.

Cook under the top broiler for approximately 8 minutes, until they begin to colour slightly, turning when half done.

Remove the baking sheet from the oven, season with salt and pepper to taste, and serve immediately.

 Richard Béliveau

Braised
Brussels sprouts with turmeric

Preparation time: 1 hour
Difficulty: easy

4 to 6 servings

1 kg (2 lbs) Brussels sprouts, washed and dried
60 ml (1/4 cup) olive oil
2 tsp ground turmeric
Salt and freshly ground pepper

Preheat the oven to 200°C (400°F).

With a sharp paring knife, make a cross-shaped incision in the bottom of each Brussels sprout.

Place the sprouts in a Ziploc bag, add the olive oil and the turmeric, seal the bag and shake well to coat thoroughly.

Remove from the bag and arrange in one layer on a baking sheet.

Cover with aluminium foil and cook in the oven for approximately 40 minutes, until they are tender.

 Richard Béliveau

side dishes

baked asparagus
braised Brussels sprouts

Curried spinach and pumpkin

Preparation time: 40 minutes
Difficulty: average

4 servings

1 tbsp olive oil

2 medium onions, finely sliced

2 garlic cloves, sliced

1 tbsp fresh ginger, grated

2 fresh hot cherry or bird peppers

1 tsp ground coriander

1 tsp ground cumin

1 tsp mustard seed

1 tsp ground turmeric

1 kg (2 lbs) pumpkin or squash, peeled and cut into cubes

375 ml (1 1/2 cups) chicken or vegetable stock

150 g (5 oz) fresh young spinach

Salt and freshly ground pepper

1 tbsp sliced almonds, toasted (see page 141)

7 g (1/4 cup) fresh coriander, finely chopped

Heat the oil in a saucepan. Sauté the onions and garlic over high heat, taking care not to brown.

Add the ginger, peppers, and the spices, and mix well.

Add the pumpkin and the stock, bring to a boil and let simmer for 15 minutes.

Add the spinach, stir delicately, and let simmer for another minute. Season with salt and pepper to taste.

Garnish with the almonds and fresh coriander before serving.

curried spinach
Indian cabbage
garlic-scented
curly kale

side
dishes

 Jean Vachon, Chef-Instructor at the École hôtelière de la Capitale in Quebec

Indian cabbage

Preparation time: 10 minutes
Difficulty: easy

4 servings

640 g (4 cups) cabbage, shredded

3 tbsp olive oil

1 tsp ground turmeric

1/2 tsp mustard seed

2 tbsp water

Salt and freshly ground pepper

In an ovenproof 1.5 litre (6 cups) glass dish, cook the cabbage in the microwave oven for 4 minutes on high setting.

Add the olive oil, turmeric, and the mustard seed, and mix well.

Add the water, cover, and cook for 6 minutes. Let stand for 3 minutes.

Season with salt and pepper to taste before serving.

Garlic-scented curly kale

Preparation time: 10 minutes
Difficulty: easy

4 to 6 servings

You can replace the curly kale with Swiss chard, pakchoi, or spinach

1 curly kale (kale)

3 to 4 tbsp olive oil

2 or 3 garlic cloves, minced

Rinse and dry the kale well before shredding it into 2 cm (3/4 in) strips.

Heat the olive oil in a large, heavy skillet and cook the garlic over medium heat.

Add the kale and cook, stirring constantly until it is tender.

 Richard Béliveau (top and bottom recipes)

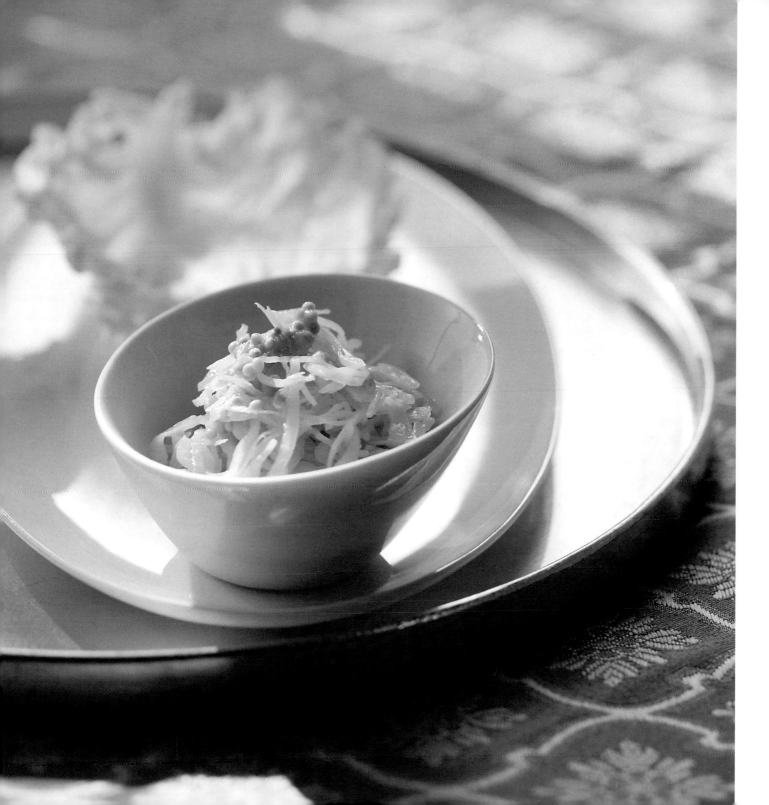

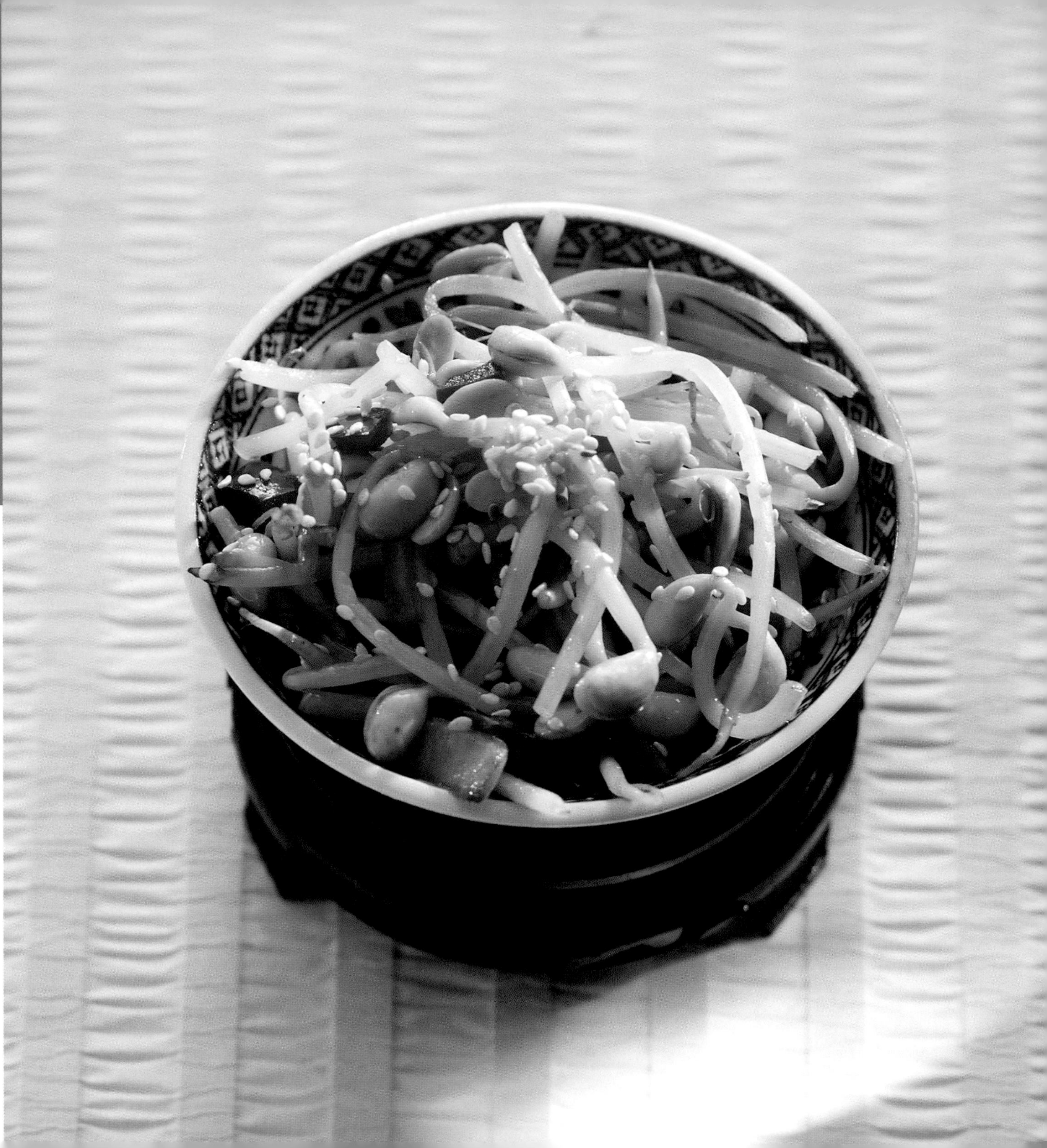

Sautéed bean sprouts

Preparation time: 25 minutes   4 to 6 servings
Difficulty: average

500 g (1 lb) fresh bean sprouts

3 tbsp olive oil

3 spring onions, chopped

2 garlic cloves, crushed

2 tbsp fresh ginger, chopped

1/2 green pepper, diced

1/2 red pepper, diced

Salt and freshly ground pepper

2 tbsp soy sauce

1 tbsp sesame oil

1 tbsp sesame seeds, toasted (see page 141)

Thoroughly wash the bean sprouts. Drain and pat dry with paper towels.

Heat the olive oil in a skillet. Sauté the onions, garlic, and ginger. Add the peppers and mix well.

Incorporate the bean sprouts and mix well. Season with salt and pepper to taste.

Add the soy sauce and cook over high heat for approximately 2 minutes, stirring constantly.

Remove from the heat, add the sesame oil and sprinkle with the sesame seeds. Serve immediately.

 Jean Vachon, Chef-Instructor at the École hôtelière de la Capitale in Quebec

Cauliflower au gratin

Preparation time: 45 minutes   4 servings
Difficulty: easy

300 g (2 cups) cauliflower, separated into florets

175 ml (3/4 cup) 35 % whipping cream

1 egg yolk

1 pinch of ground nutmeg

50 g (1/3 cup) favourite cheese, grated (Gruyère, Emmenthal, cheddar, etc.)

50 g (1/3 cup) Parmesan, freshly grated

Salt and freshly ground pepper

Cook the cauliflower in boiling salted water for 12 to 15 minutes, taking care not to overcook. Drain well and place in a buttered au gratin dish.

Mix the remaining ingredients in a bowl. Season with salt and pepper to taste, and pour over the cauliflower.

Cook in the oven under the broiler for approximately 15 minutes, until the cheese is a golden brown.

 Jean-Pierre Cloutier, Chef-proprietor of Café-restaurant du Musée in Quebec

side dishes

sautéed bean sprouts
cauliflower au gratin

Chinese-style
spinach

Preparation time: 30 minutes
Difficulty: average

6 servings

1 kg (2 lbs) fresh spinach, washed, stems removed

3 tbsp olive oil

2 medium onions, sliced into rounds

1 garlic clove, crushed

1 tbsp cornstarch

4 tsp soy sauce

Salt and freshly ground pepper

Salt the spinach, and cook over high heat for 1 to 3 minutes in a skillet without adding water.

Heat the olive oil in a heavy skillet. Sauté the onions and garlic over medium heat for 6 to 7 minutes, until the onions are tender and translucent.

In a small bowl, mix the cornstarch well in the soy sauce. Pour over the onions and stir. Cook over low heat for 1 to 2 minutes, until the mixture thickens.

Season with salt and pepper to taste.

Drain the spinach, and mix together with the sauce.

 Jean Vachon, Chef-Instructor at the École hôtelière de la Capitale in Quebec

Chinese-style spinach

Japanese-style spinach

side dishes

Japanese-style
spinach

Preparation time: 30 minutes
Difficulty: average

4 servings

500 g (1 lb) very fresh spinach

VINAIGRETTE

30 g (1/4 cup) walnuts

1 tbsp flaxseed

1 tbsp sugar

2 tbsp rice wine vinegar

2 tbsp Japanese soy sauce

Carefully wash the spinach, and cook in boiling salted water for approximately 2 minutes, until their colour begins to change.

Rinse immediately in cold water. Drain in a sieve, pressing down firmly to remove all the water, and pat dry with paper towels.

Shape the spinach into 4 sausage shapes. Cut into 2.5 cm (1 in) lengths and arrange on 4 individual serving plates.

Blend all the vinaigrette ingredients in a food processor until they form a thick paste. Pour over the spinach chunks and serve at room temperature.

 Richard Béliveau

Cabbage duet

Preparation time: 45 minutes
Difficulty: easy

4 servings

If you want to increase the nourishment value of this hearty dish, add a can of rinsed and drained legumes a few minutes before the end of cooking. If you prefer, you may add brown rice, barley, or another cooked cereal.

1 tbsp olive oil

1 onion or 1 medium leek, chopped

12 Brussels sprouts

160 g (1 cup) Scotch kale, chopped

160 g (1 cup) pakchoi, chopped

3 garlic cloves, minced

1 tsp ground turmeric

1 tsp curry powder

Freshly ground pepper

1 litre (4 cups) soy milk nature

2 tbsp soy sauce

Almonds, walnuts, or hazelnuts, coarsely chopped

Heat the olive oil in a large saucepan. Sauté the onion until it is slightly coloured.

Add the Brussels sprouts, kale, pakchoi, and garlic, and stir several minutes over medium heat. Add the turmeric, curry, and pepper.

Pour in the soy milk and let simmer slowly for approximately 20 minutes, until the vegetables are cooked.

Add the soy sauce and almonds just before serving.

 Marlène Gagnon, Chef-Instructor at the École hôtelière de la Capitale in Quebec

Pearl onion
preserve

Preparation time: 2 hours
Difficulty: easy

Approximately 750 ml

As pearl onions are very difficult to peel, soaking them in very hot water before peeling will make the task a lot easier. This onion preserve is especially delicious with a terrine or vegetable pâté.

300 g (2 cups) pearl onions

50 g (1/4 cup) raisins

160 ml (2/3 cup) maple syrup

1 tsp tomato paste

1 tsp whole coriander seeds

3 tbsp extra virgin olive oil

175 ml (3/4 cup) white wine

80 ml (1/3 cup) cider vinegar

1 bay leaf

1 pinch of thyme

Salt

Place all ingredients in a saucepan. Bring to a boil, reduce the heat and let simmer slowly for approximately 1 1/2 hours until desired consistency.

Transfer to Mason jars and store in the refrigerator.

 Christophe Alary, Chef-Instructor at the École hôtelière de la Capitale in Quebec, elected Chef of the Year 2004 by his peers

side
dishes

cabbage duet
pearl onion
preserve

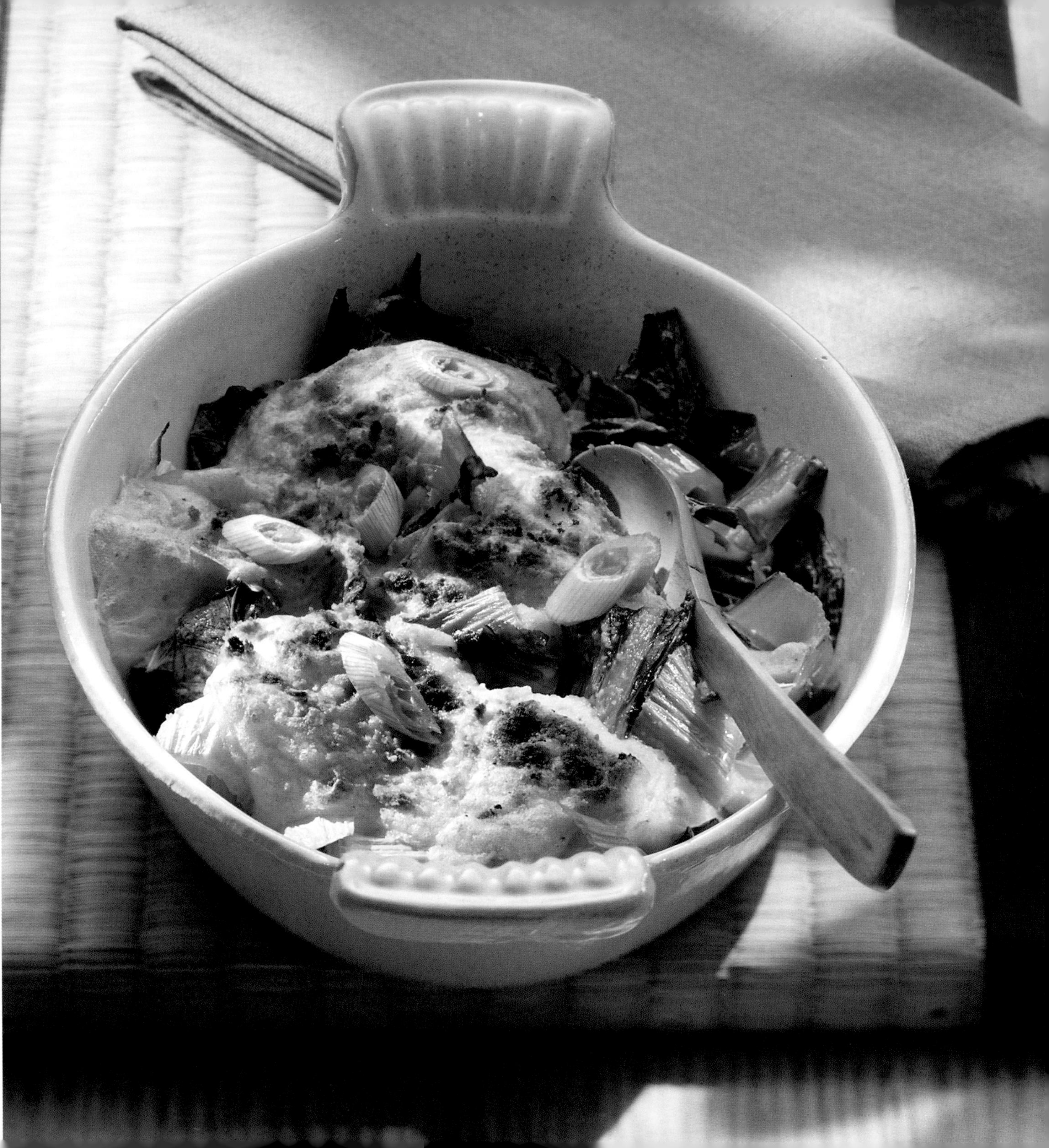

Pakchoi au gratin

Preparation time: 45 minutes
Difficulty: average

4 servings

480 g (3 cups) pakchoi, coarsely chopped

1 green onion, finely chopped

1 garlic clove, finely chopped

1 tbsp fresh ginger, chopped

CASHEW-FLAVOURED BÉCHAMEL

500 ml (2 cups) vegetable stock or milk

60 g (1/2 cup) cashew nuts, ground

2 tbsp wheat flour

2 tbsp butter

Salt and freshly ground pepper

Sear the pakchoi in a very hot non-stick skillet to colour lightly. Remove from the heat.

Add the green onion, garlic, and the ginger, and transfer to a buttered au gratin dish.

To make the béchamel sauce, combine all the sauce ingredients well with a mixer. Cook over low heat in a saucepan, stirring constantly until desired thickness. Pour this sauce over the vegetables.

Cook in the oven at 180°C (350°F) for 20 to 30 minutes.

 Marlène Gagnon, Chef-Instructor at the École hôtelière de la Capitale in Quebec

Grilled or sautéed oyster mushrooms

Preparation time: 40 minutes
(with waiting time)
Difficulty: easy

2 servings

500 g (1 lb) oyster mushrooms, sliced

80 ml (1/3 cup) olive oil

1 onion, finely chopped

1 garlic clove, minced

125 ml (1/2 cup) chicken stock

Coarse salt and freshly ground pepper

Fresh flat-leaf parsley, finely chopped

GRILLED OYSTER MUSHROOMS

Cut the largest mushrooms in half, leaving the smaller ones whole.

Brush with the olive oil. Add the garlic, coarse salt, and pepper. Cover and set aside for 20 to 30 minutes in the refrigerator.

Cook under a very hot grill for 3 minutes each side, remove and serve immediately.

SAUTÉED OYSTER MUSHROOMS

Heat the olive oil in a skillet and sauté the onion and garlic. Add the mushrooms and stir as soon as they begin to release their juices.

Pour in the stock and season with salt and pepper to taste.

Reduce the liquid and serve immediately, garnished with the parsley.

 Mohand Yahiaoui, Chef-proprietor of Les rites berbères in Montreal

side dishes · pakchoi au gratin · grilled oyster mushrooms

Moroccan
-roasted root vegetables

Preparation time: 1 hour
Difficulty: easy
4 servings

(4 cups) favourite root vegetables (mix of carrots, turnips, parsnips, potatoes, Jerusalem artichokes, etc.), cut in 2 cm (3/4 in) cubes

1/2 tsp ground turmeric

1 tsp ground cumin

2 tsp dried parsley

Salt and freshly ground pepper

60 ml (1/4 cup) olive oil

Preheat the oven to 220°C (425°F).

In a small bowl, mix together the turmeric, cumin, parsley, salt, pepper, and olive oil.

Place the vegetables in a large Ziploc bag and pour in the spiced olive oil. Seal well and shake delicately to coat the vegetables with the oil.

Remove from the bag and arrange the vegetables in one layer on a baking sheet covered with waxed paper.

Cook uncovered for 40 to 50 minutes, depending on the vegetables chosen. The vegetables must be turned from time to time to ensure even cooking.

 Richard Béliveau

Ratatouille
provençale

Preparation time: 1 h 30
Difficulty: easy
4 servings

250 g (1 1/4 cup) eggplant, sliced

250 g (1 1/4 cup) zucchini, sliced

4 tsp coarse salt

Stream of olive oil

200 g (1 1/3 cups) red onions, finely sliced

2 garlic cloves, minced

240 g (2 cups) red pepper, cubed

500 g (3 1/3 cups) ripe tomatoes, peeled (see page 142) and diced

12 fresh basil leaves, chopped

4 sprigs of fresh thyme

1 bay leaf

Salt and freshly ground pepper

Arrange the eggplant and zucchini in a sieve. Sprinkle with the coarse salt and let stand for 30 minutes to release the excess water.

Rinse the slices under cold water and pat dry with paper towel. Cut into quarters.

Heat the olive oil in a saucepan. Sauté the onions over medium-high heat. Add the garlic, eggplant, zucchini, and peppers. Cook several minutes to soften the peppers.

Add the tomatoes and the fines herbes. Season with salt and pepper to taste, and simmer approximately 30 minutes over low heat.

 Jean-Pierre Cloutier, Chef-proprietor of Café-restaurant du Musée in Quebec

Moroccan-roasted root vegetables

ratatouille provençale

side dishes

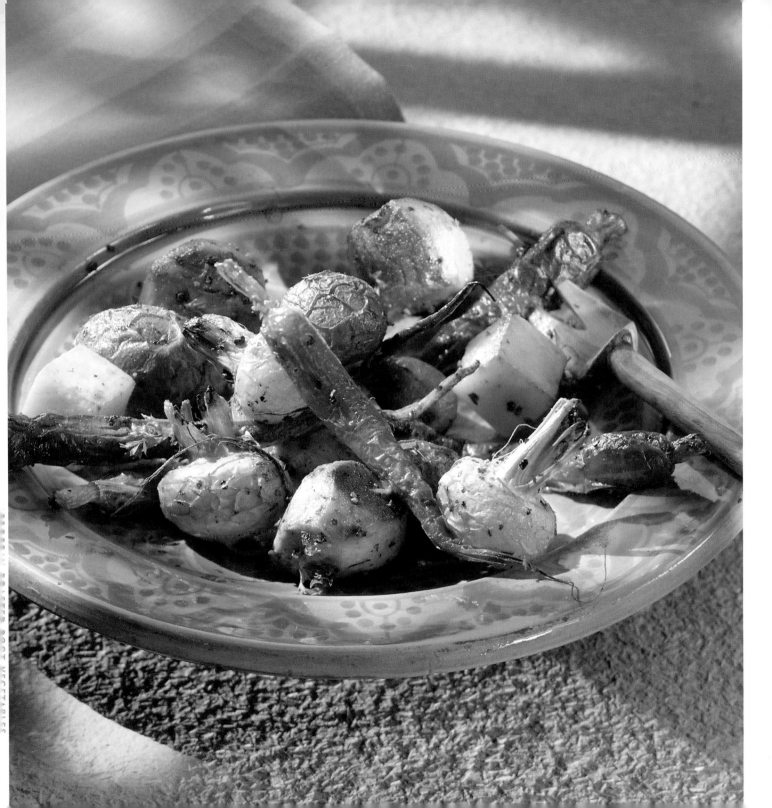

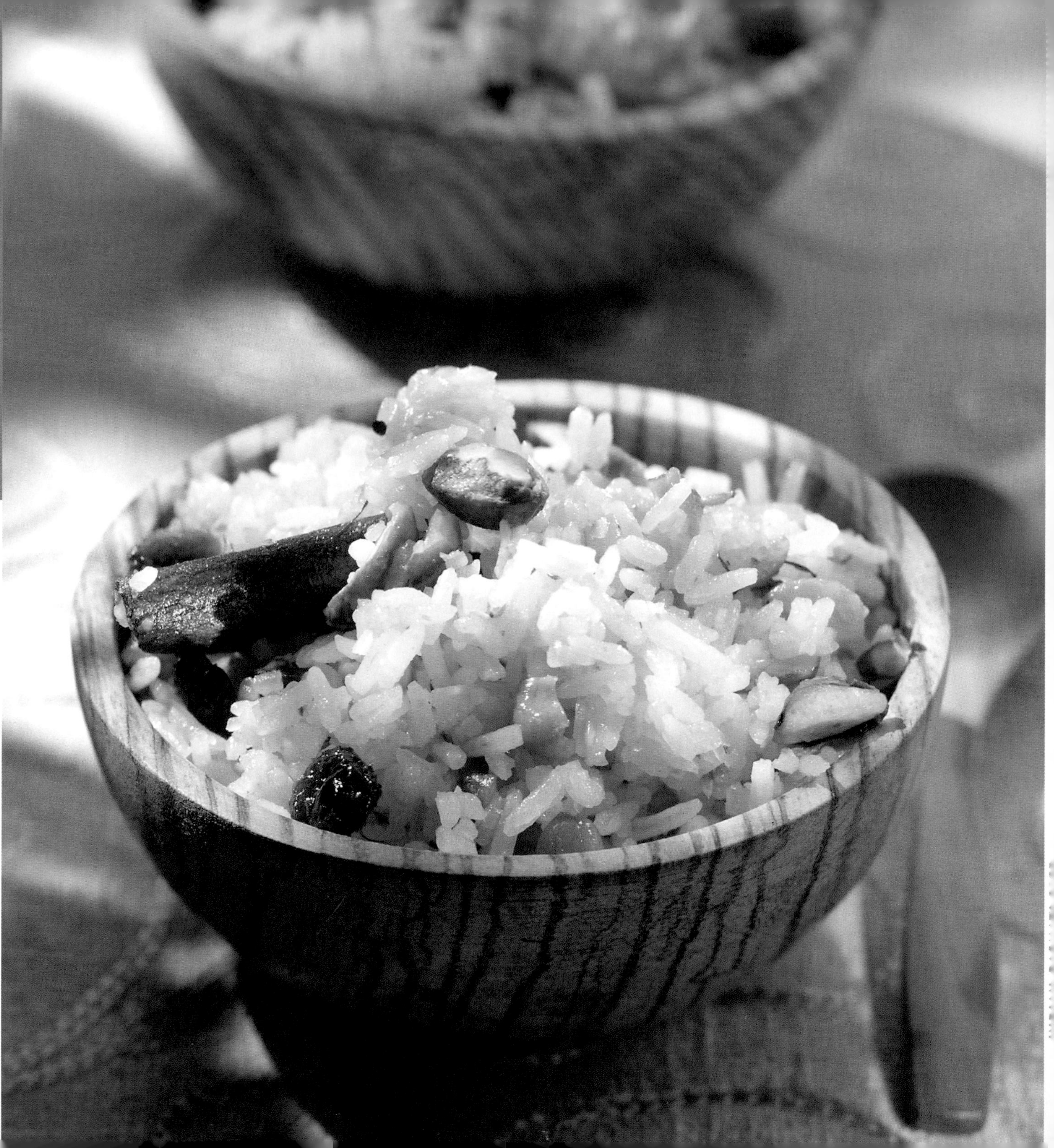

Indian basmati rice

Preparation time: 1 hour
Difficulty: easy

10 servings

1 kg (5 cups) basmati rice
125 ml (1/2 cup) olive oil
1 tbsp garlic, finely chopped
160 g (1 cup) onions, finely chopped
1 tbsp cumin seed
1 tbsp caraway seeds
1 tbsp coriander seeds
6 cardamom seeds
1 cinnamon stick
1 pinch of saffron
1 l (4 cups) chicken or vegetable stock
50 g (1/4 cup) dried apricots
50 g (1/4 cup) raisins
3 tbsp cashew nuts
2 tbsp unsalted pistachio nuts, shelled
Salt and freshly ground pepper

Rinse the rice under cold running water until the water runs clear, and let stand to drain for 30 minutes.

Heat the olive oil in a heavy saucepan, and sweat the garlic and the onions over low heat until they are translucent.

Add the cumin, caraway, coriander, cardamom, and the cinnamon. Stir well and cook for 1 minute.

Add the rice and stir until all the grains become translucent.

Add the saffron and stock, and bring to a boil. Reduce the heat, cover, and cook slowly for approximately 20 minutes.

Incorporate the dried fruit, walnuts, and pistachio nuts. Cover and cook for another 10 minutes over very low heat.

Season with salt and pepper to taste before serving.

 Susan Sylvester, Chef-Instructor at the École hôtelière de la Capitale in Quebecc

Tasty turmeric rice

Preparation time: 1 h 30
Difficulty: average

4 servings

If you don't have a fitted lid for your pot, you can use aluminium foil to seal the pot before placing in the oven.

60 ml (1/4 cup) extra virgin olive oil
1 onion, diced
1 red pepper, diced
1 green pepper, diced
250 g (1 2/3 cups) green peas, still frozen
400 g (2 cups) white or long grain rice
2 bay leaves
2 tbsp ground turmeric
Coarse salt and freshly ground pepper
Approximately 1 l (4 cups) chicken stock

Heat the olive oil in a Dutch oven. Sauté the onion and peppers over medium-high heat.

As soon as the vegetables begin to brown, add the green peas. Cook while stirring for approximately 3 minutes.

Add the rice, reduce the heat, and continue to stir. Add the bay leaves and turmeric, and season with the coarse salt and pepper to taste.

Pour in just enough stock to cover the rice. Cover and cook in the oven at 180°C (350°F) for approximately 1 hour.

Remove from the oven and let stand covered for 10 minutes before serving.

 Mohand Yahiaoui, Chef-proprietor of Les rites berbères in Montreal

side
dishes

Indian
basmati rice

tasty turmeric
rice

Rice pilaf
with green peas and almonds

Preparation time: 1 hour
Difficulty: average

4 servings

200 g (1 cup) Basmati rice

2 tbsp olive oil

80 g (1/2 cup) Spanish onions, coarsely chopped

15 cardamom seeds

1/2 tsp black peppercorns

3 whole cloves

3/4 tsp ground cumin

2 cinnamon sticks

3/4 tsp ground turmeric

500 ml (2 cups) chicken stock, hot

50 g (1/4 cup) sultana raisins

50 g (1/3 cup) frozen green peas

2 tbsp sliced almonds, toasted (see page 141)

This rice is a good side dish for all curries, as well as meat and fish recipes. Try it with the spicy Indian-style lamb (see recipe on page 177).

Rinse the rice under cold running water until the water runs clear, and let stand to drain.

Heat the olive oil in a large saucepan. Cook the onions and the spices approximately 1 minute over medium-high heat. Add the rice and stir to coat the grains with the oil.

Pour in the stock and bring to a boil. Reduce the heat and simmer for 15 minutes covered.

Remove from the heat. Add the dried raisins, frozen green peas, and the almonds, and let stand 15 minutes covered before serving.

rice pilaf with green peas and almonds

vegetable tian

side dishes

Jean Vachon, Chef-Instructor at the École hôtelière de la Capitale in Quebec

Mediterranean
vegetable tian

Preparation time: 2 h 15
Difficulty: easy

4 servings

This vegetable tian is especially recommended with fish and meat dishes.

150 ml (2/3 cup) olive oil

1 medium onion, sliced

1 medium zucchini, sliced

1 bunch fresh basil, chopped

1 small eggplant, sliced

2 Italian tomatoes, halved

Salt and freshly ground pepper

Brush an au gratin dish with olive oil, and place the onion in the dish. Season with salt and pepper to taste.

Cover the onions with the zucchini and sprinkle with 2 1/2 tablespoons of the olive oil. Season with salt and pepper to taste.

Cover with the basil and sprinkle with 2 1/2 tablespoons of the olive oil.

Cover with the eggplant and sprinkle with 2 1/2 tablespoons of the olive oil. Season with salt and pepper to taste.

Cover with the tomatoes and sprinkle with 2 1/2 tablespoons of the olive oil. Season with salt and pepper to taste.

Cook in the oven at 135°C (275°F) for 2 hours.

Philippe Castel, elected health-conscious chef by his peers in 2004

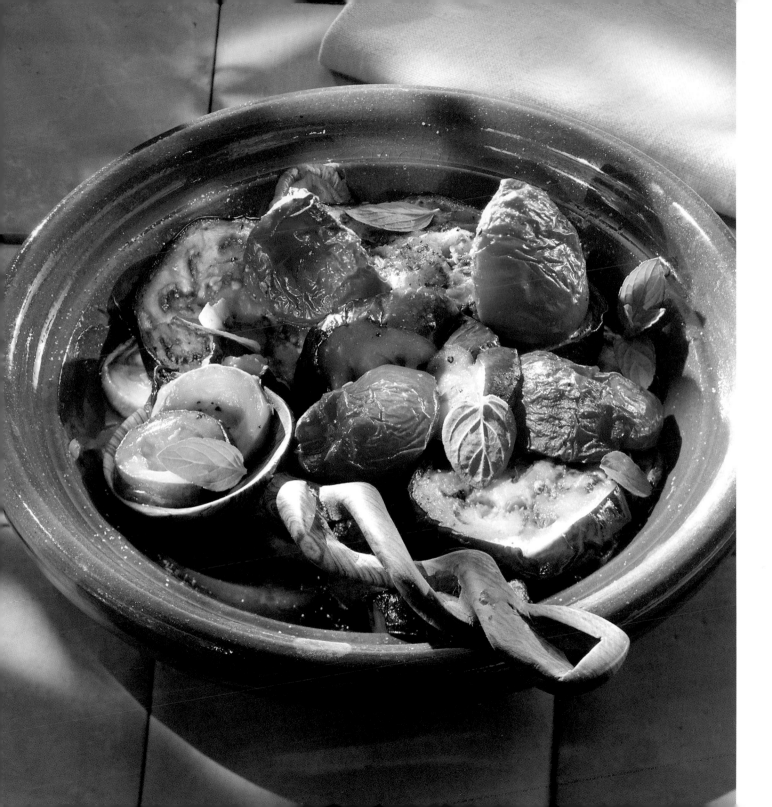

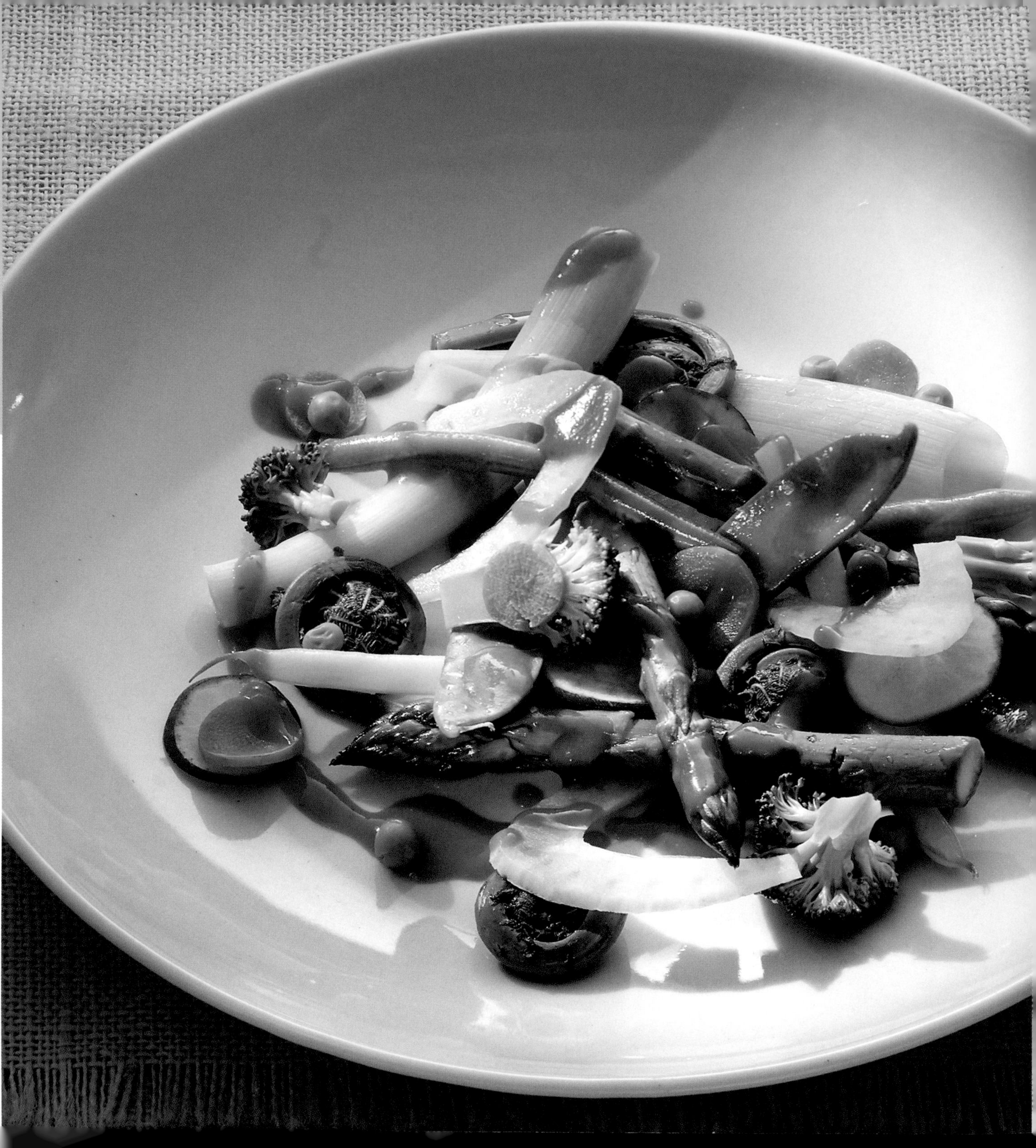

Raw/cooked vegetable
in tomato essence salad

4 servings

Preparation time: 45 minutes
Difficulty: average

Espelette pepper is grown in the Espelette commune, and in a few other Basque communes. At the end of summer, the peppers are picked and threaded onto swags (garlands). Then they are hung to dry on house facades for a month or two. To vary this essence recipe, replace the tomatoes with carrot juice. The taste will be entirely different, but just as interesting.

COOKED VEGETABLES
Green or white asparagus

Green or yellow beans

Young leeks

Snow peas

Fiddleheads

Salt and freshly ground pepper

RAW VEGETABLES
Broccoli

Fennel

Baby carrots

Fresh green beans

Radishes

Red or yellow cherry tomatoes

Salt and freshly ground pepper

TOMATO ESSENCE
3 tomatoes

2 tbsp olive oil

Juice of half a lemon, freshly squeezed

Salt and freshly ground pepper

FINES HERBES
Fresh mint, basil, and chervil

SEASONINGS
Coarse salt

Espelette pepper

Cooked vegetables: wash, stem, and peel the vegetables as required. Cook for several minutes in a large quantity of boiling salted water. Ensure the vegetables remain crunchy. Cool under cold running water and set aside.

Raw vegetables: peel the carrots, radishes, and fennel. Leave the snow peas whole. Separate the broccoli into florets and slice the cherry tomatoes.

Tomato essence: peel, seed, and quarter the tomatoes. Process them in a food mixer with the olive oil and lemon juice. Season with salt and pepper to taste.

Fines herbes: keep the fines herbes whole, removing only the largest stems.

In a bowl, carefully mix all the raw and cooked vegetables together with the tomato essence. Arrange decoratively on a serving dish, alternating sizes, shapes, and forms.

Sprinkle with the coarse salt and Espelette pepper, and decorate with a small bouquet of fresh fines herbes.

 Jean Soulard, President of the Fondation Serge-Bruyère and Executive Chef at the Fairmont Le Château Frontenac in Quebec City

salads

raw/cooked vegetable in tomato essence salad

Avocado and shrimp citrus salad

Preparation time: 20 minutes
Difficulty: easy

4 servings

1 grapefruit

1 orange

2 avocados, cubed

250 g (1/2 lb) shrimp, cooked and peeled

Stream of olive oil

Several drops of walnut oil

2 tbsp flaxseed

6 sprigs of chervil, chopped

Salt and freshly ground pepper

Lamb's lettuce or fresh lettuce

With a sharp knife, remove the peel and white skin from the grapefruit and orange, and quarter them over a bowl, reserving the juice.

Mix all ingredients together in a large bowl, except the lettuce. Add the reserved citrus juice.

Season with salt and pepper to taste.

Serve on a bed of lamb's lettuce or your favourite lettuce

 Jean-Pierre Cloutier, Chef-proprietor of Café-restaurant du Musée in Quebec

Vietnamese chicken and cabbage salad

Preparation time: 15 minutes
Difficulty: easy

4 servings

You will enjoy this salad served with shrimp crisps, easy to find in all Asian grocery stores and many supermarkets.

SALAD

300 to 400 g (10 to 14 oz) chicken, cooked and sliced

300 g (1 3/4 cups) white head cabbage, shredded

1 medium onion, cut in fine strips

2 carrots, coarsely grated

1/2 bunch fresh mint, chopped

30 g (1 cup) fresh coriander, chopped

VINAIGRETTE

4 garlic cloves, sliced

1 hot red pepper (or to taste), chopped

2 tbsp white vinegar

60 ml (1/4 cup) lime juice, freshly squeezed

60 ml (1/4 cup) vegetable oil

1 tbsp fish sauce (nuoc-mâm or nam pla)

2 1/2 tbsp sugar

Mix all the vinaigrette ingredients together in a small bowl.

Place all the salad ingredients in a large bowl, except the coriander.

Add the vinaigrette.

Garnish with the coriander and serve.

 Florence Albernhe, Chef-proprietor of Le Grain de riz in Quebec

avocado and shrimp salad

chicken and cabbage salad

salads

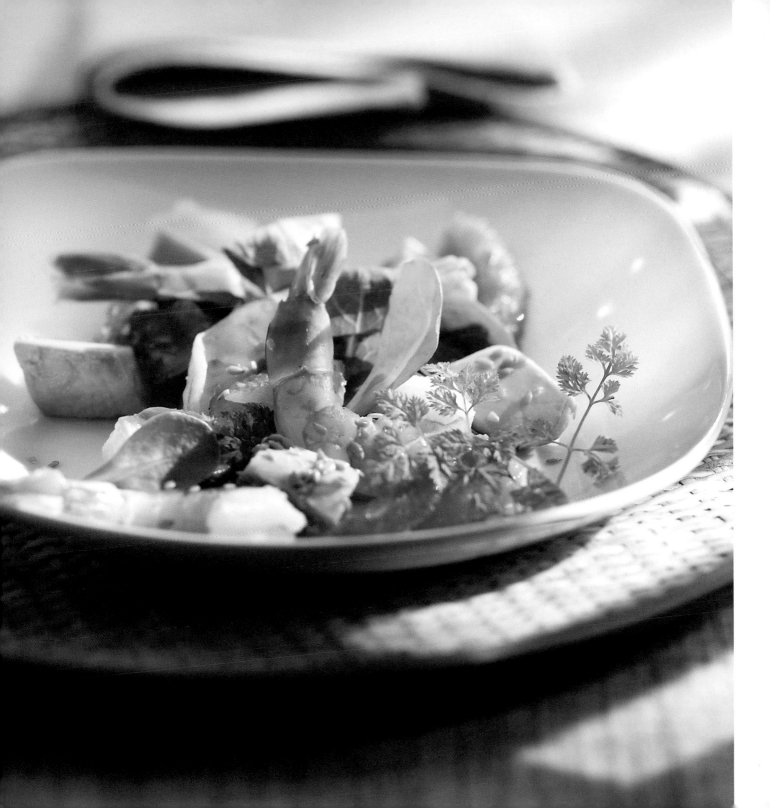

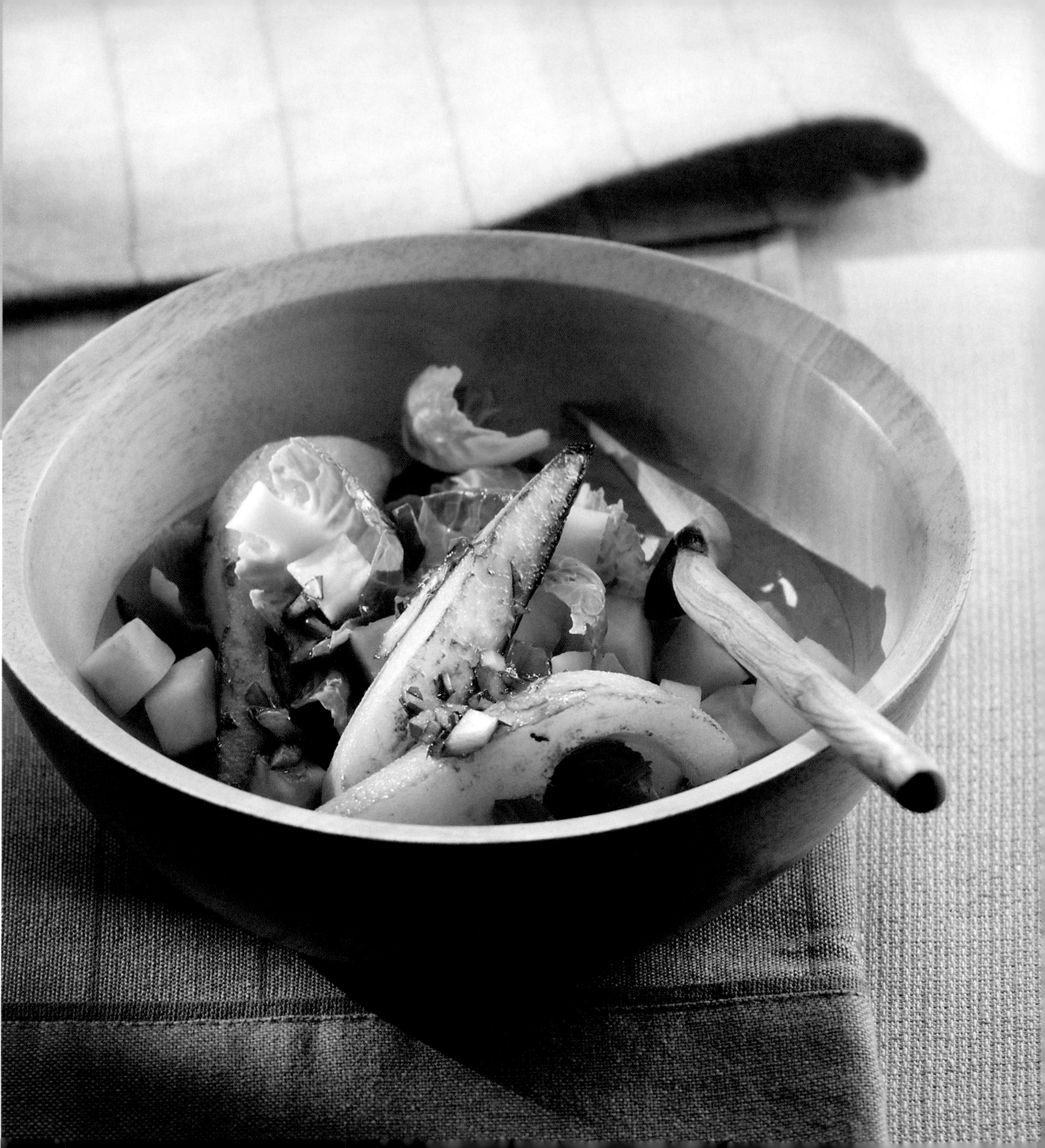

Brussels sprout salad

Preparation time: 35 minutes
Difficulty: average

4 servings

SALAD

350 g (12 oz) Brussels sprouts

100 g (1/2 cup) celery root, cut into small cubes

3 very ripe pears

2 tbsp olive oil

1 tbsp sugar

VINAIGRETTE

1/2 red onion, chopped

6 tbsp grapeseed oil

2 tbsp soy sauce

2 tbsp rice wine vinegar

1 garlic clove, minced

1 bunch basil (Thai basil, preferably), chopped

1 tsp sesame oil

Separate the Brussels sprout leaves and wash carefully. Cook in boiling salted water for 1 minute. The leaves must remain crunchy.

Cook the celery root in boiling water for 1 or 2 minutes.

Peel and core the pears, and cut them into quarters. Sear the pears in olive oil in a skillet. Add the sugar and cook to caramelize slightly.

Prepare the vinaigrette, mixing all vinaigrette ingredients together.

Arrange the Brussels sprout leaves, celery root, and pears in 4 individual serving plates, sprinkle with the vinaigrette and serve.

 Éric Villain, Chef-co-owner of the Bistro Le Clocher Penché in Quebec

Watercress and goat cheese salad

Preparation time: 25 minutes
Difficulty: easy

4 servings

2 very ripe pears

600 g (1 1/3 lbs) fresh watercress, rinsed and dried

100 g (3 1/2 oz) fresh goat cheese

VINAIGRETTE

80 ml (1/3 cup) walnut oil

2 tbsp red wine vinegar

1 tbsp old style Dijon mustard

Salt and freshly ground pepper

Prepare the vinaigrette by mixing the walnut oil and vinegar in a small bowl. Add the mustard and season with salt and pepper to taste. Whisk well to emulsify.

Peel and core the pears, and cut them into thin slices.

Arrange the pear slices in a shallow dish and add the watercress. Crumble the goat cheese on top of the salad and sprinkle with the vinaigrette. Serve immediately.

 Christophe Alary, Chef-Instructor at the École hôtelière de la Capitale in Quebec, elected Chef of the Year 2004 by his peers

salads

Brussels sprout salad

watercress salad

Watercress
salad with raspberries and tomatoes

Preparation time: 15 minutes
Marinade : 1 to 2 hours
Difficulty: easy

4 servings

Even if you don't have any watercress handy, you can still make this refreshing salad, using any of your favourite leaf vegetables.

1 mango
300 g (2 cups) ripe tomatoes
150 g (1 cup) raspberries
400 g (14 oz) fresh watercress

VINAIGRETTE

Fresh basil, chopped

Garlic to taste

5 tbsp olive oil

4 tsp raspberry vinegar

Salt and freshly ground pepper

Cut the mango and tomatoes into 1 cm (1/2 in) cubes and place in a large bowl with the raspberries.

Prepare the vinaigrette, mixing the basil, garlic, olive oil, and vinegar together in a small bowl. Season with salt and pepper to taste. Pour over the fruit and mix carefully.

Cover and marinate for 1 to 2 hours in the refrigerator.

Serve on a bed of watercress.

 Philippe Coudroy, Chef-Instructor at the École hôtelière de la Capitale in Quebec

Coleslaw

Preparation time: 20 minutes
Marinade: 1 to 2 hours
Difficulty: easy

4 servings

Use a food processor or grater to grate the cabbage.

300 g (1 3/4 cups) Scotch kale, grated
100 g (2/3 cup) red cabbage, grated
150 g (3/4 cup) carrots, grated

VINAIGRETTE

150 ml (2/3 cup) olive oil

50 g (1/4 cup) honey

3 tbsp lemon juice, freshly squeezed

2 1/2 tbsp red wine vinegar

1 tsp powdered mustard

2 1/2 tsp salt

2 1/2 tsp freshly ground pepper

2 1/2 tsp dried thyme

2 1/2 tsp dried parsley

2 1/2 tsp garlic, finely chopped

1 tsp fresh ginger, grated

Mix the vegetables in a large bowl.

Mix all the vinaigrette ingredients together in a small bowl.

Pour the vinaigrette over the vegetables, cover, and marinate for several hours in the refrigerator before serving.

 Florence Albernhe, Chef-proprietor of Le Grain de riz in Quebec

watercress salad with raspberries
coleslaw
salads

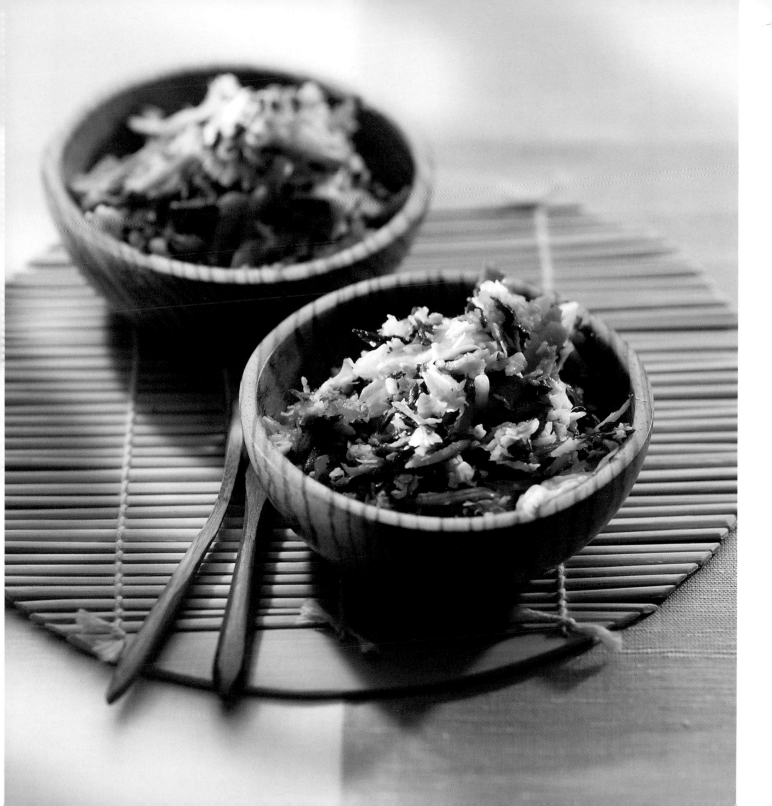

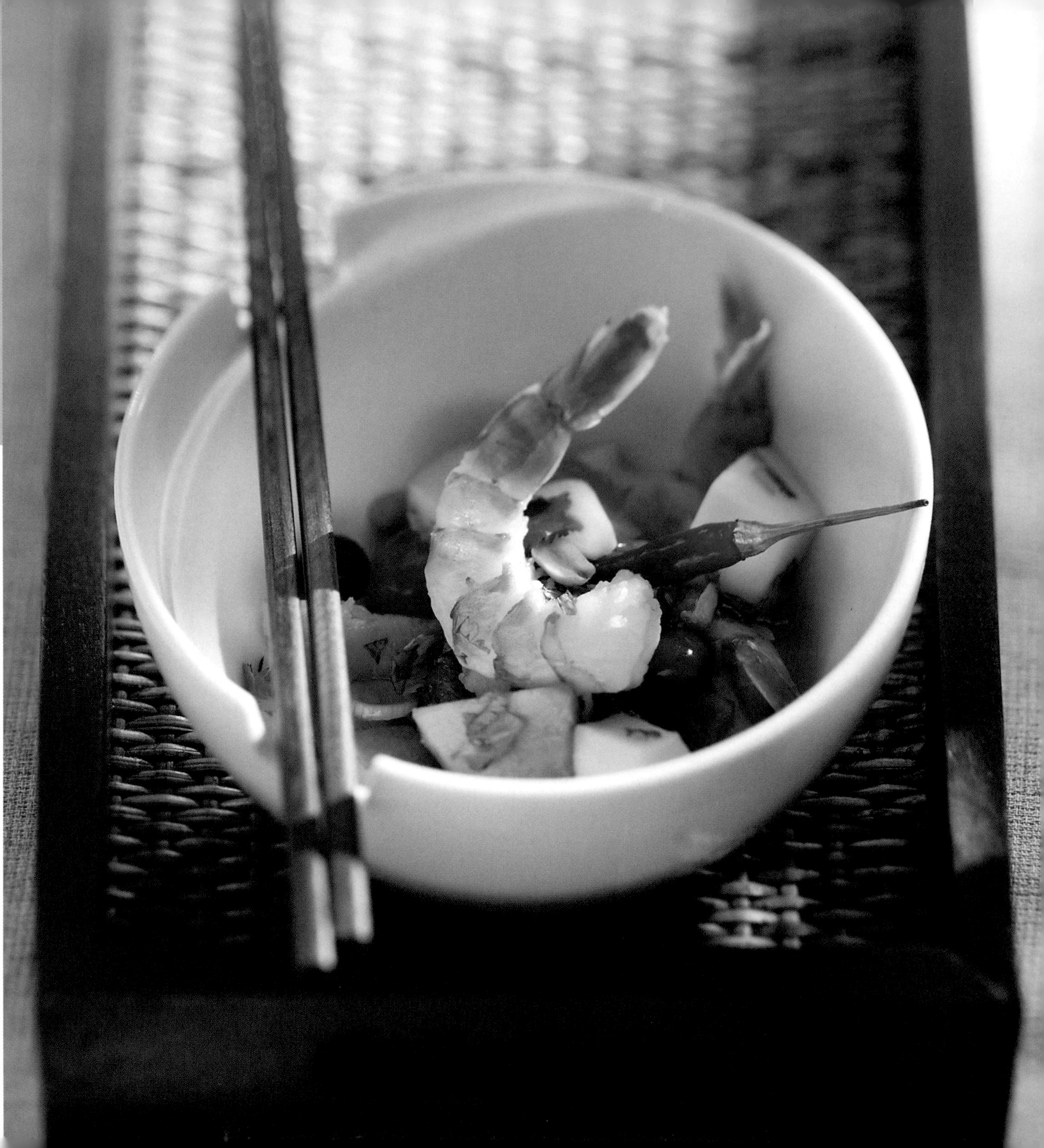

Thai shrimp and fruit salad

Preparation time: 25 minutes   **4 to 6 servings**
Difficulty: average

400 g (2 cups) favourite fruit (mango, papaya, green apple, pear, mandarin, grapefruit, pomelo, strawberry, grape, etc.)

2 tbsp vegetable oil

1 shallot, finely sliced

1 garlic clove, finely sliced

Juice of one lime, freshly squeezed

Zest of one lime

Fish sauce (nuoc-mâm or nam pla) or salt

Approximately 1 tsp sugar (optional)

100 g (3 1/2 oz) shrimp, cooked

2 tbsp peanuts, toasted, chopped

Fresh fines herbes (mint, coriander, Thai basil, etc.), chopped

Red or green hot pepper, minced

Prepare the fruit, cutting into cubes, slices, or strips. If you are using apples, sprinkle them with a bit of lemon juice to stop them from discolouring.

Heat the oil in a skillet, and sweat the shallot and garlic over medium-low heat, taking care not to brown.

In a bowl, mix together the lime juice and zest, fish sauce, sugar, shallots, and their cooking oil.

Add the fruit and the shrimp. Toss carefully and verify the seasoning.

Garnish with the peanuts, fines herbes, and hot pepper to taste.

 Susan Sylvester, Chef-Instructor at the École hôtelière de la Capitale in Quebec

Green bean and arame seaweed salad

Preparation time: 25 minutes   **4 servings**
Difficulty: easy

300 g (2 cups) fine green beans

2 tbsp dried arame seaweed

60 ml (1/4 cup) warm water

1 1/2 tbsp rice wine vinegar

2 tsp sesame oil

40 g (1/4 cup) red onions, finely sliced

1/2 tsp sea salt

Cook the beans in a saucepan of boiling water, uncovered, until they are tender and still crunchy. Rinse quickly under cold water to stop cooking.

Soak the seaweed in a bowl of warm water for approximately 5 minutes.

In a bowl, mix together the vinegar, half the water that the seaweed was soaked in, and the sesame oil.

Add all the other ingredients and stir delicately. Season with salt to taste.

 François Rousseau, Chef-Instructor at the École hôtelière de la Capitale in Quebec

salads   Thai shrimp and fruit salad / green bean salad

Green curried
legume salad

Preparation time: 15 minutes
Difficulty: easy   **4 servings**

This salad is delicious as is, but you can also use it as a stuffing for artichokes.

475 g (2 1/4 cups) canned legumes, your choice, rinsed and drained

75 g (2/3 cup) multicoloured peppers, diced

2 tbsp onions, finely chopped

50 g (1/4 cup) cucumber, diced

1/2 red apple, diced

1/2 tsp fresh ginger, grated

1 tbsp green curry paste

60 ml (1/4 cup) lemon juice, freshly squeezed

1 tbsp honey

80 ml (1/3 cup) olive oil

Salt and freshly ground pepper

Mix all ingredients together, except the olive oil.

Season with salt and pepper to taste, and add the oil. Mix well, cover, and refrigerate for several hours until ready to serve.

 Benoît Dussault, Chef-Instructor at the École hôtelière de la Capitale in Quebec

Lobster and
Savoy cabbage salad

Preparation time: 1 hour
Difficulty: average   **4 servings**

SALAD

2 lobsters, approximately 700 g (1 1/2 lbs) each

1 small Savoy cabbage

2 oranges, peeled and sectioned

VINAIGRETTE

3 tbsp orange juice, freshly squeezed

Juice of one lemon, freshly squeezed

3 tbsp olive oil

1 tsp Dijon mustard

Sprigs of fresh chives, chopped

Salt and freshly ground pepper

Mix all the vinaigrette ingredients together in a small bowl.

Cook the lobster for 15 minutes in boiling salted water.

Remove and discard the outside leaves of the cabbage. Separate the cabbage leaves, removing any stems that are too large. Cut the leaves into thin strips and blanch for 5 minutes in boiling salted water. Rinse under cold water to stop cooking, and drain well.

Season the cabbage strips with a third of the vinaigrette.

Remove the meat from the lobster. Cut the tails into medallions; break the claws and remove the meat. Brush the lobster meat with the vinaigrette.

Place the cabbage on a serving plate, add the orange sections and garnish with the lobster chunks on top.

Serve with the remaining vinaigrette in a sauce bowl.

 Jean Soulard, President of the Fondation Serge-Bruyère and Executive Chef at the Fairmont Le Château Frontenac in Quebec City

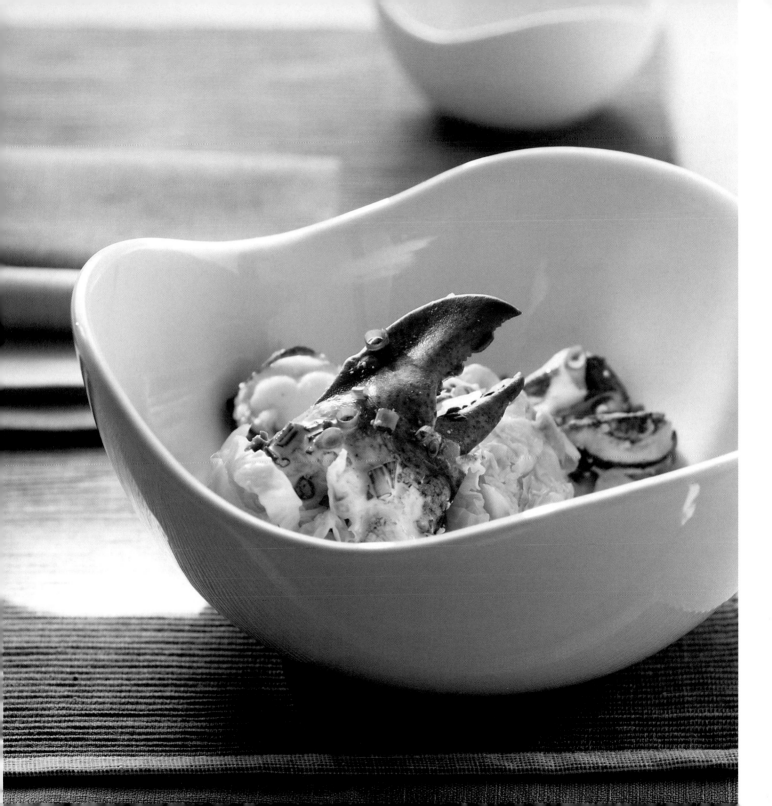

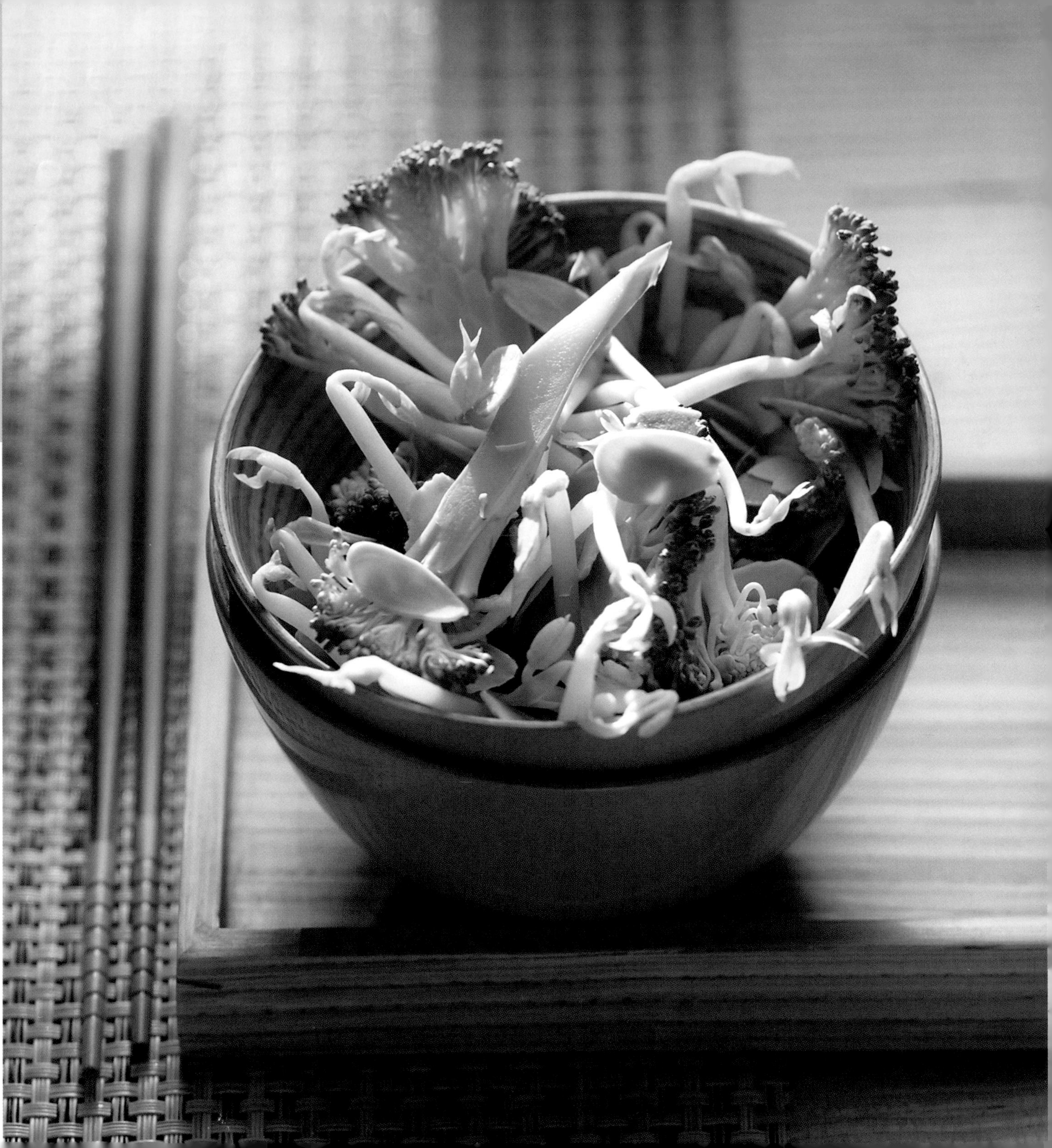

Broccoli, almond, and bean sprout salad

Preparation time: 1 h 15   **3 or 4 servings**
Difficulty: easy

Keep the broccoli stems to make a soup or other side dish.

SALAD

1 broccoli, broken into florets and finely sliced

250 g (1/2 lb) bean sprouts

2 tsp sliced almonds, toasted (see page 141)

VINAIGRETTE

3 tbsp soy sauce

1 garlic clove, minced

1 tbsp fresh ginger, minced

Salt and freshly ground pepper

80 ml (1/3 cup) olive oil

Prepare the vinaigrette, mixing the soy sauce, garlic, and ginger together. Season with salt and pepper to taste. Incorporate the oil slowly, whisking constantly.

Arrange the broccoli slices on a plate and sprinkle with the vinaigrette. Cover and marinate for 1 hour in the refrigerator.

Add the bean sprouts and toss well. Garnish with the toasted almonds and serve.

 Philippe Castel, elected health-conscious chef by his peers in 2004

Mexican corn salad

Preparation time: 15 minutes   **4 servings**
Difficulty: easy

4 corn on the cob, cooked, kernels removed, or 2 cups canned niblet corn, drained

1 green onion, sliced

80 g (2/3 cup) sliced almonds

1 red pepper, diced

1 celery stalk, diced

2 tbsp fresh coriander, chopped

2 tbsp fresh oregano, chopped

Juice of one lime, freshly squeezed

1 garlic clove, chopped

80 ml (1/3 cup) olive oil

50 g (1/3 cup) black olives, sliced

500 g (2 1/4 cups) red kidney beans, canned, rinsed, and drained

Tabasco or jalapeno pepper, chopped

Salt

Mix all ingredients together in a large bowl.

Cover and refrigerate for 1 hour before serving.

 Éric Harvey, Chef-Instructor at the École hôtelière de la Capitale in Quebec

salads — bean sprout salad / Mexican corn salad

Green papaya
salad

Preparation time: 20 minutes　　　　**4 servings**
Difficulty: easy

This salad is usually served accompanied with small diced raw vegetables, sticky rice, and roast chicken.

300 g (1 1/2 cups) green papaya, peeled and cut in sticks

7 small fresh hot peppers

6 garlic cloves, coarsely chopped

50 g (1/3 cup) long green beans, cut in sections

60 g (1/2 cup) unsalted peanuts, toasted

30 g (1 oz) small shrimp, cooked and peeled

6 cherry tomatoes, quartered

3 tbsp lemon or lime juice, freshly squeezed

1 tbsp sugar

1 tbsp fish sauce (nuoc-mâm or nam pla)

Crush and blend a piece of the green papaya, hot peppers, and the garlic in a food processor or with a mortar.

Transfer to a large bowl and add the beans, peanuts, shrimp, tomatoes, and the remaining papaya.

Whisk together the lemon juice, sugar, and fish sauce, pour over the papaya mixture, and toss well.

 Jean Vachon, Chef-Instructor at the École hôtelière de la Capitale in Quebec

Green mango
salad

Preparation time: 25 minutes　　　　**4 servings**
Difficulty: average

Green mango is a slightly sweet variety that is very popular in Asia and the West Indies. Serve this salad with your favourite steamed rice.

4 green mangoes

2 tbsp lime juice, freshly squeezed

3 tbsp small shrimp, cooked and peeled

2 tbsp untoasted nuts, unsalted, ground

2 tbsp sugar

60 ml (1/4 cup) fish sauce (nuoc-mâm or nam pla)

2 tbsp sambal oelek (see page 142)

1 bunch fresh mint, chopped (set aside a few sprigs)

2 shallots, chopped

1 bunch fresh coriander, chopped (set aside a few sprigs)

1 or 2 cherry or bird peppers, finely chopped

4 large lettuce leaves, fresh and crispy

Peel the mangoes and slice into very thin strips with a sharp knife or mandoline.

In a bowl, mix the mangoes together with the lime juice, shrimp, peanuts, sugar, fish sauce, and the sambal oelek.

Add the mint, shallots, coriander, and peppers.

Verify the seasoning and add sugar and lime juice as required.

Serve each portion in a large lettuce leaf. Garnish with a few sprigs of mint and coriander.

 Jean Vachon, Chef-Instructor at the École hôtelière de la Capitale in Quebec

green papaya
salad

green mango
salad

salads

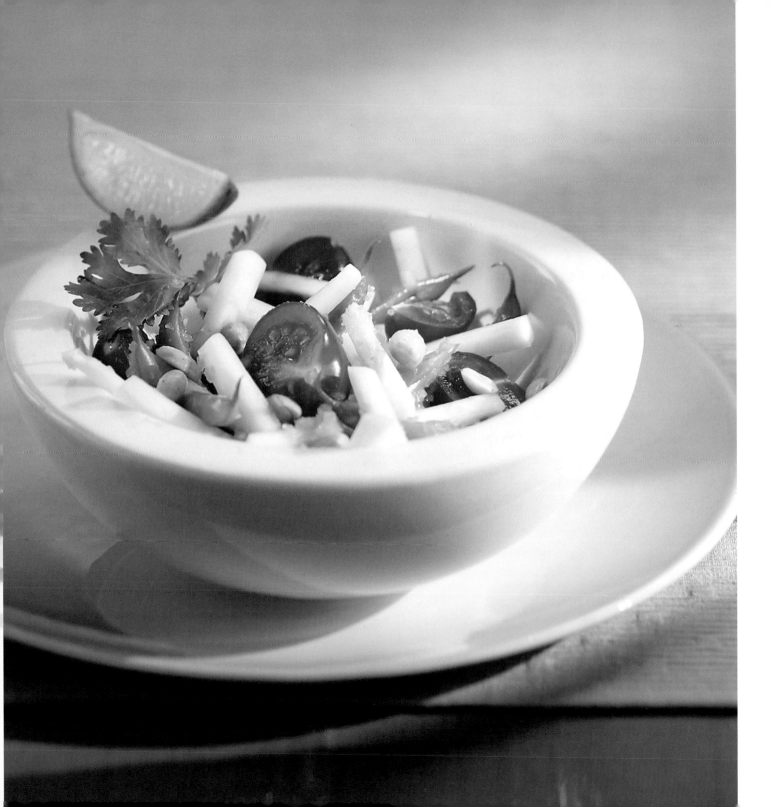

Cheese and vegetable salad

Preparation time: 30 minutes   **4 to 6 servings**
Difficulty: average

This salad will keep for 5 to 6 days in the refrigerator. You can liven it up by adding toasted pine nuts or flaxseed to taste. It will be even tastier if you make it the day before, as all the flavours will have time to marry. The vinaigrette is also delicious with a spinach salad. Keep any leftover in the refrigerator for later use. Chilli oil can be kept in an airtight jar in the refrigerator. Try it with salads, pizza, sandwiches, and sautéed dishes. Broccoflower is a cross between broccoli and cauliflower.

CHILLI OIL

125 ml (1/2 cup) olive oil

1 tbsp chilli flakes

VINAIGRETTE

1 tbsp sesame oil

80 ml (1/3 cup) rice wine vinegar

3 tbsp soy sauce

1 1/2 tsp garlic, minced

1 tbsp fresh ginger, minced

SALAD

1 medium carrot, julienned

1 medium onion, cubed

2 celery stalks, cubed

40 g (1/4 cup) green beans, cut in half

1 bouquet of broccoflower, finely sliced

1 bouquet of cauliflower, finely sliced

30 g (1/4 cup) Swiss cheese, diced

Make the chilli oil by heating the olive oil over medium heat until it is quite hot. Remove from the heat and add the chilli flakes. Let cool.

Whisk the chilli oil together with all the vinaigrette ingredients and set aside.

Steam the vegetables until they are tender, but still al dente. Cool under cold running water and drain well.

Mix all the vegetables together in a large bowl. Sprinkle with 60 ml (1/4 cup) of the vinaigrette, and garnish with the cheese.

Salad: Philippe Castel, elected health-conscious chef by his peers in 2004

Vinaigrette: Susan Sylvester, Chef-Instructor at the École hôtelière de la Capitale in Quebec

cheese and vegetable salad   salads

Pakchoi and spinach salad

Preparation time: 15 minutes
Difficulty: easy

4 servings

If you can't find baby spinach, buy regular spinach and coarsely chop with a sharp knife. If you are not going to use all the salad at one meal, serve the vinaigrette on the side.

SALAD
150 g (2 cups) baby spinach

2 celery stalks, finely chopped

80 g (1 cup) bean sprouts

1 red pepper, cut into small cubes

160 g (1 cup) pakchoi, sliced

120 g (1 cup) cashew nuts, lightly grilled, coarsely chopped

2 tbsp fresh chives, chopped

VINAIGRETTE
60 ml (1/4 cup) soy sauce

125 ml (1/2 cup) grapeseed oil

1 garlic clove, minced

1 tbsp fresh ginger, minced or fincly grated

Mix all the salad ingredients together in a large bowl.

Mix all the ingredients for the vinaigrette in a small bowl.

Pour the vinaigrette over the salad and mix well. Cover and refrigerate for 1 hour before serving.

 Marlène Gagnon, Chef-Instructor at the École hôtelière de la Capitale in Quebec

Legume salad

Preparation time: 15 minutes
Difficulty: easy

4 servings

SALAD
475 g (2 1/4 cups) canned legumes, rinsed and drained

1 green onion, chopped

1 red pepper, diced

50 g (1/4 cup) celery, diced

VINAIGRETTE
110 g (3/4 cup) silken tofu

30 g (1/4 cup) flaxseed, ground

1 tbsp lemon juice, freshly squeezed

1 tbsp grapeseed oil

2 tbsp water

1 garlic clove, chopped

1 tbsp hot mustard

GARNISH
Lettuce leaves

60 g (1/2 cup) almonds, chopped

Mix the legumes with the green onion, pepper, and the celery.

Using a mixer or a food processor, blend all the vinaigrette ingredients together into a mayonnaise texture.

Pour over the legumes and mix well.

Serve on a bed of lettuce, and garnish with the almonds.

Marlène Gagnon, Chef-Instructor at the École hôtelière de la Capitale in Quebec

salads

pakchoi and spinach salad

legume salad

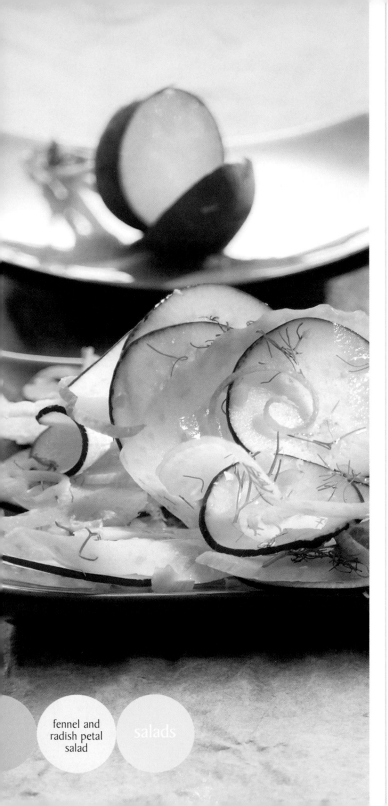

fennel and radish petal salad

salads

Fennel and radish petal salad

Preparation time: 25 minutes   **4 servings**
Difficulty: average

If you do not have a mandoline, a well-sharpened knife will do the job of slicing very fine fennel and radish "petals."

SALAD

500 g (1 lb) radishes, finely sliced with a mandoline

1 fennel bulb, finely sliced with a mandoline

100 g (2/3 cup) walnuts, finely chopped

VINAIGRETTE

Zest of 2 oranges, tangerines, or mandarins

Juice of 2 oranges, tangerines, or mandarins, freshly squeezed

3 tbsp balsamic vinegar

Salt and freshly ground pepper

150 ml (2/3 cup) extra virgin olive oil

Mix the radishes, fennel, and walnuts together in a bowl.

Blanch the citrus zest in boiling water for approximately 1 minute. Rinse under cold water to stop the cooking.

In a small bowl, prepare the vinaigrette, mixing together the zest, citrus juice, and vinegar. Season with salt and pepper to taste. Whisk in the oil very slowly with a fork or whisk to emulsify the mixture.

Pour the vinaigrette over the salad, cover and chill for 1 hour in the refrigerator before serving.

 Philippe Castel, elected health-conscious chef by his peers in 2004

Warm sherry
and salmon salad

Preparation time: 30 minutes   4 servings
Difficulty: average

*This salad is even more remarkable when
served with ripe tomatoes or glazed tomatoes in
olive oil (see page 172).*

SALAD

4 salmon escalopes, 60 g (2 oz) each

3 tbsp olive oil

600 g (1 1/4 lbs) very fresh mixed greens

Fresh fines herbes to taste (parsley, chives,
tarragon, basil)

120 g (2/3 cup) cucumber, seeded and sliced

60 g (1/3 cup) radishes, finely sliced

VINAIGRETTE

1 tbsp shallots, chopped

2 tbsp Dijon mustard

4 tbsp Meaux or old style Dijon mustard

1 tbsp honey (preferably unpasteurized)

60 ml (1/4 cup) sherry vinegar

375 ml (1 1/2 cups) soybean oil

Salt and freshly ground pepper

*Prepare the vinaigrette, mixing the shallots,
mustards, honey, and vinegar together in a bowl.
Gradually incorporate the soybean oil. Season
with salt and pepper to taste.*

*Season the salmon with salt and pepper, and place
on a lightly greased roasting pan. Brush the
salmon with the olive oil and grill in the oven.*

*Arrange the salmon escalopes on a bed of mixed
greens. Add the fines herbes, cucumber, and the
radishes, sprinkle with the vinaigrette, and serve
immediately.*

 **François Rousseau, Chef-Instructor at the
École hôtelière de la Capitale in Quebec**

Spring salad

Preparation time: 15 minutes   4 servings
Difficulty: easy

SALAD

600 g (3 cups) artichoke hearts, whole or sliced,
canned

2 medium tomatoes, quartered

1 bunch fresh watercress, washed and patted dry

100 g (2/3 cup) old cheddar, grated

2 tbsp fresh chives, chopped

30 g (1/4 cup) whole hazelnuts, toasted and chopped
(see page 141)

VINAIGRETTE

4 tbsp Dijon mustard

3 tbsp white wine or maple vinegar

3 tbsp maple syrup (preferably dark amber)

150 ml (2/3 cup) good quality hazelnut oil
(preferably)

Grapeseed oil

Salt and freshly ground pepper

*Prepare the vinaigrette, mixing the mustard,
vinegar, and syrup together in a bowl. Add the oil,
whisking constantly. Season with salt and pepper
to taste.*

*Mix all the salad ingredients except the hazelnuts
together in a large bowl.*

*Add the vinaigrette at the last moment. Garnish
with the hazelnuts and serve.*

 **Marlène Gagnon, Chef-Instructor at the
École hôtelière de la Capitale in Quebec**

salads

warm sherry
and salmon
salad

spring salad

Nepalese salad

Preparation time: 40 minutes
Difficulty: easy
4 servings

250 g (1/2 lb) baby potatoes

1 tbsp ground turmeric

60 g (1/2 cup) sesame seeds

Juice of one lemon, freshly squeezed

15 g (1/2 cup) fresh coriander, chopped

125 ml (1/2 cup) water

Salt and freshly ground pepper

3 tbsp olive oil

2 green peppers, finely sliced

1 jalapeno pepper, finely chopped

1 tbsp cumin seed

Cook the potatoes whole until they are slightly soft in the centre. Cool rapidly in cold water and cut into rounds.

In a large bowl, mix the potatoes, turmeric, sesame seeds, lemon juice, coriander, and the water. Season with salt and pepper to taste.

Heat the olive oil in a sauté pan and sauté the peppers, jalapeno, and the cumin over medium-high heat.

Add the potatoes, mix well and serve warm.

 Jean-Pierre Cloutier, Chef-proprietor of Café-restaurant du Musée in Quebec

Nepalese salad

spinach and blood orange salad

salads

Spinach and blood orange salad

Preparation time: 15 minutes
Difficulty: easy
4 servings

Two vinaigrettes for one recipe, to alternate. The blood oranges can be replaced by regular oranges.

SALAD
2 oranges

200 g (7 oz) spinach leaves

VINAIGRETTE
2 tbsp soy sauce

1 garlic clove, chopped

1 1/2 tbsp fresh ginger, minced

Salt and freshly ground pepper

80 ml (1/3 cup) olive oil

2 tsp sesame oil

VINAIGRETTE (VARIANT)
1 tbsp sherry vinegar

Salt and freshly ground pepper

4 tsp orange juice, freshly squeezed

60 ml (1/4 cup) olive oil

With a sharp knife, remove the peel and white skin from the oranges, and quarter them over a bowl, reserving the juice.

Wash and remove the stems from the spinach.

Prepare the vinaigrette, mixing all ingredients together in order. Add the orange juice.

Mix the spinach and oranges together in a large bowl. Add the vinaigrette at the last minute, and mix well.

 Philippe Castel, elected health-conscious chef by his peers in 2004

Olivier Neau, Chef-Instructor at the École hôtelière de la Capitale in Quebec

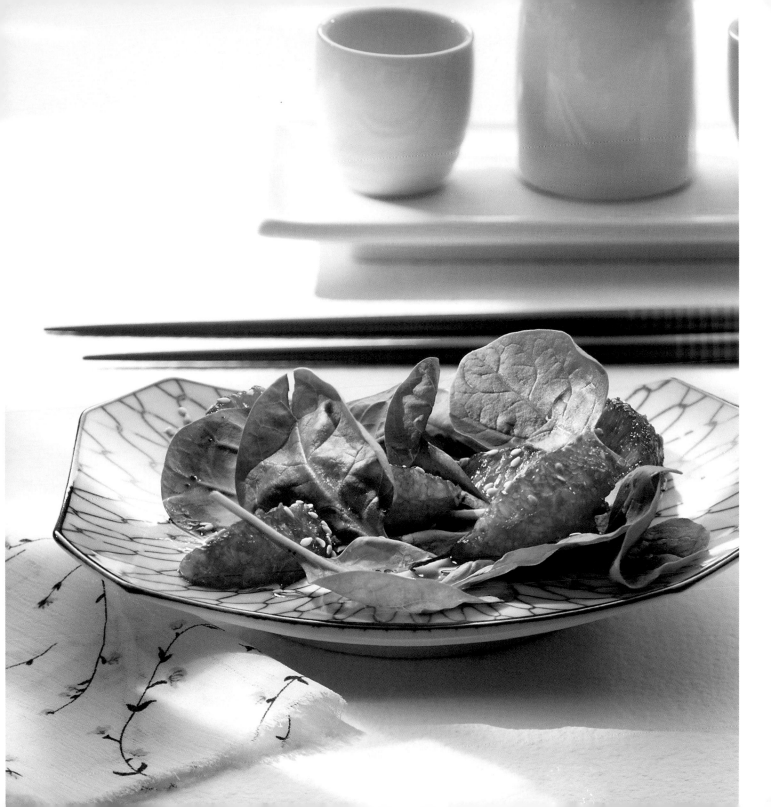

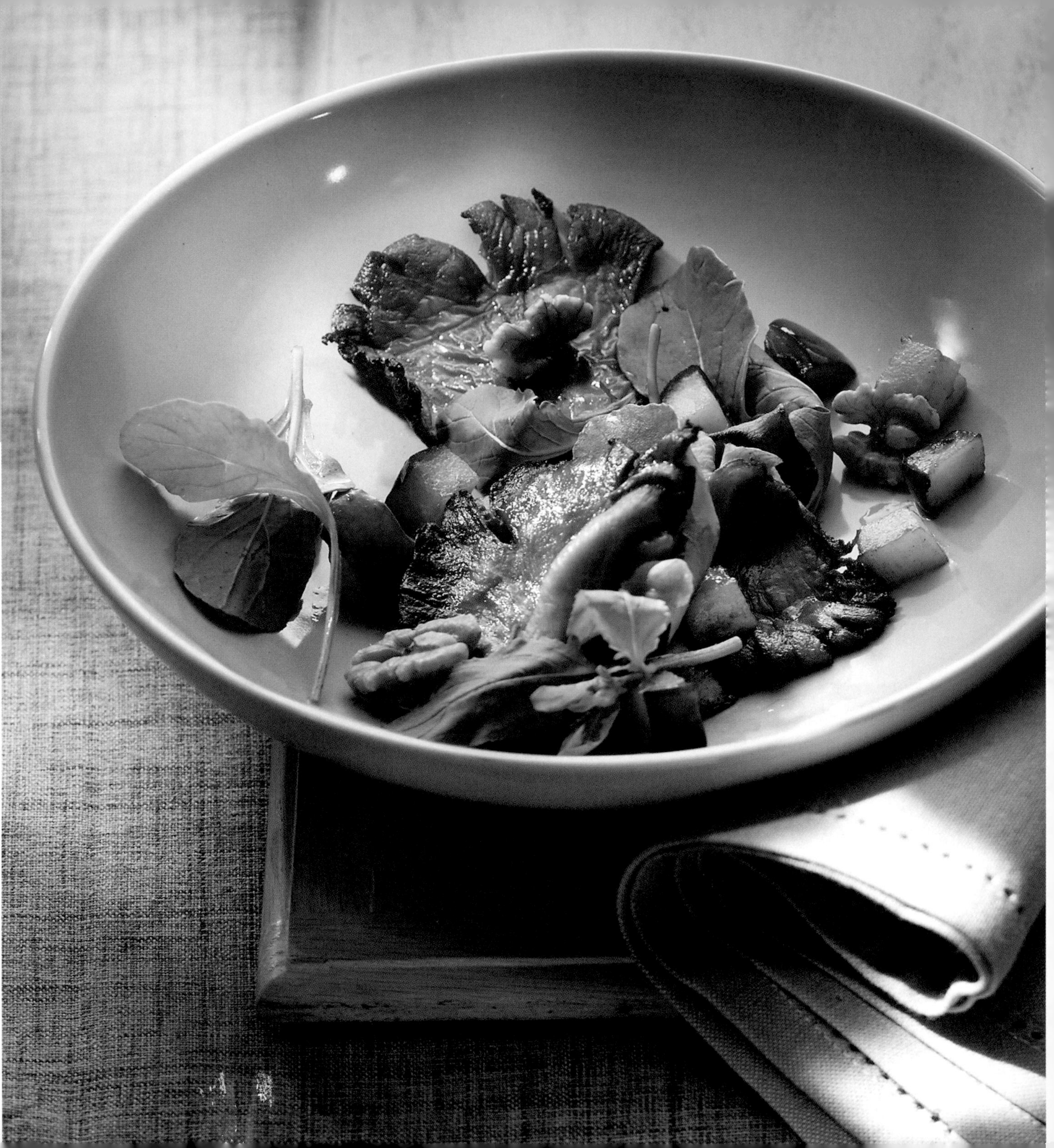

Apple and oyster mushroom salad

Preparation time: 30 minutes
Difficulty: easy

4 servings

2 tbsp butter

3 apples, cubed

375 g (3/4 lb) oyster mushrooms

2 tbsp cider vinegar

60 ml (1/4 cup) olive oil

Salt and freshly ground pepper

400 g (5 cups) fresh arugula

60 g (1/2 cup) walnuts

Cook the apples and the oyster mushrooms separately in the butter for 1 to 2 minutes over medium-high heat.

In a small bowl, mix the vinegar and the olive oil together. Season with salt and pepper to taste.

Toss the arugula with the vinaigrette in a large bowl. Add the apples, mushrooms, and walnuts, mix well and serve warm.

 Jean-Pierre Cloutier, Chef-proprietor of Café-restaurant du Musée in Quebec

Warm Brussels sprouts salad

Preparation time: 40 minutes
Difficulty: average

4 servings

320 g (11 oz) Brussels sprouts

3 tbsp vegetable oil

2 green onions, finely sliced

Salt and freshly ground pepper

2 tbsp tarragon vinegar

2-3 tbsp Indian cress buds (nasturtium flower-buds) or capers

1/2 pack of fresh chives, chopped

With a sharp paring knife, make a cross-shaped incision in the bottom of each Brussels sprout. Steam for approximately 12 minutes.

Heat the oil in a saucepan, and add the sprouts and green onions. Season generously with salt and pepper, cooking for barely a minute.

Deglaze the pan with the vinegar, stirring well. Incorporate the nasturtium flower-buds and the chives.

 Jean-Pierre Cloutier, Chef-proprietor of Café-restaurant du Musée in Quebec

salads

apple and mushroom salad

warm Brussels sprouts salad

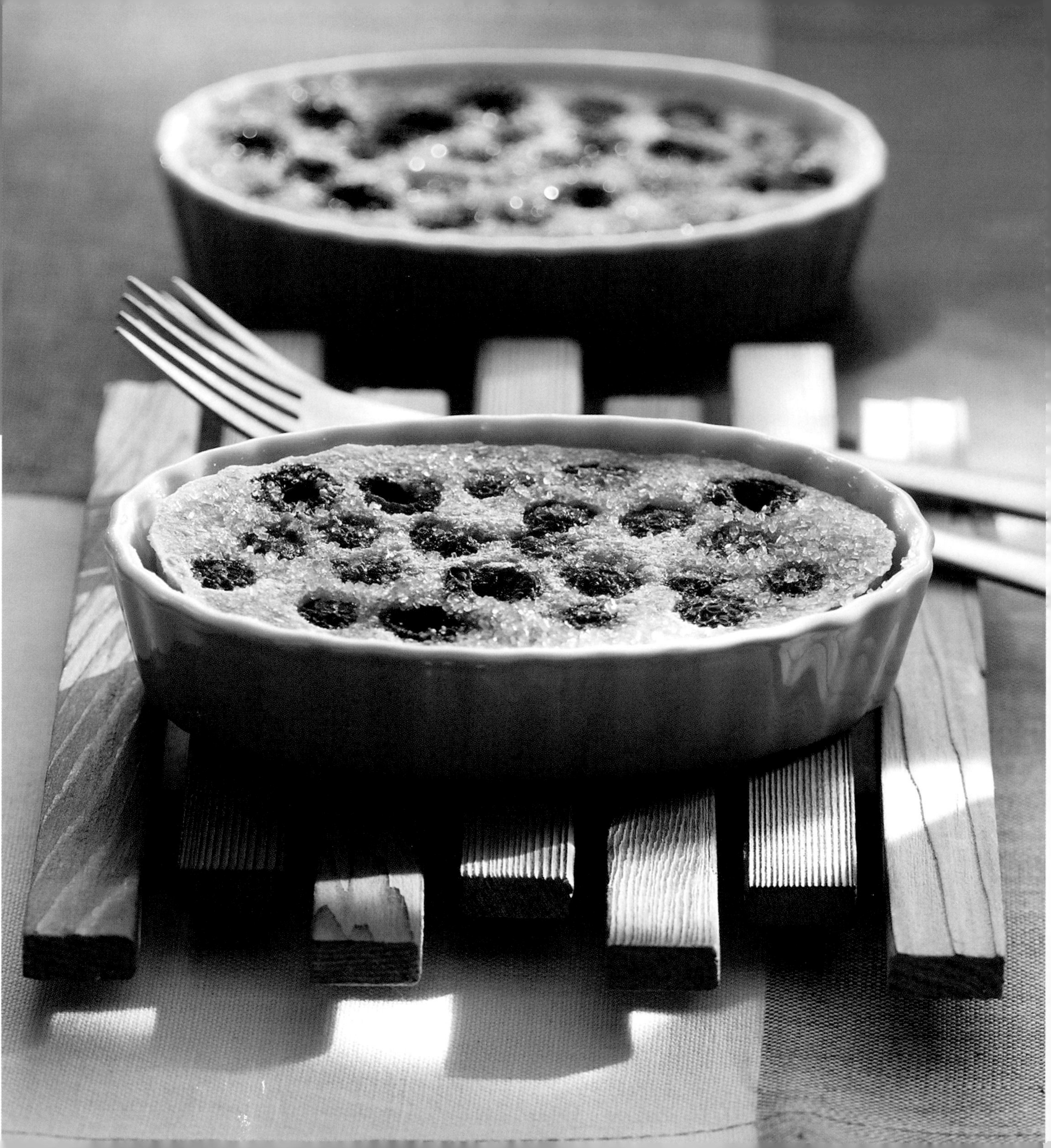

Sweet chestnut brownies

Preparation time: 1 h 30
Difficulty: average

24 brownies

You will find toasted chestnut flakes in Italian grocery stores, natural food stores, and specialized boutiques. These brownies are even better the day after they are cooked. Store them at room temperature in an airtight container.

100 g (3 1/2 oz) 72 % dark chocolate

120 g (1/2 cup) butter

80 g (1/3 cup) sugar

4 eggs, separated

30 g (1/4 cup) walnuts

30 g (1/4 cup) pecans

60 g (1/2 cup) toasted chestnut flakes, or almond, or hazelnut powder

Melt the chocolate with the butter and the sugar in a double boiler, uncovered.

Add the egg yolks one at a time, whisking vigorously after each yolk.

Using a mixer, and in a clean bowl, whip the egg whites until stiff peaks form, and fold delicately into the chocolate mixture.

Add the walnuts, pecans, and chestnut flakes.

Line a 25 x 30 cm (10 x 12 in) cake mould with waxed paper.

Transfer the brownie mixture to the mould and bake in the oven at 190°C (375°F) for 25 to 30 minutes.

Remove and let stand 10 minutes before turning out and cutting into squares.

 Philippe Castel, elected health-conscious chef by his peers in 2004

Raspberry clafouti

Preparation time: 1 h 15
Difficulty: average

8 servings

60 g (1/2 cup) unbleached flour

60 g (1/2 cup) oatmeal

60 g (1/2 cup) ground almonds

3 eggs

125 ml (1/2 cup) maple syrup

100 g (1/2 cup) granulated maple sugar

150 ml (2/3 cup) 35 % whipping cream

150 ml (2/3 cup) soy milk

250 g (1 2/3 cups) fresh raspberries

Grease and flour a 25 x 30 cm (10 x 12 in) mould.

Mix the unbleached flour, oatmeal, and almonds together in a bowl.

Beat the eggs in another bowl. Add the syrup and the maple sugar, mixing well. Incorporate the dry ingredients.

Add the cream and the soy milk delicately, and transfer to the mould. Cover the top with the raspberries.

Bake in the oven at 200°C (400°F) for 30 to 40 minutes.

Remove from the oven and turn out immediately.

 Jean Vachon, Chef-Instructor at the École hôtelière de la Capitale in Quebec

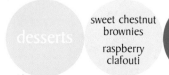

desserts

sweet chestnut brownies

raspberry clafouti

Yogurt and fresh fruit cup

Preparation time: 45 minutes
Difficulty: average

4 servings

200 g (1 1/3 cup) fresh raspberries

200 g (1 1/3 cup) fresh cranberries

200 g (1 1/3 cup) red plums, quartered

100 g (1/2 cup) rhubarb, chopped

400 g (1 2/3 cups) unrefined brown sugar

300 g (1 1/4 cups) plain yogurt

300 g (1 1/4 cups) plain kefir

150 g (1 cup) granola nuts

Several fresh mint leaves

Place the fruit and sugar in a saucepan. Bring to a boil, stirring occasionally to keep from sticking. Let simmer approximately 15 minutes, until the cranberries burst and the rhubarb is cooked.

Transfer to a bowl and allow to cool in the refrigerator.

Mix the yogurt and kefir together in a bowl. Cover and set aside in the refrigerator.

Fill a glass cup (highball or other) two-thirds with the chilled fruit, and add a dollop of the yogurt.

Garnish with the granola and fresh mint leaves just before serving.

 Steve McCandless, Chef-co-owner of the Bistro Le Clocher Penché in Quebec

Fieldberry and dark chocolate surprise

Preparation time: 1 h 15
Difficulty: easy

4 servings

2 tbsp blueberries

2 tbsp raspberries

2 tbsp blackberries

2 tbsp strawberries

60 g (1/4 cup) sugar

300 ml (1 1/4 cups) 35 % whipping cream

180 g (6 oz) 72 % dark chocolate

Fresh mint leaves, shredded

Purée the fruit and the sugar in a mixer.

Spoon into icecube trays and freeze for 1 hour.

Divide the cream into equal quantities.

Melt the chocolate in a double boiler, and stir in one half of the cream, whisking rapidly to avoid forming crystals.

Whisk the other half of the cream until slightly firm, and incorporate it into the melted chocolate.

Half fill 4 dessert cups with the chocolate mixture.

Place a fruit cube in the middle of each cup and cover with the remaining mousse.

Garnish each cup with several mint leaves.

 Philippe Castel, elected health-conscious chef by his peers in 2004

yogurt
cup
dark chocolate
surprise

desserts

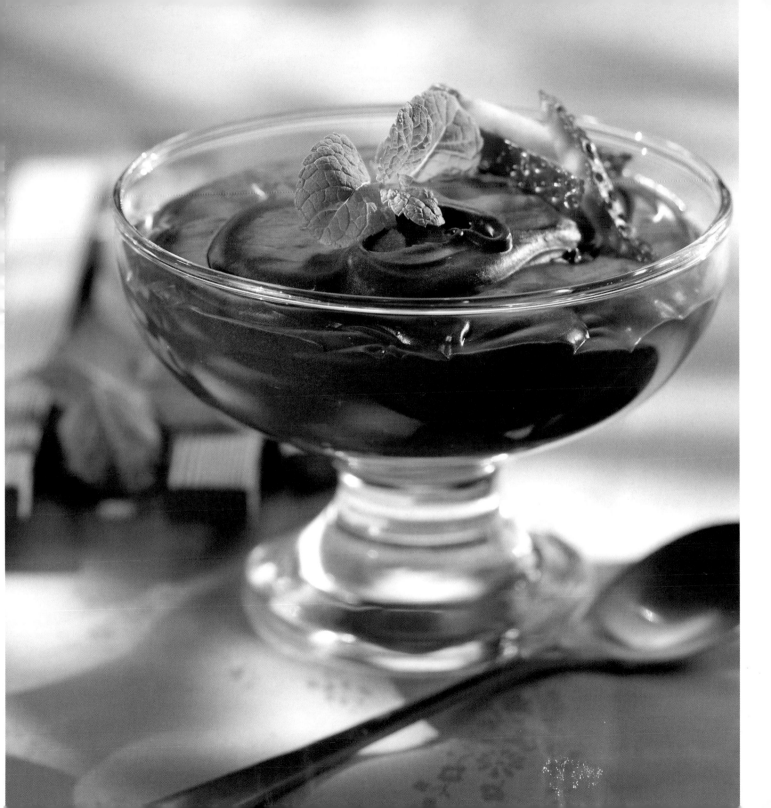

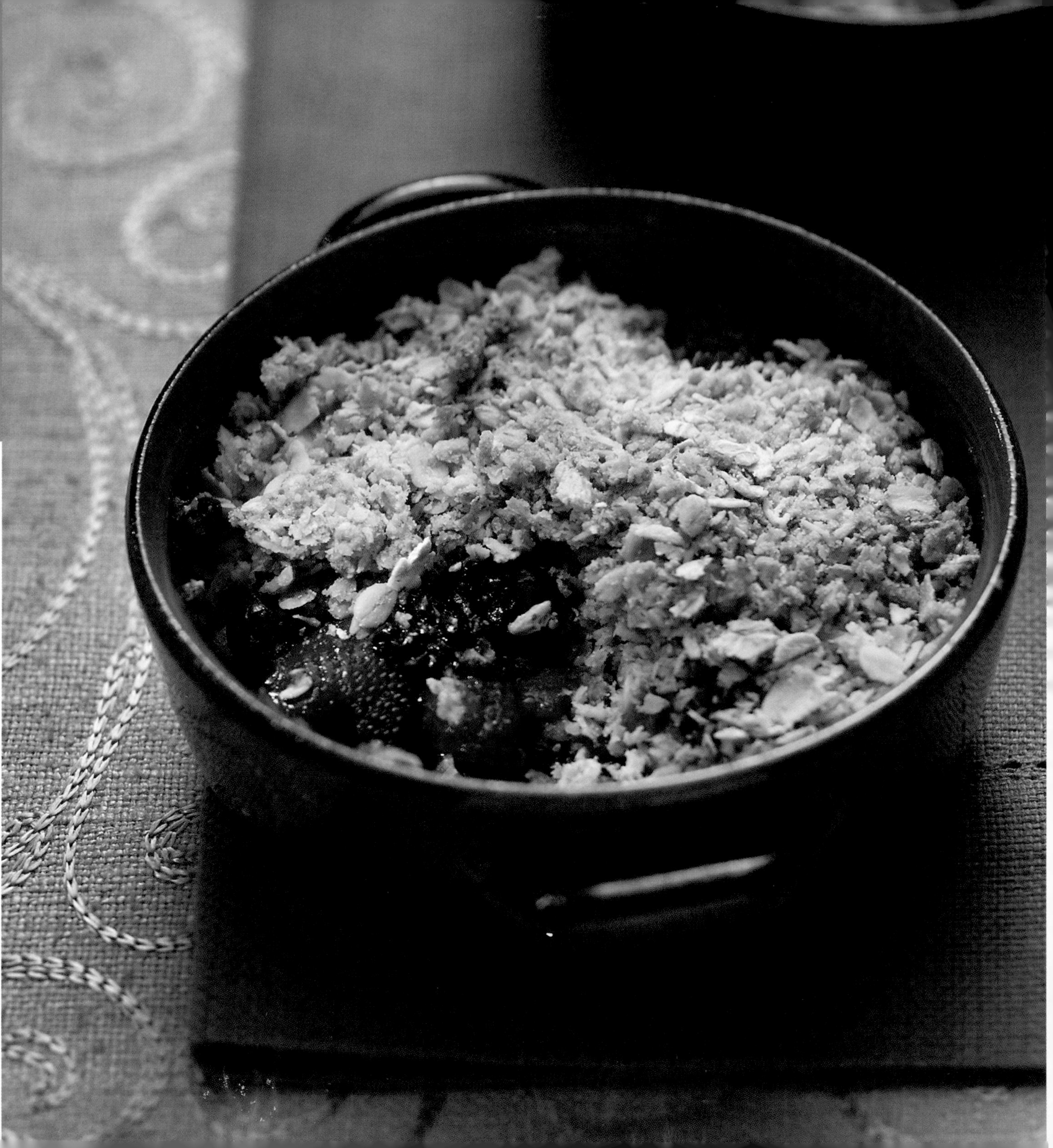

Dark chocolate and silken tofu pudding

Preparation time: 25 minutes   4 servings
Difficulty: easy

Silken almond tofu is a dessert that is sold in natural food stores and most supermarkets.

375 g (2 1/2 cups) silken almond tofu

300 g (10 oz) 70 % dark chocolate

Selection of small fieldberries

Process the tofu in a mixer for approximately 30 seconds, until smooth.

Melt the chocolate in a double boiler.

Add the melted chocolate to the tofu.

Using a mixer, beat the tofu and chocolate mixture for 1 minute on low speed.

Transfer the pudding to 4 ramekins and garnish with the fieldberries.

 Éric Harvey, Chef-Instructor at the École hôtelière de la Capitale in Quebec

Fieldberry croustade

Preparation time: 1 hour   6 to 8 servings
Difficulty: easy

If you are using frozen berries, do not thaw them beforehand for this recipe. Berries are an excellent source of a wide variety of anti-cancer agents, and everyone should eat them regularly. This croustade is delicious with French vanilla ice cream.

90 g (1 cup) rolled oats

120 g (1/2 cup) brown sugar, packed well

35 g (1/4 cup) all-purpose flour

3 tbsp cold butter

600 g (4 cups) variety of berries, fresh or frozen (strawberries, raspberries, blueberries, and blackberries)

Preheat the oven to 180°C (350°F).

Mix the rolled oats, brown sugar, flour, and butter together to obtain a homogenous mixture.

Arrange the fruit in a 20 x 20 cm (8 x 8 in) pyrex dish and cover with the mixture.

Cook in the oven for 30 to 45 minutes, uncovered, until the fruit begins to boil and the centre is properly cooked. Serve warm.

 Richard Béliveau

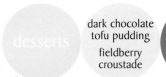

desserts

dark chocolate tofu pudding

fieldberry croustade

Clementine–
green tea infusion

Preparation time: 20 minutes   **5 servings**
Difficulty: easy

250 ml (1 cup) water

60 g (1/4 cup) sugar

2 tsp green tea

10 clementines, peeled and separated into sections

40 g (1/4 cup) fresh bilberries or blueberries, or cranberries

Boil the water and sugar for 3 minutes. Add the tea and steep for 5 minutes.

Strain the tea. Add the clementines and the blueberries (or cranberries) and let simmer 2 minutes.

Cover and let macerate for 12 hours in the refrigerator.

 Christophe Alary, Chef-Instructor at the École hôtelière de la Capitale in Quebec, elected Chef of the Year 2004 by his peers

Hot chocolate
tartlets

Preparation time: 45 minutes   **10 tartlets**
Difficulty: easy

This recipe from Belgium can also be made with equal parts of wheat flower and all-purpose flour. You can add small berries in the centre and flavour them with finely chopped fresh basil.

180 g (3/4 cup) soft butter

300 g (1 1/2 cups) granulated maple sugar

190 g (6 1/3 oz) semi-sweet dark chocolate, melted

6 eggs

100 g (2/3 cup) all-purpose flour, sifted

Butter 10 small tart moulds.

Melt the butter and transfer to a bowl. Add the maple sugar and whisk well.

Add the chocolate and mix well.

Incorporate the eggs one at a time, and then add the flour.

Pour into the moulds and cook in the oven at 150°C (300°F) for approximately 10 minutes. Serve immediately.

 Isabelle Légaré, Chef-Instructor at the École hôtelière de la Capitale in Quebec

clementine infusion

hot chocolate tartlets

desserts

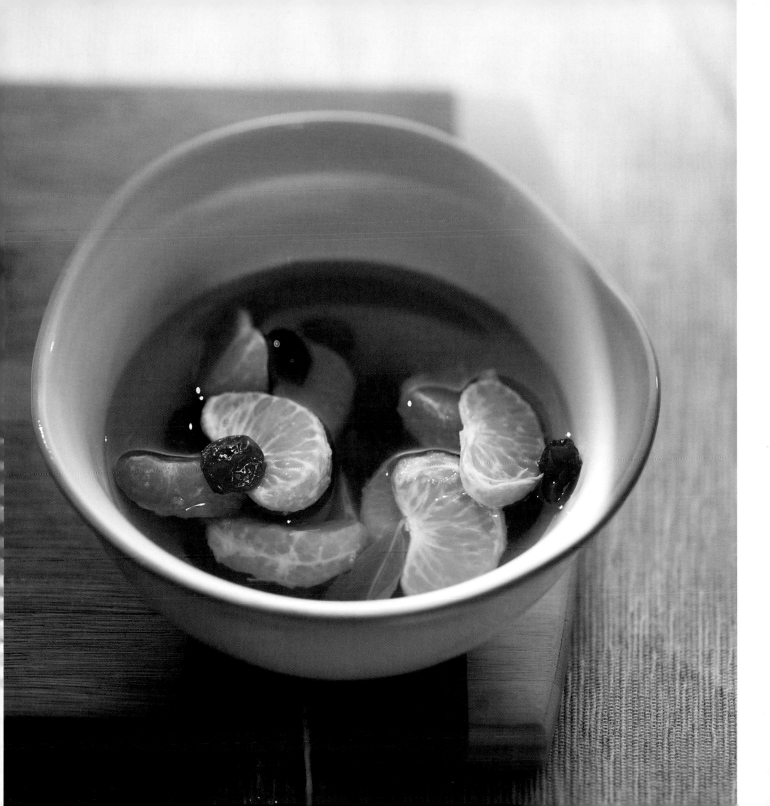

Tropical
fruit salad

Preparation time: 15 minutes **4 servings**
Difficulty: easy

100 g (1/2 cup) honey

1/2 tsp fresh ginger, finely chopped

100 g (1/2 cup) pineapple, diced

2 oranges, sectioned

1 lime, sectioned

2 mangoes, diced

1 mandarin, sectioned

Heat the honey and the ginger for approximately 2 minutes.

In a large bowl, mix all the fruit together and coat with the hot honey.

Cover and allow to macerate for 12 hours in the refrigerator before serving.

 Éric Harvey, Chef-Instructor at the École hôtelière de la Capitale in Quebec

Burgundy
fieldberry soup

Preparation time: 20 minutes **4 servings**
Difficulty: easy

150 g (3/4 cup) honey

175 ml (3/4 cup) red Burgundy wine

1 cinnamon stick

Freshly ground pepper

100 g (2/3 cup) blueberries

100 g (2/3 cup) raspberries

100 g (2/3 cup) strawberries

100 g (2/3 cup) blackberries or cranberries

Boil the honey for 8 minutes.

Add the wine and the cinnamon stick. Pepper to taste and let boil for another 5 minutes.

Add to the fruit and allow to cool in the refrigerator.

Serve in fancy dessert bowls.

 Éric Harvey, Chef-Instructor at the École hôtelière de la Capitale in Quebec

tropical
fruit salad

burgundy
fieldberry
soup

desserts

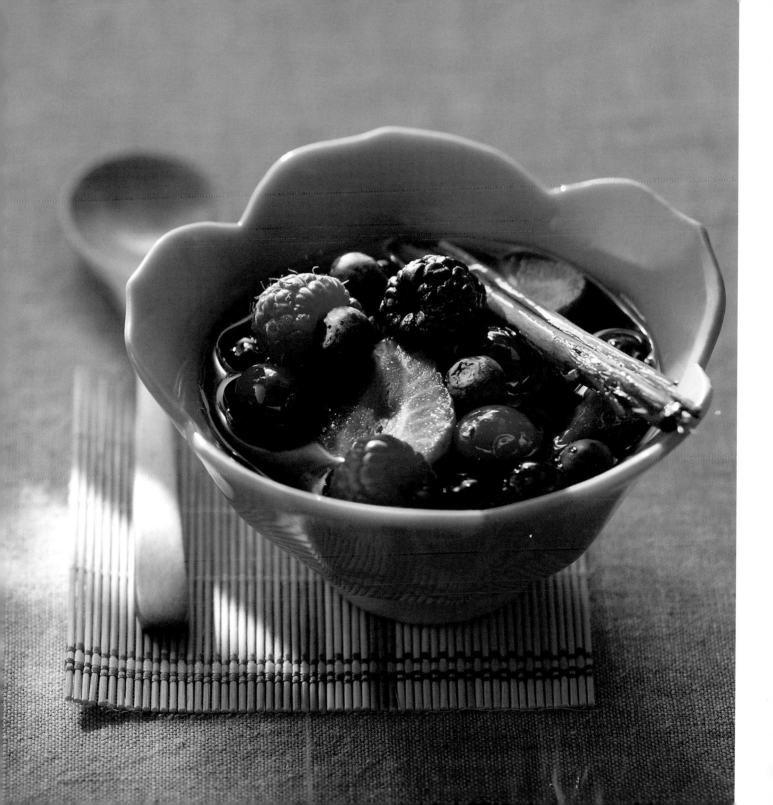

Green
tea–infused tapioca

Preparation time: 45 minutes   **10 servings**
Difficulty: easy

Green tapioca is easy to find in Asian grocery stores, and is especially prized by the Vietnamese. Its colour comes from the leaves of the pandanus, or screw-pine plant. Pistachio paste is made in the same manner as almond paste. It is easy to find in Arab grocery stores.

500 ml (2 cups) soy milk

1 bag green tea

75 g (1/3 cup) tapioca, rinsed and drained

120 g (1/2 cup) sugar

1 tbsp pistachio paste

20 fresh cherries, pitted and chopped

4 tbsp sour cream or plain yogurt

Heat the soy milk and steep the tea bag for 10 minutes.

Remove the tea bag.

Transfer the tapioca to the milk and cook for 15 to 20 minutes, stirring occasionally. Add the sugar and pistachio paste at the end of cooking.

Garnish 10 liqueur glasses with the tapioca.

Process the cherries and the sour cream in a food processor and pour over the tapioca.

 Christophe Alary, Chef-Instructor at the École hôtelière de la Capitale in Quebec, elected Chef of the Year 2004 by his peers

Green tea and
soy milk truffles

Preparation time: 30 minutes   **30 truffles**
Rest time: 2 hours
Difficulty: easy

250 ml (1 cup) vanilla soy milk

2 green tea bags

250 g (1/2 lb) 70 % dark chocolate

90 g (3/4 cup) unsalted pistachio nuts, shelled

Slowly bring the soy milk to a boil with the tea bags.

Remove the tea bags and pour the boiling milk on the chocolate. Stir for 2 minutes and let cool for 2 hours at room temperature.

Meanwhile, grind the pistachio nuts in a food processor.

Shape 30 truffles with the cooled chocolate and roll the balls to coat in the pistachio grounds.

 Éric Harvey, Chef-Instructor at the École hôtelière de la Capitale in Quebec

green tea tapioca

green tea and soy milk truffles

desserts

Dried fruit
and carrot cake

Preparation time: 2 hours　　　　　　　**10 servings**
Difficulty: average

375 ml (1 1/2 cups) boiling water

200 g (1 cup) dried fruit (cranberries, plums, apricots, figs, dates, grapes, etc.), chopped

1 tbsp allspice

1 tsp ground ginger

1 pinch of ground nutmeg

1/2 tsp salt

225 g (1 1/2 cups) whole-wheat flour

60 g (3/4 cup) wheat bran

1 tsp baking powder

1 tsp baking soda

200 g (1 cup) carrots, grated

60 ml (1/4 cup) flaxseed or other first cold pressed oil

2 tbsp honey

125 ml (1/2 cup) maple syrup

Preheat the oven to 180°C (350°F).

Pour the boiling water over the dried fruit and let steep for 10 minutes.

In a bowl, mix together the allspice, ginger, nutmeg, salt, flour, wheat bran, baking powder, and baking soda.

In another bowl, mix together the carrots, dried fruit, and their soaking water, flaxseed oil, honey, and maple syrup.

Add the dry ingredients to the moist ingredients, and stir until blended.

Transfer to a 23 x 13 cm (9 x 5 in) non-stick loaf pan and cook in the oven for approximately 1 hour 15 minutes. The cake is cooked when a toothpick inserted into the centre comes out clean.

 Susan Sylvester, Chef-Instructor at the École hôtelière de la Capitale in Quebecc

desserts　　dried fruit and carrot cake

Thanks and Acknowledgements

The inspiration essential to the writing of this book came to us from the remarkable courage shown by cancer patients both young and old who engage in a daily struggle against this terrible disease. We wish to honour them and to express our deep admiration for their determination and will to fight.

Thank you to the Charles Bruneau Foundation, whose encouragement and financial support allowed us to develop the nutratherapy research program established in the Hemato-Oncology Division at the CHU Sainte-Justine Research Centre.

Thank you to the UQAM Foundation and its generous donors, who supported us by endowing the Chair in Cancer Prevention and Treatment. We thank them for their vision and their unfailing support.

Thank you to The Cancer Research Society, whose considerable research grants have supported our projects from the beginning of the program.

Thank you to Dr. Claude Bertrand, neurosurgeon, for his generosity with regard to the endowment of the Claude Bertrand Chair in Neurosurgery at the CHU, of which I am honoured to be the first holder (R.B.).

Thank you to all of our clinician colleagues at the Hemato-Oncology Division at the CHU Sainte-Justine Research Centre for their incredible devotion in the fight against children's cancer.

Thank you to all the members of the Division – nurses, pharmacists, volunteers, therapists – for their tremendous commitment and their generous involvement in the lives of young cancer patients.

Thank you to all the scientists in the Molecular Medicine Laboratory, whose research work is at the heart of the first discoveries in nutratherapy, for their extraordinary enthusiasm in furthering medical knowledge.

Thank you to all the talented chefs who contributed to the preparation of this book, and especially those of the Fondation Serge-Bruyère. Upon being challenged, they repeatedly rose to the occasion by creating delicious meals that met our strict criteria. A special thank you to Jean-Pierre Cloutier, of the Musée national des Beaux-arts du Québec's Café-Restaurant, and to the Fondation's Guylaine Boisvert, for their enthusiastic project supervision.

Thank you to Dr. Serge Carrière, without whom none of this would have been possible, for his wisdom, his humanity, the clarity of his vision, and his unending efforts in bettering the human condition.

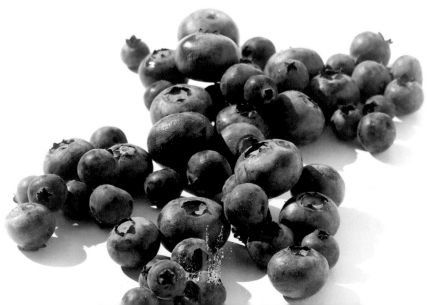

Bibliography

Chapter 1

To learn more about . . .

. . . the prevention of cancer through diet:
- World Cancer Research Fund/American Institute for Cancer Research. *Food, Nutrition and the Prevention of Cancer: A Global Perspective.* 1997, 670 pages.
- R. Doll, R. Peto. "The causes of cancer : quantitative estimates of avoidable risks of cancer in the United States today." *J. Natl Cancer Inst.* 1981; 66 : 1196-1265.
- W.C. Willett. "Diet and cancer." *Oncologist* 2000; 5 : 393-404.
- B.N. Ames, L.S. Gold, W.C. Willett. "The causes and prevention of cancer." *Proc. Natl Acad. Sci. U.S.A.* 1995; 92 : 5258-5265.

. . . tumoral microfoci:
- J. Folkman, R. Kalluri. "Cancer without disease." *Nature* 2004; 427 : 787.
- W.C. Black, H.G. Welch. "Advances in diagnostic imaging and overestimation of disease prevalence and the benefits of therapy." *N. Eng. J. Med.* 1993; 328 : 1237-1243.

. . . the puzzle of cancer:
- D. Hanahan, R.A. Weinberg. "The hallmarks of cancer." *Cell* 2000; 100 : 57-70.

. . . anti-cancer phytochemical compounds:
- Y.-J. Surh. "Cancer chemoprevention with dietary phytochemicals." *Nature Reviews on Cancer* 2003; 3 : 768-780.
- T. Dorai, B.B. Aggarwal. "Role of chemopreventive agents in cancer therapy." *Cancer Lett.* 2004; 215 : 129-140.

Chapter 2

To learn more about . . .

. . . the role of inflammation in the development of cancer:
- L.M. Coussens, Z. Werb. "Inflammation and cancer." *Nature* 2002; 420 : 860-867.
- F. Balkwill, K.A. Charles, A. Mantovani. "Smoldering and polarized inflammation in the initiation and promotion of malignant disease." *Cancer Cell* 2005; 7 : 211-217.

. . . the NFκB protein:
- M. Karin. "Nuclear factor-κB in cancer development and progression." *Nature* 2006; 441 : 431-436.

. . . omega-3 fatty acids:
- D.P. Rose, J.M. Connolly. "Omega-3 fatty acids as cancer chemopreventive agents." *Pharm. Ther.* 1999; 83 : 217-244.
- S.C. Larsson, M. Kumlin, M. Ingelman-Sundberg, A. Wolk. "Dietary long-chain n-3 fatty acids for the prevention of cancer : a review of potential mechanisms." *Am. J. Clin. Nutr.* 2004; 79 : 935-945.

Chapter 3

To learn more about . . .

. . . the negative impact of obesity on health:
- D.W. Haslam, P.T. James. "Obesity." *Lancet* 2005; 366 : 1197-1209.
- D.B. Allison, K.R. Fontaine, J.E. Manson, J. Stephens, T.B. VanItalie. "Annual deaths attributable to obesity in the United States." *JAMA* 1999; 282 : 1530-1538.

. . . the impact of meal (food) portion size on obesity:
L.R. Young. *The Portion Teller: Smartsize Your Way to Permanent Weight Loss.* New York : Morgan Road Books, 2005, 256 pages.

. . . the relationship (link) between obesity and cancer:
- E.E. Calle, R. Kaaks. "Overweight, obesity and cancer : epidemiological evidence and proposed mechanisms." *Nature Reviews on Cancer,* 2004; 4 : 579-591.

- A. McTiernan. "Obesity and cancer : the risks, science and potential management strategies." *Oncology* 2005; 19 : 871-886.

Chapter 5

To learn more . . .
- E. Kotake-Nara, M. Kushiro, H. Zhang, T. Sugawara, K. Miyashita, A. Nagao. "Carotenoids affect proliferation of human prostate cancer cells." *J. Nutrition* 2001; 131 : 3303-3306.
- C.F. Skibola, J.D. Curry, C. VandeVoort, A. Conley, M.T. Smith. "Brown kelp modulates endocrine hormones in female Sprague-Dawley rats and in human luteinized granulosa cells." *J. Nutrition* 2005; 135 : 296-300.

Chapter 6

To learn more . . .
- S.P. Wasser. "Medicinal mushrooms as a source of antitumor and immunomodulating polysaccharides." *Appl. Microbiol. Biotechnol.* 2002; 60 : 258-274.
- A.T. Borchers, C.L. Keen, M.E. Gershwin. "Mushrooms, tumors and immunity : an update." *Exp. Biol. Med.* 2004 : 229 : 393-406.

Chapter 7

To learn more . . .
- A.L. Webb, M.L. McCullough. "Dietary Lignans : potential role in cancer prevention." *Nutrition and Cancer* 2005; 51 : 117-131.
- H. Adlercreutz. "Phyto-oestrogens and cancer." *Lancet Oncology* 2002; 3 : 364-373.

Chapter 8

To learn more . . .
- B.B. Aggarwal, S. Shishodia. "Suppression of the nuclear factor kappa-B activation pathway by spice-derived phytochemicals : reasoning for seasoning." *Ann. N.Y. Acad. Sci.* 2004; 1030 : 434-441.
- J.W. Lampe. "Spicing up a vegetarian diet : chemopreventive effects of phytochemicals." *Am. J. Clin. Nutr.* 2003; 78 : 579S-583S.
- Y.J. Surh, K.S. Chun, H.H. Cha, S.S. Han, Y.S. Keum, K.K. Park, S.S. Lee. "Molecular mechanisms underlying chemopreventive activities of anti-inflammatory phytochemicals : down-regulation of COX-2 and iNOS through suppression of NF-kappa-B activation." *Mutation Res.* 2001; 480-481 : 243-268.

Chapter 9

To learn more about . . .

. . . the importance of intestinal bacteria:
- R.E. Ley, D.A. Peterson, J.I. Gordon. "Ecological and evolutionary forces shaping microbial diversity in the human intestine." *Cell* 2006; 124 : 837-848.
- F. Bäckhed, R.E. Ley, J.L. Sonnenberg, D.A. Peterson, J.I. Gordon. "Host-bacterial mutualism in the human intestine." *Science* 2005; 307 : 1915-1920.
- F. Guarner, J.-R. Malagelada. "Gut flora in health and disease." *Lancet* 2003; 360 : 512-519.

. . . the beneficial effects associated with probiotics:
- J. Ezendam, H. von Loveren. "Probiotics : immunomodulation and evaluation of safety and efficacy." *Nutrition Rev.* 2006; 64 : 1-14.
- S.C. Leahy, D.G. Higgins, G.F. Fitzgerald, D. van Sinderen. "Getting better with bifidobacteria." *J. Appl. Microbiol.* 2005; 98 : 1303-1315.
- I. Wollowski, G. Rechkemmer, B.L. Pool-Zobel. "Protective role of probiotics and prebiotics in colon cancer." *Am. J. Clin. Nutr.* 2001; 73 : 451S-455S.
- J. Saikali, C. Picard, M. Freitas, P. Holt. "Fermented milks, probiotic cultures and colon cancer." *Nutr. Cancer* 2004; 49 : 14-24.

Subject Index